Canyon Ranch
Nourish

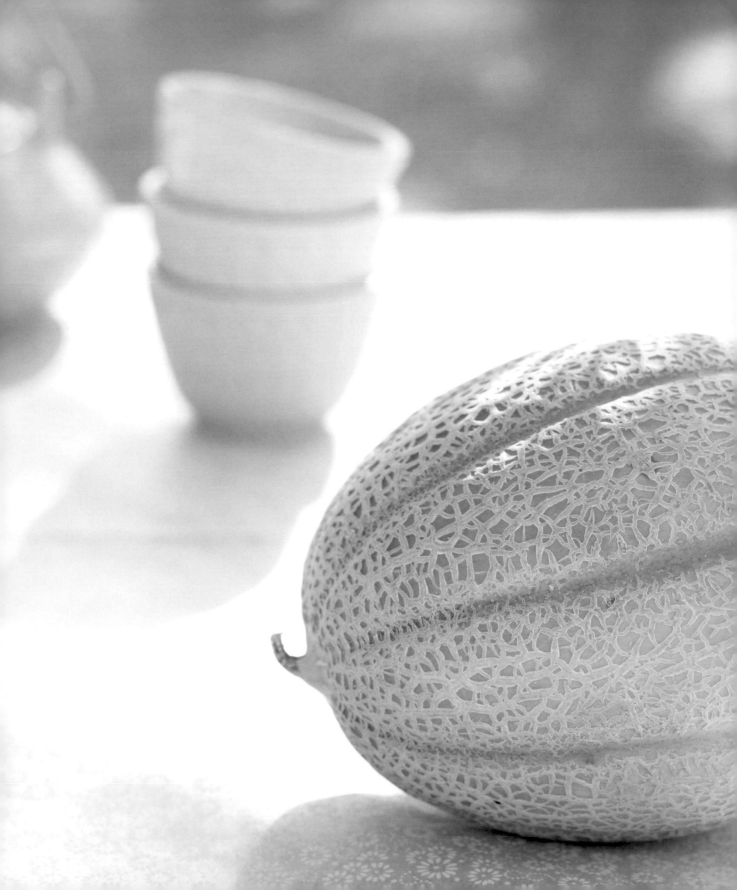

Canyon Ranch
Nourish

indulgently healthy cuisine

Scott Uehlein *and* Canyon Ranch

CANYONRANCH®

The Power of Possibility®

VIKING STUDIO

VIKING STUDIO
Published by the Penguin Group
Penguin Group (USA) Inc., 375 Hudson Street, New York, New York 10014, U.S.A.
Penguin Group (Canada), 90 Eglinton Avenue East, Suite 700, Toronto, Ontario, Canada M4P 2Y3
(a division of Pearson Penguin Canada Inc.)   ·   Penguin Books Ltd, 80 Strand, London
WC2R 0RL, England   ·   Penguin Ireland, 25 St. Stephen's Green, Dublin 2, Ireland (a division
of Penguin Books Ltd)   ·   Penguin Books Australia Ltd, 250 Camberwell Road, Camberwell,
Victoria 3124, Australia (a division of Pearson Australia Group Pty Ltd)   ·   Penguin Books
India Pvt Ltd, 11 Community Centre, Panchsheel Park, New Delhi – 110 017, India   ·
Penguin Group (NZ), 67 Apollo Drive, Rosedale, North Shore 0632, New Zealand (a division
of Pearson New Zealand Ltd)   ·   Penguin Books (South Africa) (Pty) Ltd, 24 Sturdee Avenue,
Rosebank, Johannesburg 2196, South Africa

Penguin Books Ltd, Registered Offices: 80 Strand, London WC2R 0RL, England

First published in 2009 by Viking Studio, a member of Penguin Group (USA) Inc

10   9   8   7   6   5

Photographs by Julie Toy

LIBRARY OF CONGRESS CATALOGING IN PUBLICATION DATA
Uehlein, Scott.
Canyon Ranch: nourish : indulgently healthy cuisine / Scott Uehlein and Canyon Ranch.
p. cm.
Includes index.
ISBN 978-0-670-02073-7
1. Cookery (Natural foods) 2. Canyon Ranch. I. Canyon Ranch. II. Title.
TX741.U34 2009
641.5'636—c22   2008035491

Printed in China
Set in DIN

Designed by Vertigo Design New York

To Enid and Mel Zuckerman, whose vision and dedication have inspired thousands to live healthier lives.

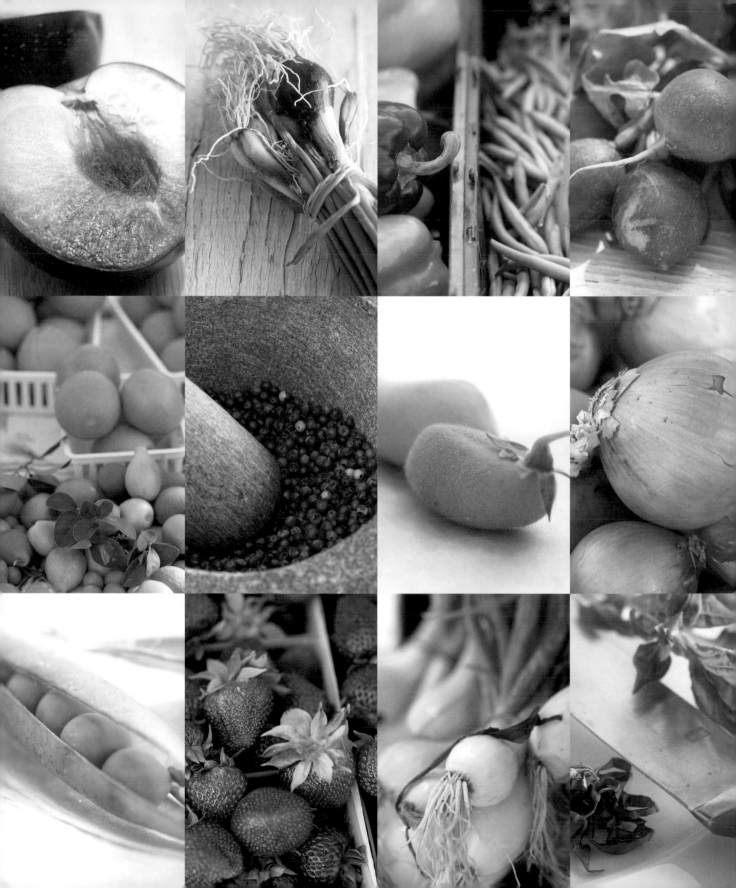

CONTENTS

IT'S ABOUT TASTE

From its beginning thirty years ago, Canyon Ranch has been a leader in the development of "spa cuisine." We've fought that label all along—the Ranch is immeasurably more than what most people think of as a spa, and, frankly, we think of our food as simply great, healthy cuisine. Back in the 1980s, though, we probably deserved every bad thing associated with those two words. Fortunately, we've come a long way since the days of tofu and sprouts and "reinvented classics" like low-fat beef Wellington. Spa is now a grown-up cuisine of its own. I only half laugh when people tell me how surprised they are at just how flavorful our food is. It's *all* about flavor.

When we begin to build a menu item, we build it from the ground up, so our dining guests do not have any preconceived notions as to what the dish will taste like. No longer do we reinvent lower-fat versions of dishes that have already been done, as we can only disappoint you with the outcome. (There are exceptions to every rule. . . . More recently, I began playing with some "classics," so I have amended my "never" stance to "OK, but only if it's better than the original." The recipes here for Pot Roast, Macaroni and Cheese, and Classic Egg Salad Sandwich are three exceptions that really prove the rule.) But for the most part, I try not to reinvent.

As the dish takes shape, we look for key elements. Those elements are sweet, sour, bitter, and salty. Of course, now we also pay homage to the "fifth sense" of umami, but more on that later. Sweet, sour, bitter, and salty can come from many sources. Sweetness in a savory dish might be captured as a taste element through caramelization, the addition of a fruit, or even a natural sweetener such as honey, maple syrup, or sugar. Sweet is easy to overdo, so we use it in savory dishes as a counterpoint to sour. Sour is incorporated through the introduction of an acid, generally citrus or vinegar. Bitter is kind of dicey because many people do not care for this taste, but bitter elements are actually easier to incorporate than you might think. Bitter may be very subtle, such as the slight bitter taste you get from marking a piece of fish on the grill, or more bold, in the form of a bitter green vegetable. Either way, without bitter, the balance of the dish will be off. Salty simply means a properly seasoned dish, not salty like potato chips are salty.

All of these elements need to be present for the dish to be properly balanced. Throw too much of one element into the mix and you will have a dish that is out of balance and fails to satisfy. Forget to incorporate everything, and you end up with a dish that is "missing something." All the elements have to be there. Because we are creating dishes that are lower in fat, we must make sure we are satiating the palate—but don't worry, we *will* satiate your palate. In fact, the taste of the food will be more vibrant than ever: Without so much butter and cream, which just mute your sense of taste, flavors really come alive.

The most recent addition to the flavor fold is umami. Umami is the sensation of "savoriness," which is almost a mouth-feel as much as a taste, but it is widely recognized as our fifth sense of taste. Umami is perceived by certain receptors on the tongue and is found naturally in higher concentrations in foods such as soy sauce, mushrooms, and meats. While we do not go out of our way to include items higher in umami in our cuisine, you won't be surprised to see umami-rich foods appearing in many of our recipes.

I have to insert a word about subtleties. You will notice that many of our recipes include key ingredients such as freshly ground black pepper or grated fresh ginger or even strange instructions such as "toast the spices." We do this purposefully as each of these elements adds subtle flavors that would otherwise not be present. For example, if you use pepper out of a shaker, it tastes completely different from the freshly ground stuff—you can even tell the difference by smelling it. Try it sometime. The toasting of spices introduces a subtle nutty flavor, and by crushing or bruising spices in a mortar and pestle, you bring out their natural oils and therefore increase their flavor.

Texture is another element we consider in composing a dish. Everything on the plate can't be crunchy, nor should everything be soft: Again, balance is key. Crunch may come from a raw vegetable such as cucumber, but it also may come from a cooked vegetable, such as bok choy. It can come from very obvious sources such as shoestring potatoes or more subtle sources such as the slight crunch of the perfectly crisp exterior of our sautéed Grits Cake. Soft might be a sweet strawberry in among the crunchy arugula of our Strawberry, Chicken, and Arugula Salad. For sure, both elements are present.

The last consideration is eye appeal. We eat with our eyes first! This means each recipe we prepare must be visually appealing.

I hope this gives a bit of an overview of flavor, texture, and eye appeal, three key elements in cooking in a lighter, healthier, and more natural manner, the way we do at Canyon Ranch. I wish you happy and healthy cooking!

—Chef Scott Uehlein

ACKNOWLEDGMENTS

PROJECT COORDINATORS
Morey Brown
Marilyn Majchrzak, M.S., R.D.

EXECUTIVE CHEFS
James Boyer
Steve Betti
Justin Morrow

THE KITCHEN STAFF OF CANYON RANCH
Canyon Ranch in Tucson
Canyon Ranch in Lenox
Canyon Ranch Living Miami Beach
Canyon Ranch SpaClub in Las Vegas

FOOD DEVELOPMENT STAFF
Haley Trego
Lara Kirtley

NUTRITIONISTS
Lisa Powell, M.S., R.D.
Megan Mullin, M.S., R.D.
Lori Reamer, R.D.

RECIPE TESTERS
Tricia Owen
Ron Gilson
Mary Paganelli
Lois Friedman

NUTRITION WRITER
Kathleen Johnson, M.S., R.D.

EDITOR
Renée Downing

SENIOR ART DIRECTOR
Teri Bingham

PHOTOGRAPHER
Julie Toy

FOOD STYLIST
Valerie Aikman-Smith

PHOTOGRAPHY ASSISTANT
Ed Rudolph

INTRODUCTION

Canyon Ranch is a byword for health, luxury, and comfort because for nearly thirty years we've made it our business to make guests feel loved and cared for. We've been very successful because our efforts come from the heart: We truly care about our guests. They feel it, and most of them return again and again.

A big part of our caring is in the food we serve. We don't just feed our guests, we *nourish* them. Meals are included in a Canyon Ranch resort vacation, and those meals must be extraordinary. Our guests tend to be very particular, and we are extremely careful about what we give them. Our food meets both the highest culinary and nutritional standards, which makes it unique. We prepare every dish, every meal not just to please our guests, but also to contribute to their health, well-being, and vitality. Our food, in short, is made with love. This book is filled with great recipes and helpful techniques and information, all motivated by the fervent wish to help you live well and long.

And because our concept of health and well-being has expanded over the years to encompass a healthy environment, we have come to insist that the food we serve be not only clean and wholesome, but also organic, seasonal, and local or regional, insofar as possible. These issues are of increasing interest to our guests, and we urge you to become part of the great awakening to the importance of knowing where food comes from and how it's produced. To that end, in this book we provide plentiful advice about what to look for when you shop.

Please, enjoy these recipes. And cook with love.

CHAPTER ONE | *For us, nutrition is a wide, deep, broad, exciting subject that reaches into every aspect of life. We don't believe in dieting. We do believe in balance, in moderation, and in savoring all the pleasures of eating well. We believe in food that nourishes body and soul.*

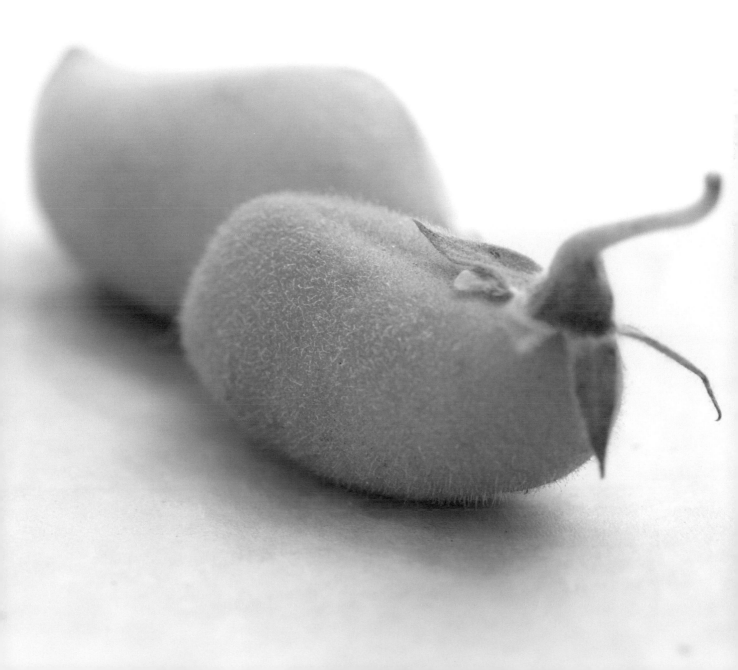

canyon ranch
nutrition basics

OUR BALANCED APPROACH TO EATING WELL

Canyon Ranch's gifted chefs work with a brilliant staff of nutritionists to ensure that every luscious meal that comes out of our kitchens meets an exacting set of nutritional standards. **Our recipes emphasize:**

- **A wide variety of ingredients from plants,** since vegetables, fruits, whole grains, beans, nuts and seeds, and herbs and spices are delicious and satisfying, and they are the foods with the most power to prevent disease.

- **Plenty of fiber from a wide variety of plant foods,** because the good news about fiber's health benefits appears to be never ending.

- **Minimal added sugar and no artificial sweeteners.** Our recipes call for a variety of natural sweeteners, including sugar, honey, and molasses, in moderate quantities. Our preferred noncaloric sweetener for table use is stevia, a natural herbal sweetener.

- **Balanced portions of protein and carbohydrate,** and small amounts of healthy fat. Because this combination satisfies both nutritional needs and appetite, we strive to provide in each of our meals, including our vegetarian options, some protein rich food. Our protein offerings include beans—we love beans of all kinds, for being so versatile, tasty, and nourishing—soy foods, fish, eggs, low-fat dairy products, and the leanest cuts of poultry and red meat.

- **Healthy fats in moderation.** In the old days, spa food meant no fat. We're long past that idea, and our food could now probably best be described as being rich in "good fat," since we use special care in selecting fats and oils that are beneficial to health. Organic extra virgin olive oil and organic expeller-pressed canola oil, rich in flavor and antioxidants, are our preferred choices. We also emphasize omega-3 fatty acids (found mainly in fish and flaxseeds) and fats from other plant sources, including avocados and nuts. We minimize saturated fats and never use trans fats.

A FEW GREAT RULES OF THUMB FOR EATING WELL

Many people feel overwhelmed by the often confusing, seemingly contradictory information about nutrition that floods the media, but you really don't have to worry about how every new study might apply to you. Here are a few of the simple, easy-to-remember rules that our nutritionists—who follow and understand all those research findings—give our guests.

About Salt

Our foods are seasoned with an array of herbs and spices, with moderate use of salt. Research that we find very exciting shows that spices contain compounds with astounding benefits for body and brain—yet another reason to spice it up. We keep a careful eye on sodium, however, because most Americans regularly consume more salt than is recommended. This is a concern because excessive sodium intake is associated with high blood pressure and is a risk factor for heart disease, stroke, some cancers, and kidney disease. We encourage you to become more aware of the amount of sodium contained in what you eat and to consider using less salt.

Canyon Ranch chefs try to keep total daily salt to less than the recommended guideline for healthy individuals: about 2,300 mg of naturally occurring and added sodium per day. (This is equivalent to about a teaspoon of salt.) Does this mean our food lacks flavor? Absolutely not. Our chefs creatively season the highest quality, freshest, most flavorful ingredients with small amounts of salt along with delectable, health-promoting herbs and spices. Their goal is always to allow the natural flavors of the foods to shine.

You'll notice that our recipes call for sea salt. Sea salt is a little lower in sodium and higher in other minerals than table salt, and we love the subtle flavors it brings to our dishes. When purchasing sea salt, the less refined, the better: The best sea salt is actually still a bit damp and may not be completely white. And while we encourage you to use local or regional foods, here is one area where we happily ignore this principle: We use only Mediterranean sea salt, which we think is the best.

The good news about reducing the salt in your diet is that a preference for excessive saltiness is an acquired taste. If you start cutting down, you'll notice within a month or so that your desire for salt has diminished. We humans are highly adaptable: You'll gradually get used to a lower-sodium diet, just as you adapted to an overly salty one. Try it and see.

Splurge on color, color, color.

Red, purple, green, orange, yellow, and the blue of blueberries—the brilliant colors of fruits and vegetables come from phytochemicals, a varied class of miracle nutrients that scientists are just beginning to appreciate. You don't need to know a thing about biochemistry, though, to get maximum benefit from eating fruits and vegetables: Just choose a variety of intense colors every day.

Limit white (except for cauliflower, onions, and garlic).

Simple carbohydrates such as white flour, pasta, rice, and potatoes act almost like sugar on your blood-sugar levels, sending them way up and then letting them drop. Over time, this pattern can contribute to insulin resistance and type 2 diabetes and is associated with heart disease and other serious chronic illnesses. Switch to whole grain products: The germ and fiber that are removed in processing to whiteness make a huge nutritional difference.

Don't eat anything your great-grandmother didn't.

This rule reflects the fact that the healthiest foods are those that humans have been eating since the dawn of time: Our bodies evolved to make use of the substances they contain. Because your ancestors almost certainly ate diets rich in whole grains, legumes, fruits, and vegetables—and didn't eat processed, packaged, or junk food for the simple reason that it didn't exist—the grandma rule can greatly simplify your decision making about what to buy. Sugar-coated cereal with freeze-dried fruit and marshmallow bits? Nope. Crackers made with partially hydrogenated vegetable oil and artificial flavorings? Not those, either. Carbonated soft drinks sweetened with high-fructose corn syrup? The dear woman never touched them, so neither should you.

Speed-read food labels: Check out the first four ingredients on any nutrition label and don't eat anything you can't pronounce.

You could go blind reading food labels. Here are two shortcuts: Look at the first three or four ingredients. Ingredients are always listed according to quantity: The predominant ingredient comes first, the second comes next, etc. So if you're trying to cut down on, say, sugar in your diet, look at the labels of products you're considering to see if there's some form of sweetener (sugar, sucrose, fructose, high-fructose corn syrup, or other ingredients ending in -ose, and manitol, and other sugar alcohols ending in -ol, etc.) among the first four ingredients. If there is, put the item back. The second trick is to skim quickly for polysyllables. If you don't know what it is, or even how to say it, do you really want to eat it?

Choose foods that are in a state as close as possible to the way they grew.

Less processed is better than highly processed; simpler is better than complicated; whole is better than refined. Better a tomato than a can of tomato juice; better a baked potato (with the peel) than potato chips; better fish than fishsticks. Whole grains are a good example of this principle: You'll see the words *whole grain* on labels all over the supermarket, and products made with whole grain flour certainly are better than those made with more highly processed flours. But the most wholesome type of whole grain food is the entire kernel cooked in liquid until it's tender: Oatmeal, especially made with steel-cut oats, is a wonderful food, as are so many of our terrific salads, soups, and sides that showcase nutty, delicious whole grains.

Eat mostly plants.

Plant-based foods are less calorie dense than animal products; they're loaded with fiber, vitamins, and other important nutrients; and growing them has much less impact on the environment than producing meat, eggs, and dairy foods. Filling most of your plate with fruits, vegetables, whole grains, and beans is a good way to start improving both your health and that of the planet.

Never skip breakfast, and don't let yourself get overly hungry.

Body and brain function best when they're fueled regularly with a balanced combination of quality carbohydrates, protein, and healthy fats. Eat a balanced breakfast and small healthy snacks midmorning and in the late afternoon to keep from becoming ravenous. Some hummus with a couple of whole grain crackers, a few olives and a slice of cheese, a handful of almonds and an apple—these are snacks that keep your energy up and your blood sugar steady, and that make it easier to eat reasonably later on.

THE BASICS OF SELECTING FOOD

At Canyon Ranch we go to immense trouble to find the best food available: We quiz our vendors, send fish out to labs for analysis, and attend food expositions looking for healthy new products and sources of supply. It's necessary that we ensure that we serve only the best.

In this section, we give you the tools *you* need to find the type of food that our chefs and nutritionists select for our guests: *Real* food that is *fresh, clean,* and *wholesome.* We'll discuss these adjectives, all of which are interrelated with the principle of sustainability, one at a time.

the food you want is real

Food and beverages that are *real* do not contain chemically altered or man-made ingredients such as trans fats (partially hydrogenated vegetable oils), artificial sweeteners, high-fructose corn syrup, genetically modified ingredients, artificial colors or flavors, or preservatives. If you buy a lot of processed or packaged food and bottled beverages, or if you eat out a great deal, it's difficult to be sure that the food you're eating is real. It's easy to avoid all of these undesirable ingredients, however, if you shop for whole foods and cook from scratch, which is what our chefs do.

Of course, few of us have the time (or inclination) to bake all our own bread, cook all our beans from scratch, or boil up chicken bones every time we need a cup of stock. If you live in a town of any size, though, you'll have access to a good bakery, or stores that carry artisanal whole grain breads, organic canned beans, and organic low-sodium chicken stock. Homemade is best, but these will do just fine.

the food you want is fresh

Fresh used to mean food that hadn't been frozen, canned, or dried. At Canyon Ranch, we've changed that definition a bit in our desire to promote foods that are local and regional, seasonal, and from sustainable sources.

Food that's local and seasonal is the best choice for a number of reasons. Yes, it's lovely to have asparagus in October and berries year-round, but they aren't as appealing once you begin to recognize the hidden costs of raising crops in greenhouses or shipping produce for thousands of miles. For example, much winter fruit comes from South America, where American demand for out-of-season produce has triggered the widespread clearing of forests and the use of pesticides prohibited in the United States. This trend is having distressing environmental effects right here at home. Many North American songbirds, for instance, have suffered precipitous population

fresh food is:

- Seasonal

- Healthy and delicious

- Grown close to home, ideally, within a day's drive or so

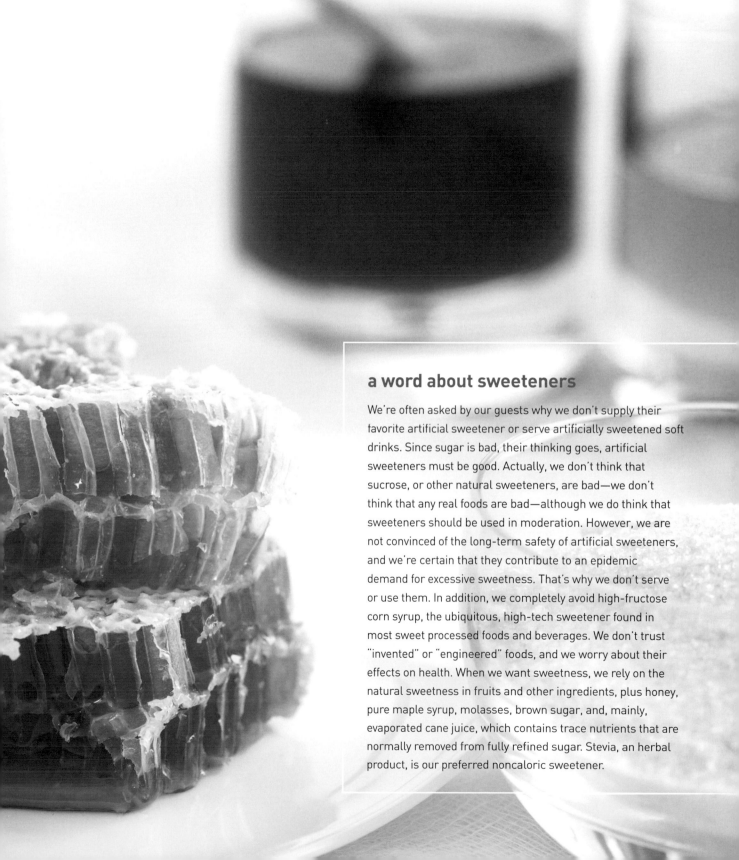

a word about sweeteners

We're often asked by our guests why we don't supply their favorite artificial sweetener or serve artificially sweetened soft drinks. Since sugar is bad, their thinking goes, artificial sweeteners must be good. Actually, we don't think that sucrose, or other natural sweeteners, are bad—we don't think that any real foods are bad—although we do think that sweeteners should be used in moderation. However, we are not convinced of the long-term safety of artificial sweeteners, and we're certain that they contribute to an epidemic demand for excessive sweetness. That's why we don't serve or use them. In addition, we completely avoid high-fructose corn syrup, the ubiquitous, high-tech sweetener found in most sweet processed foods and beverages. We don't trust "invented" or "engineered" foods, and we worry about their effects on health. When we want sweetness, we rely on the natural sweetness in fruits and other ingredients, plus honey, pure maple syrup, molasses, brown sugar, and, mainly, evaporated cane juice, which contains trace nutrients that are normally removed from fully refined sugar. Stevia, an herbal product, is our preferred noncaloric sweetener.

drops in recent years: These birds winter in Latin America, and the loss of habitat and poisoning by pesticides are thought to be the reasons for their decline. Fresh strawberries in December are tempting, but they carry hidden environmental and health costs that many of us are simply not willing to pay. (The pesticides that kill orioles and bobolinks aren't good for humans, either, and cannot be washed off strawberries.)

In addition, produce that has been bred to be shipped over long distances is not as tasty or nutritious as older strains and is typically picked green and then chemically ripened. Such produce may look beautiful—eye appeal is what moves inventory—but it is inferior in flavor and nutrition to locally produced, naturally ripened fruits and vegetables. For example, the supermarket tomato has rightly become a byword for disappointment. Our recommendation is that you look for high-quality frozen (and in some cases, such as tomato products, canned) fruits and vegetables out of season, or wait until the season swings around to indulge in fresh local produce.

Of course, we serve bananas and pineapples at Canyon Ranch, and salads in winter. Rather than making local and seasonal a hard-and-fast rule, we encourage you to learn where your food is coming from and make the freshest, most responsible choices you can. We find that there's actually a great deal of satisfaction in eating with the rhythm of the seasons: Butternut squash just seems to taste best when the weather's cold, and blueberries are extra special when we wait for summer to enjoy them. And is there anything better than a vine-ripened tomato still warm from the summer sun?

A few fresh ideas:

- Grow a few simple things yourself. Tomatoes, squash, chard, beans, and herbs are easy. Grow them in containers if you don't have a yard.

- Learn about the seasonality of various vegetables and fruits. This is information that your grandmother knew in her bones but that you may have lost.

- Buy produce that's grown locally or regionally—or at least in your own hemisphere. If something isn't labeled as to origin, ask your produce manager where it comes from. He or she should know.

- When there's a local bumper crop of something you like, buy in quantity and freeze it yourself.

- Explore farmers' markets in your area. You'll find the freshest locally grown foods there, and you can meet the people who produce them. Farmers' markets benefit small farmers and strengthen communities, and they're fun. For more information on farmers' markets and community-supported agriculture, visit www.localharvest.org.

what does organic mean?

- **100% Organic**
  According to the USDA, organic food is produced without using synthetic pesticides, petroleum or sewage-sludge-based fertilizers, bioengineering, or ionizing radiation. Organic meats, poultry, eggs, and dairy products come from animals that have been fed organic feed and given no antibiotics or growth hormones.

- **Organic**
  At least 95 percent of the ingredients are organically produced and the food does not contain sulfites.

- **Made with organic ingredients**
  At least 70 percent of the ingredients are organic; the remaining 30 percent must come from the USDA's approved list and cannot contain sulfites.

the food you want is clean

We define clean foods as those free from pesticide and herbicide residues, hormones and antibiotics, unnecessary additives and preservatives, undesirable ingredients, contaminants, and food-borne pathogens.

Worrying excessively about the food you eat takes the joy out of eating, and we don't want that. (Our nutritionists explicitly urge our guests not to be "food fussers.") Rather than worrying, we suggest that you make clean choices and let your consumer preferences reflect your concerns. Know that in the huge feed-back system that is the food industry, every dollar you spend on food can be a vote for a cleaner food supply and a healthier world.

Why organic?

One of the simplest and most powerful choices you can make is to buy organic, whenever possible. Many people are understandably skeptical about the value of the organic label. This is due in part to confusion between *organic* and *natural*, a marketing word that means essentially nothing. But in the United States and Europe, *organic* actually means a lot.

When you buy food that's organic, the U.S. government is guaranteeing that it is real, clean, and sustainably produced, which is a great start. And research has shown that organic produce contains more antioxidants than conventionally grown fruits and vegetables. So you're not just getting cleaner food, you're getting more nourishing food when you buy organic.

Organic foods tend to be more expensive than conventionally produced ones. If you have to choose, we suggest that you prioritize the following types of food in order to buy organic: dairy, eggs, poultry, beef and lamb, produce, corn and soy products, and coffee and tea.

A label calling any of these foods organic guarantees that the foods are free from undesirable ingredients, including those from genetically modified crops. For detailed, up to date information on organic priorities, we suggest that you visit the Web sites of the Institute for Agriculture and Trade Policy, Environmental Working Group, and the Organic Trade Association (see the Resources list on pages 12–13.

Organic, though, is not the whole story. Some exceptionally clean, nutritionally valuable foods, including wild-caught Pacific salmon and wild boreal blueberries, are not labeled organic because they grow entirely outside the food-production system. It's also the case that many small farmers and ranchers who use admirable methods are not certified organic. On the other hand, organic foods that are produced at a great distance may be environmentally extravagant because of the shipping. And organic may not fully capture another concern people have about their food: The humane treatment of animals. To sum up, organic is good, but there can be trade-offs. It is important to consider many different factors when choosing the food that fits your needs.

You also want your food to be, literally, clean, in the plain sense of "not dirty." Always wash produce properly to remove pesticide and herbicide residues, bacteria, and dirt. To wash food properly:

- Use one teaspoon mild soap in one gallon of water, or purchase a prepared produce wash solution. Always clean produce before cutting it.
- Use a vegetable brush on hard produce the skin of which you plan to eat.
- Peel wax-coated nonorganic produce such as cucumbers.
- Discard the outer leaves of cabbage and head lettuce.

the food you want is wholesome

Wholesome is a word we love for the way it captures an old-fashioned sense of goodness. All real, fresh food that's been cleanly grown and handled is wholesome, and eating it is an excellent way to support your health and increase your longevity.

Of course, some people have intolerances or reactions to certain foods, such as dairy or wheat products, and sensitive individuals should avoid these foods. Significantly, the foods that cause the greatest problems vary from culture to culture and tend to be among the most-consumed foods: Rice is a problem for many people in China, for instance. This suggests that eating a wide variety of foods is a key to avoiding sensitivities.

When we speak about wholesomeness, however, we are especially concerned about one type of food—genetically modified crops—for a number of reasons. The introduction of DNA from one organism into the DNA of another is a troubling thing, and current research indicates that genetic modification may create unexpected new allergens or may contaminate foods in unexpected ways. Genetic modification may also create ecological damage, creating insecticide-resistant insects and herbicide-resistant superweeds. In addition, genetically modified crops are owned by the chemical companies that produce them, and these companies

wholesome food is:

- Whole and real
- Not genetically modified
- Nutritionally dense
- Exquisitely flavored
- Appropriately portioned
- Eaten in serenity

own the seeds and control the crops, so that farmers cannot select the seeds that do best in their fields. We also fear that genetically modified organisms (GMOs) will contaminate traditional seed stocks and land and that all these factors will lead to a loss of genetic diversity and may damage small farmers around the world.

For all these reasons, we feel that genetically modified foods are fundamentally unwholesome. The foods and food products most likely to be affected are corn and corn products, soybeans and soybean products and canola oil. Since current food labeling laws do not require that manufacturers disclose the use of genetically modified ingredients, the only way to guarantee that these foods are not genetically modified is to buy organic. (Genetically modified produce is required to have a price look-up (PLU) code that starts with 8. When in doubt, check the item's supermarket sticker.)

Much of the supply of feed grains for animals is genetically modified, which means that in order to fully avoid these foods, it's important to select organic eggs, dairy products, poultry, and meat: The USDA organic standard forbids the use of this type of feed and the use of hormones or antibiotics in raising animals. When it comes to eggs and chicken, we prefer organic and free-range selections; in beef and lamb, we look for organic and grass-fed varieties, which are leaner, tastier, cleaner, and more nourishing than grain fed; for dairy, we buy organic products.

dairy basics

- Buy organic dairy foods when you can and those certified "r-BGH free," if organic is not available. R-BGH is the moniker for recombinant bovine growth hormone, which is frequently given to dairy cattle to improve milk production. It's particularly important to select organic or r-BGH-free high-fat dairy products such as whole milk, cream, and butter because contaminants concentrate in fat.

- Consider buying artisan cheeses made in traditional ways. These can be found at many cheese shops, online, and at natural foods stores. The cheese makers who produce these treasured cheeses are generally using milk from local dairies that don't use hormones.

- If you have the opportunity, try dairy foods from grass-fed cows. Milk carries the flavors of the feed given to the cow, so the taste may be a little different from what you are used to. But, as with grass-fed beef, milk from grass-fed cows is lower in inflammatory fatty acids and higher in omega-3 fatty acids than that from grain-fed animals.

Nutritional density is another important aspect of wholesomeness. The words refer to the amount and quality of nutrients in a food. Processing destroys nutrients, and reliance on highly refined sugar, flour, cornstarch, and processed oils results in foods with little flavor, few surviving nutrients, and lots of calories.

Resources

We've found the following online resources invaluable in selecting the cleanest and healthiest food.

PRODUCE
Environmental Working Group
www.ewg.org
Check out their "Shopper's Guide to Pesticides in Produce," which features regular updates on the vegetables and fruits with the most and least pesticide residue. This is very valuable information when you're trying to decide which produce to buy organic and which conventionally grown fruits and vegetables are safe. EWG also lists tips for safe handling of produce.

SEAFOOD
Monterey Bay Aquarium
www.montereybayaquarium.org/cr/seafoodwatch.asp
Learn all you ever wanted to know and then some about sustainable seafood choices. Download regional U.S. pocket guides to eating seafood that is responsibly caught.

Environmental Defense Fund
www.edf.org/seafood
Look up fish choices that are good for you and the ocean in EDF's "Pocket Seafood Selector," a comprehensive list that you can easily tuck in your purse or wallet to take along when you shop for seafood or eat out.

FOOD ADDITIVES TO AVOID
Center for Science in the Public Interest
www.cspinet.org
Although our advice is to eat fresh and natural as much as possible, canned or packaged foods may sometimes be a more convenient choice. So take a few minutes to review the center's Nutrition Action Newsletter and its "Chemical

Some wholesome foods, on the other hand, are high in calories but rich in flavor and vital nutrients. Nuts and olive oil, for example, are high in calories, but vitamins, minerals, flavonoids, antioxidants, and marvelous flavor come along with every calorie. We think you'll find that nutrition-packed, flavorful foods are more satisfying.

Cuisine," a guide to food additives. This site also features other practical food and nutrition advice.

RED MEAT, POULTRY, AND DAIRY PRODUCTS
www.eatwild.com
Review this comprehensive guide to grass-fed and organic beef, lamb, bison, poultry, and dairy products. This is a great resource with an extensive list of suppliers of pasture-raised products.

LOCAL FOODS
www.localharvest.org
Source local foods where you live by searching online by map, city/state, and zip code for farmers' markets, restaurants, Community Supported Agriculture (CSA) groups, and more.

SEASONAL PRODUCE
www.fieldtoplate.com/guide.php
Check out this seasonal lookup guide by state on this useful site.

GENERAL INFORMATION
Consumers Union
www.consumersunion.org/food.html; www.greenerchoices.org/eco-labels.
Research up-to-date food and food product advice as well as updated eco-label information.

Institute for Agriculture and Trade Policy
www.iatp.org/
Download consumer Smart Guides to healthy choices for meat and dairy, produce, fish, as well as plastics.

HOW TO GET TO REAL, FRESH, CLEAN, AND WHOLESOME

- Commit to real food: Check to see if your pantry needs an overhaul. Although real, wholesome food often requires that you spend some time in the kitchen, you'll find dozens of recipes here that can be prepared quickly and easily.

- Know where your food comes from and how it was produced.

- Begin to understand your unique food needs. Notice how you react to specific foods and adjust accordingly. You are the expert on you.

- Exercise restraint with portion sizes. Our recipes include portion sizes: Pay attention.

- Cook and eat from your own cultural tradition, and from those of others. Food with a story is uniquely satisfying.

- Cook from this cookbook! It's all here.

- Share meals with family and friends and take satisfaction in feeding them well. Nourish yourself and the people you love.

HEALTHY COOKING BASICS

These techniques and tips are the cornerstone of cooking in our Canyon Ranch kitchens.

preparing and cooking chicken, fish, and red meat

BRAISING. Braising means to brown and then simmer in a covered pan on the stove top or in the oven in a small amount of liquid over a long period of time, usually 1½ to 3 hours. When braising red meat, remove all visible fat and brown with as small an amount of canola oil as possible.

BROILING. Broiling means to cook quickly with intense, direct heat in an oven under a broiler. The high heat seals in the juices, browns the outside, and keeps meat tender.

GRILLING. Grilling means to cook food on a rack, rapidly, with dry heat over gas, wood coals, charcoal, or electric coil. Grilling is an intense, rapid cooking method that gives food a crisp exterior and moist, flavorful interior.

This is a quick, low-fat way to cook chicken, fish, and red meat. Make sure to preheat the grill hot enough so that the meat sizzles when placed on the surface. It is also advisable to lightly coat the grill rack or pan with canola oil sprays before adding meat to prevent sticking. Be careful with oil over open flame; it can flare up.

Grilling times and temperatures

	HOW LONG TO COOK ON EACH SIDE	INTERNAL TEMPERATURE
Chicken	3 to 5 minutes per inch of thickness	165°F at the center
Red Meat	3 to 5 minutes per inch of thickness	145°F at the center
Fish*	2 to 3 minutes per inch of thickness	135°F at the center

*NOTE: When cooking fish, watch carefully after 2 minutes to make sure it is not cooking too quickly: Fish becomes dry and rubbery when overcooked. Chef Scott likes to cook fish until it's not quite done, then pull it off the grill and cover for 3 minutes while it finishes carryover cooking. With this method, fish may not come quite to 135°F.

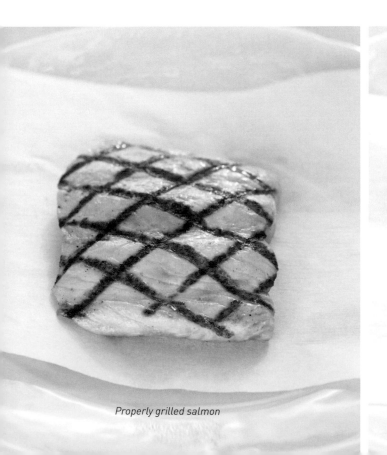

Properly grilled salmon

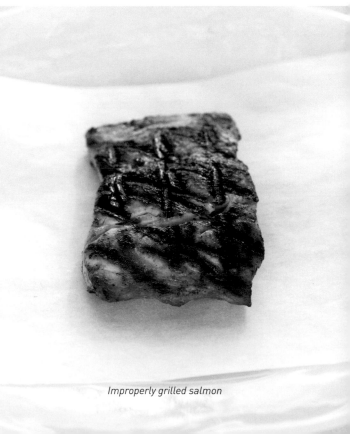

Improperly grilled salmon

Grilling Tips

- Broiling or grilling can produce char, which contains carcinogens. To minimize exposure, remove visible fat, bake for part of the cooking time, and finish on the grill.

- Turn food frequently while cooking and before eating, remove any char that forms.

- Marinate meat before cooking to seal the surface, which will minimize the formation of unhealthful compounds.

- Use lower temperatures to avoid flare-ups.

- Minimize oil in marinades.

- Use lower-temperature cooking methods such as boiling, poaching, and braising more often.

PAN GRILLING. A cast-iron grill pan works well for cooking lean grass-fed beef when you do not want the drying effects of flame but still want the nice grill marks. The grill pan is also a great choice if you've used a marinade containing oil. Preheat the grill pan for 3 to 5 minutes before adding the meat and cooking it to the desired doneness. Using the grill pan on an outside grill minimizes the mess in the kitchen—this method can involve splattering.

STIR-FRYING. Just what it sounds like: a quick, hot cooking method developed in a part of the world where fuel is precious. Use a steel wok or large sauté pan over high heat and stir and flip food constantly with a wide spatula. (Asian food specialty stores sell tools that are curved to match the slope of the wok.) Meat for stir-frying must be cut into thin pieces to cook properly. Stir-frying is not appropriate for fish because of fish's fragility.

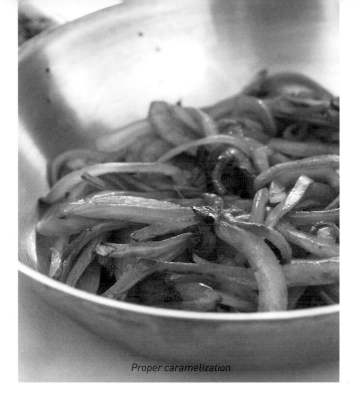
Proper caramelization

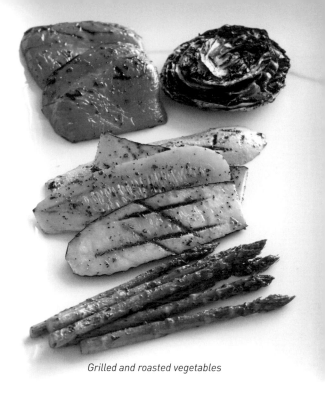
Grilled and roasted vegetables

preparing and cooking veggies

BLANCHING. Blanching involves plunging food into boiling water briefly to tenderize it and then submerging it in ice water to instantly stop the cooking process. Blanching is also used to loosen the skins of fruits such as tomatoes and peaches and to partially cook vegetables before roasting or stir-frying. It sets the color and flavor of vegetables and ensures even cooking of ingredients. To aid in loosening skin, cut an X in the bottom of a fruit or vegetable before placing it in boiling water.

CARAMELIZING. Caramelizing means to heat sugar until it liquefies and becomes a clear golden-to-dark syrup. In the case of fruits and vegetables, caramelizing refers to the process of cooking in a small amount of oil or liquid on low heat for a long period of time until the natural sugars are released and browned.

GRILLING OR ROASTING. One of our favorite ways of cooking vegetables is to grill or roast them. After you taste the caramelized sweetness of a sweet potato or zucchini cooked this way, you may never steam again. When grilling vegetables, we recommend cutting them into pieces that are large enough not to fall through the rack. However, vegetables do vary in moisture content, and when you're cooking several types at once, you will want to slice slower-cooking varieties, such as root vegetables, more thinly. Lightly spray the vegetables with canola oil spray, season with salt and pepper, and then grill until tender, about 5 minutes per side. As with meat, avoid charring.

Roasting vegetables is just as easy. Preheat the oven to 400°F and spread the vegetable pieces evenly on a baking sheet. Lightly spray the vegetables with canola oil spray and season with salt and pepper. Roast for 10 to 15 minutes, or until the vegetables are lightly browned, turning once or twice, if desired.

STEAMING. Steaming vegetables is a great way to retain all the important nutrients contained in plant foods. Bamboo steamer baskets are fine, as are metal steamer baskets that fit inside a saucepan. The bottom line on steaming is that you're just suspending vegetables over boiling water in a covered pan. Steaming takes from 5 to 8 minutes, depending on the type and size of the vegetable.

STIR-FRYING. Another quick cooking method, stir-frying retains nutrients and texture. Heat a wok or sauté pan until really hot to ensure that the food cooks quickly without sticking, then add oil. ("Hot wok, cold oil.") Use expeller-pressed canola oil, which can tolerate higher heat temperatures. Cut vegetables into bite-size pieces. Those vegetables with the longest cooking time should be added first. Quick-cooking vegetables such as snow peas and spinach should be added at the last moment. Cook only until the vegetables are tender-crisp.

preparing and cooking grains

From amaranth to exotic rices to quinoa, we love whole grains, and cooking them is simplicity itself. Some forms, such as couscous and bulgur wheat, don't even require cooking: Just stir the grain into boiling water, cover the pan, and let sit until all the water is absorbed. Cooking times and proportions of grain to liquid vary greatly from one type to the next. Follow any package directions.

preparing and cooking beans

Dozens of varieties of dried beans—including newly available, flavorful heirloom beans from all over the world—are great for adding protein and fiber to any meal. Always pick over beans, looking for stones and dirt, and rinse them in a colander before soaking.

We recommend soaking rinsed, picked-over beans for 6 to 8 hours (or overnight) before cooking. Place them in a bowl, add enough water to cover plus 3 inches, and let sit in a cool place, or quick-soak them by placing the beans in a large saucepan, covering them with 3 inches of water, and bringing them to a boil for 1 minute. Remove from the heat and soak for 1 hour.

Whichever method you use, pour off the soaking water, rinse the beans again, and add abundant fresh water before cooking. Bring the water to a boil, reduce the heat, and simmer uncovered. Consult the package or the Internet for cooking times.

Canned beans are great time-savers. Look for low-sodium organic varieties with minimal added ingredients. Drain and rinse them thoroughly before using.

selecting and cooking pasta

We like whole grain and multigrain pastas. Any kind of pasta should be cooked al dente, which means just until the uncooked core disappears. Properly cooked pasta not only tastes better, but the carbohydrate content is also absorbed more slowly, helping to balance blood sugar. Always add pasta to a large quantity of salted water at a full, rolling boil. Most dried pasta is cooked for 8 to 10 minutes (always follow package instructions). However, if you are fortunate enough to have fresh pasta available to you, 2 to 3 minutes is usually adequate. Check fresh pasta for doneness constantly.

preparing herbs and spices

MAXIMIZING THE FLAVOR OF HERBS. We use both fresh and dried herbs in our cuisine. Generally, dried herbs are used in applications that have longer cooking times, and fresh ones are used in uncooked preparations or are added at the very end of the cooking process. There are times when we may use fresh herbs in a longer-cooking recipe, and sometimes we even use the stems, such as parsley stems in a soup or stock and cilantro stems in an Asian broth, but these are exceptions. Dried herbs are more potent per volume than fresh ones: When substituting dried herbs for fresh, use about a quarter of the quantity called for.

Note: Most common herbs are easy to grow. Even if you don't plan to try to keep them around, it's often cheaper to buy a small pot of living basil, oregano, or dill than a package of cut fresh herbs. Just water the pot every day until you're ready to use your absolutely fresh herbs.

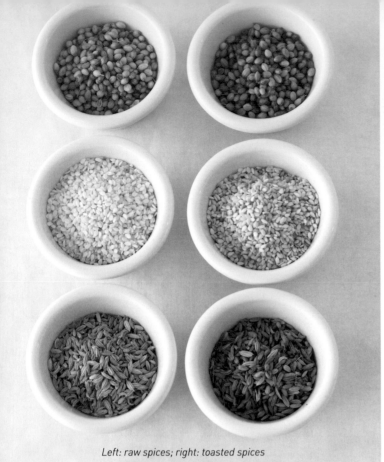

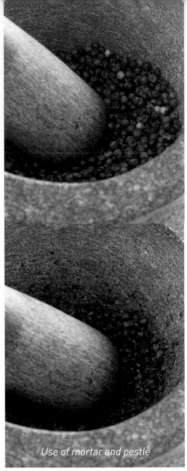

Left: raw spices; right: toasted spices

Use of mortar and pestle

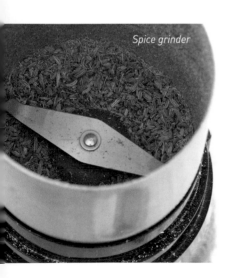

Spice grinder

TOASTING SPICES, NUTS, AND SEEDS. Toasting spices, nuts, and seeds to release flavor and aroma is a secret of great cooks the world over: Try toasting whole fennel, cumin, and coriander, for example, and experience the difference for yourself. A small toaster oven allows for more even toasting, but a conventional oven works, too. Spread whole spices, nuts, or seeds on a baking sheet and place in a 400°F oven. Start by setting the timer for 5 minutes, and then watch closely to make sure they don't burn. As our chefs say in our demo kitchen, "Not done . . . not done . . . oops, burned." If you don't want to heat up the oven, you may also dry-sauté spices.

GRINDING SPICES. Buy whole spices and grind them just before using them to maximize their flavors. A small coffee grinder or spice grinder works well for this. A mortar and pestle also work fine, especially when a very small quantity is called for.

ROASTING GARLIC. Roasted garlic lends a subtle, mellow flavor to a number of our dishes. To roast a head of garlic, lightly drizzle the whole head with extra virgin olive oil and wrap it in aluminum foil. Bake at 400°F until soft when pieced with the tip of a pointed knife, about 1 hour. Or peel garlic cloves, toss them with a little extra virgin olive oil, wrap them in aluminum foil, and roast as above. This method works well when a larger amount of garlic is called for. Roasted garlic can be minced or pureed, depending upon the application.

knife skills

CHIFFONADE. Chiffonade means to slice in very thin strips or shred with a chef's knife. Flat-leaf vegetables such as spinach, basil, and leaf lettuce are good subjects. To chiffonade, tightly roll leaves lengthwise and then thinly slice crosswise to produce slender ribbons.

CHOPPING. Chopping means to cut foods, usually with a chef's knife, into reasonably uniform-size pieces, about ½ to 1 inch. Vegetables are chopped, rather than diced, when even cooking is less important.

DICING. Dicing means to cut, usually with a chef's knife, into small cubes ranging from ⅛ to 1 inch. Vegetables are diced when even cooking is important. The smaller dice is often referred to as *brunoise*.

JULIENNING. Julienning means to slice fruits or vegetables into 2- to 3-inch strips (julienne), usually ⅛ inch wide, so that they look like matchsticks. A chef's knife is the best tool for this cutting method. There's also a classic cutting device called a mandoline that produces uniform julienne easily and rapidly.

MINCING. Mincing is a technique used to dice foods such as garlic and ginger very fine. Mincing requires a very sharp knife and patience. Foods that are meant to be tasted, not seen, are minced.

SLICING. Slicing means to cut food into pieces, either crosswise or lengthwise, depending upon the intended use. Slices in a given recipe should be of uniform thickness to ensure uniform cooking.

miscellaneous techniques and terms

BAKING. Baking means to cook by free-circulating dry air. It is very important to preheat the oven, especially when you are baking breads and desserts. Do not crowd food in the oven; give it room to bake evenly. Baking can be done in two ways: standard and convection. Convection forces hot air around the baking food and generally produces a more even baked product while using less energy. Generally, foods baked in convection ovens need 25 degrees less than standard baking, or 10 minutes less baking time. Check your oven's directions for the manufacturer's recommendations.

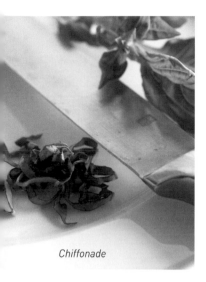

Chiffonade

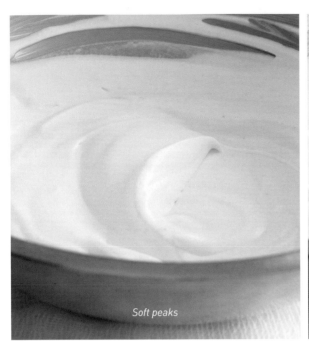

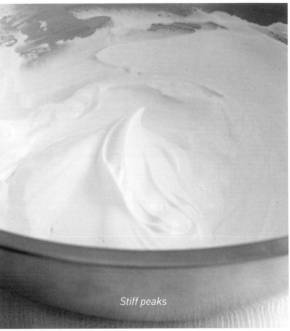

Soft peaks

Stiff peaks

BEATING UNTIL SOFT/STIFF PEAKS FORM. You can recognize how whipped a mixture is by lifting the beater or whisk. When the peaks are soft, they fall gently over themselves. When they are stiff peaks, the mixture stands straight up.

FOLDING. Folding means to incorporate one ingredient into another by gently turning one part of the mixture over the other part with a spoon or rubber spatula. Folding is a gentle way of incorporating fluffy ingredients—whipped cream and beaten egg whites, for instance—without knocking the air out of them.

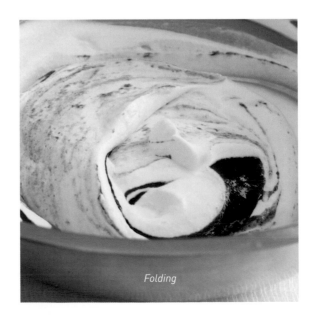

Folding

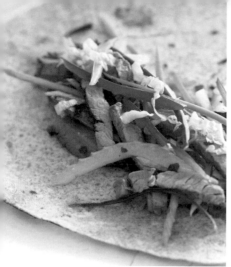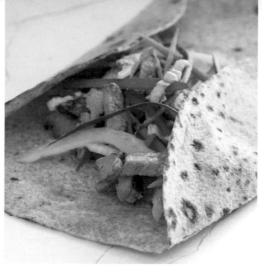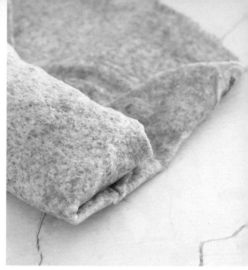

Folding burrito style

FOLDING BURRITO STYLE. To fold burrito style, warm a tortilla and lay it flat. Place the filling about 2 inches from one end of the tortilla. Tuck in the sides and roll completely to close.

MARINATING. Marinating is the process of tenderizing and flavoring food by placing it in a seasoned liquid over a period of time. It's important to pay attention to the times given for marinating: The longer meat or fish sits in a marinade, the more intense the flavor and the more sodium (if the marinade contains it) is imparted to the food. Since marinating breaks down proteins, leaving food in a marinade too long will make it unpleasantly mushy.

MAKING MEDALLIONS. Making medallions means to gently pound chicken or beef (we make two-ounce medallions) between two pieces of wax paper or plastic wrap to make it thinner and to ensure quick cooking and tenderness. Be careful not to tear the flesh.

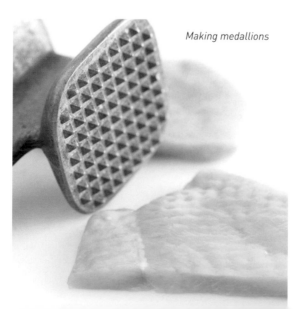

Making medallions

23

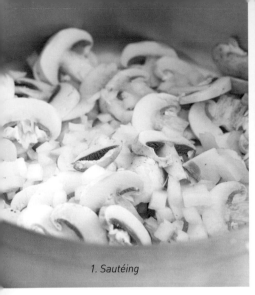

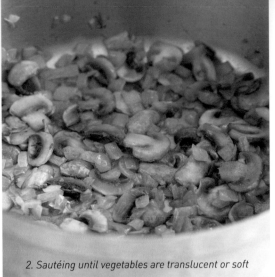

1. Sautéing

2. Sautéing until vegetables are translucent or soft

SAUTÉING. Sautéing (photo 1) means to cook food quickly in a small amount of hot oil or liquid in a skillet or sauté pan over direct heat. Sautéing seals in natural juices, sets colors, and preserves the integrity of each ingredient as well as bringing out its flavor. "Sauté onions until transculent" (photo 2) is the first step in many recipes.

DEGLAZING. Deglazing (photo 3) is when a liquid, such as stock or wine, is added to a pan in which food, usually meat or poultry, has been cooked. Cooking and stirring loosens caramelized bits from the bottom and sides of a pan, enhancing the flavor of the sauce.

REDUCING. Reducing (photo 4) means to simmer with the aim of reducing the volume of a liquid by evaporation. Reducing concentrates flavor and helps thicken the sauce.

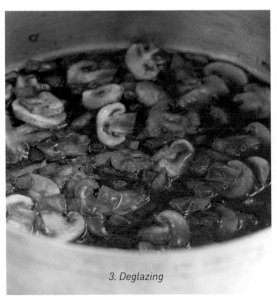

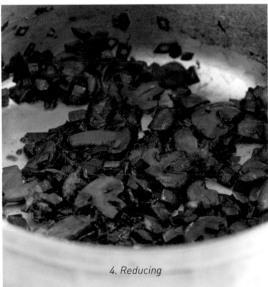

3. Deglazing

4. Reducing

SCRAPING VANILLA BEANS. To remove the seeds from a vanilla bean, cut the bean in half lengthwise. Using the tip of a sharp knife, scrape the flavorful seed paste out of the bean so the bean is clean. For ease of scraping, soak the vanilla bean in water or milk to soften it.

SIMMERING. To simmer, cook gently over low heat at a very low boil.

ZESTING. The purpose of zesting is to remove the aromatic outer peel of citrus fruit without picking up any of the bitter white pith underneath. Great tools for zesting are a citrus zester (some of our recipes will instruct you to further mince zest) or a Microplane grater (usually does not require further mincing).

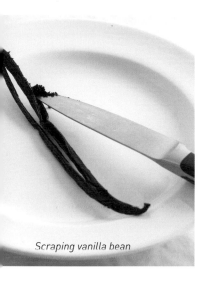

Scraping vanilla bean

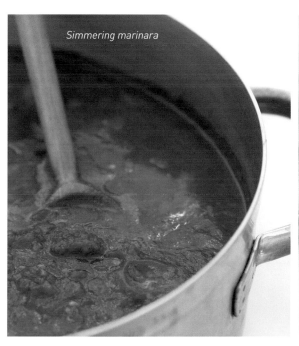

Simmering marinara

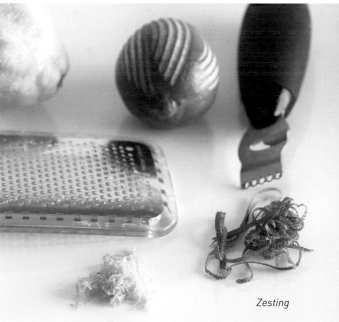

Zesting

SETTING UP YOUR KITCHEN

Having the right equipment makes cooking easier and more fun. Be sure to read a recipe through before adding it to your menu plan, and if it requires equipment you don't have, consider how often you'll use the new item before investing. For best quality at a reasonable price, visit your local restaurant supply house.

pots and pans

Baking sheet (15 x 10 x 1 inches)

Broiling or roasting pan (14 x 10 x 2 inches)

Bundt pan (10 inches)

Cake pans (8 inches and 9 inches)

Glass baking dishes or metal baking pans (8 x 8 x 2 inches and 9 x 13 x 2 inches)

Muffin tin (12 cups or two 6-cup tins)

Pie pans (9 inches and 10 inches)

Ramekins (4 ounces and 8 ounces; larger needed for Chicken Pot Pie)

Saucepans: small (1 quart), medium (1½ to 2 quarts), and large (2½ to 3 quarts)

Sauté pans: small (8 inches), medium (10 inches), and large (12 inches), with lids

Springform pan (10 inches)

Stockpot (6 quarts)

Stove-top grill pan

Tart pans (9 inches and 10 inches)

Wok

what to look for

- In sauté pans and saucepans, look for sturdy, heavy-bottomed pans that conduct heat well and can go from stove top to oven. We prefer heavy-bottomed pans because they are less likely to develop hot spots than thinner pans. Hot spots cause sticking, which, in turn, requires that you use more oil. The thickness of the sides of the pans doesn't matter. Stockpots do not need to be heavy, but they should have sturdy handles that are easy to grasp. For maximum versatility, look for one with a pasta cooker insert and steamer basket.

- Stainless steel, iron, and copper all conduct heat well.

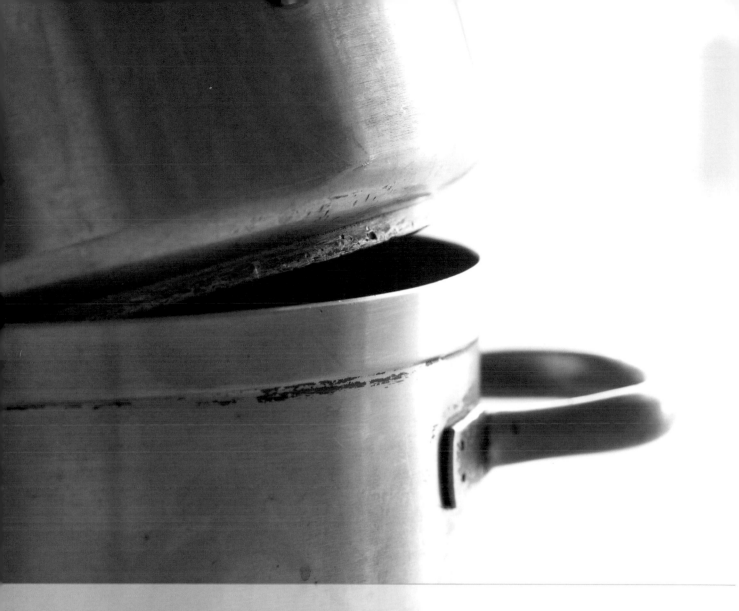

- Due to concerns about the possible toxicity of nonstick coatings when exposed to high heat, we do not use nonstick pans for any application other than cooking eggs and omelets over low heat.

- Woks should be made of steel and should *not* be nonstick. Electric woks do not work well. If an electric wok is all you have, you're better off using a large sauté pan.

- We prefer pans with cool handles. We also like glass lids, so we can see what's cooking.

- The most effective stove-top grill pans are made of cast iron.

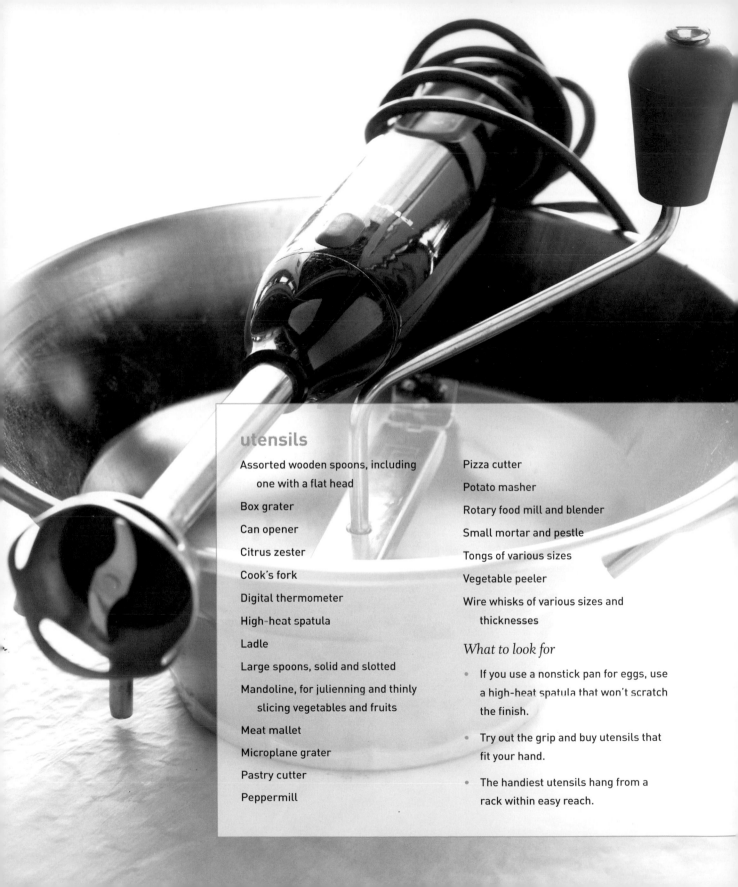

utensils

Assorted wooden spoons, including one with a flat head

Box grater

Can opener

Citrus zester

Cook's fork

Digital thermometer

High-heat spatula

Ladle

Large spoons, solid and slotted

Mandoline, for julienning and thinly slicing vegetables and fruits

Meat mallet

Microplane grater

Pastry cutter

Peppermill

Pizza cutter

Potato masher

Rotary food mill and blender

Small mortar and pestle

Tongs of various sizes

Vegetable peeler

Wire whisks of various sizes and thicknesses

What to look for

- If you use a nonstick pan for eggs, use a high-heat spatula that won't scratch the finish.

- Try out the grip and buy utensils that fit your hand.

- The handiest utensils hang from a rack within easy reach.

good knives

Boning knife, for trimming fat off chicken, duck, or meat

Chef's knife (5 to 12 inches), for slicing and chopping

Cleaver, for chopping vegetables, cutting through bone, tenderizing meat, crushing garlic cloves, and a hundred other kitchen jobs

Paring knife, for small peeling and coring jobs

Serrated knife, for cutting bread and tomatoes

Steel with guard, for sharpening

Selecting knives and keeping them sharp

- Shop where there's a good selection. A knife store is your best bet.

- Handle them to make sure they feel good and well balanced in your hand.

- Expect to pay for good cutlery. More expensive knives usually require less sharpening.

- Store knives where they don't touch each other, which will keep them sharp longer.

- Do not wash them in the dishwasher.

appliances

Blender

Crockpot

Electric mixer: handheld or stationary (stand)

Food processor with attachments; option (with a small bowl to process small quantities in recipes)

Immersion blender

Small electric spice or coffee grinder

Toaster

Vegetable juicer

What to look for

- Select a good-quality blender, with a minimum 600 revolutions per minute.

- Purchase an immersion blender that comes apart for easy cleaning.

other

Bar shaker

Cheesecloth

Colander

Cutting boards: one for raw proteins, one for other uses

Hand citrus juicer

Measuring cups and spoons

Mesh strainer

Mixing bowls: small (3 cups), medium (1½ quarts), and large (2½ quarts)

Parchment paper

Pot holders and rags

Selection of storage containers, some of which can go in the freezer

What to look for

- Mixing bowls should be stainless steel or high-fired stoneware. Steel bowls are light, practically indestructible, and can function as double boilers.

- Good-quality stainless steel measuring cups and spoons are probably more accurate and will last longer than plastic and won't retain odors. Look for a set of measuring spoons with an ⅛ teaspoon measure.

ABOUT THE RECIPES

our special ingredients

CHEESES. For the most part, we use regular full-fat cheeses: They're more fla-vorful and they melt better than reduced-fat versions. The primary exception is cream cheese, because the low-fat version is actually Neufchâtel cheese, which tastes as good as the full-fat version. We use cheese judiciously: A little grated or sliced cheese adds the finishing touch to many of our savory recipes.

COOKING SPRAYS. When we advise you to lightly coat or spray a pan with oil, the oil is not listed in the ingredients list and is not figured into the nutritional analysis because the amount of oil involved is negligible. We do mean "lightly"; a 2- to 3-second spray does the trick. Look for expeller-pressed or organic canola oil spray for higher heat applications or extra virgin olive oil spray with minimal additives and preservatives.

EVAPORATED CANE SUGAR. We've substituted organic evaporated cane sugar for sugar in all of our recipes. Evaporated cane sugar is a type of raw, less-refined sugar made from fresh cane juice that is simply evaporated and crystallized. It is straw colored with a richer, cleaner flavor than refined sugar. It has more trace minerals than regular sugar, requires less fossil fuel to produce, and is free of pesticides and residues because it's organic. We have found that it can be substituted equally for regular sugar in desserts and as a sweetener. Look for evaporated cane sugar in natural foods stores.

MULTIGRAIN BREAD. Look for breads that have whole wheat or whole grain flour as their first ingredient and that contain minimal preservatives and additives and no hydrogenated oils or high-fructose corn syrup.

STOCKS (BEEF, CHICKEN, AND VEGETABLE). While we would always encourage you to make your own stocks, we realize that stock making is a time-consuming process. Therefore, if you choose to purchase stock, choose a brand that is low sodium, natural, and organic. Our experience has been that the stocks in a box have a cleaner, richer, more homemade taste than canned varieties. Avoid powder or paste "bases" because of their high sodium levels.

TAMARI SAUCE. We use low-sodium tamari sauce because it has about a third less sodium than the regular product. We are still careful about how much we use since the sodium is concentrated. A little goes a long way to enhance the flavor of a dish.

WORCESTERSHIRE SAUCE. Some of our vegetarian recipes call for Worcestershire sauce, which traditionally contains anchovies and so, obviously, is not vegetarian. We have found a brand that does not contain any animal or fish products, nor does it have any gums, stabilizers, or preservatives; best of all, it tastes great. Look in specialty stores for similar products.

noteworthy features

RECIPE ANALYSIS. All of our recipes are analyzed for their nutritional content using Computrition software. Analyses of entrées include side dishes that appear in the ingredients list, but not those that are serving suggestions.

MEASUREMENTS. We try to use the most convenient measures in our ingredients lists. Please consult the Ingredient Conversions list (page 349) for equivalents, if you need them.

safe use of plastic wrap

We often recommend plastic wrap to cover dishes for marinating chicken, fish, or red meat or for recipe components that will be used later in a recipe that need to be refrigerated. To minimize the potential health issues related to the exposure of chemicals used in making plastics, we recommend covering a dish without letting the plastic touch the food or using a dish with a cover, preferably made of glass.

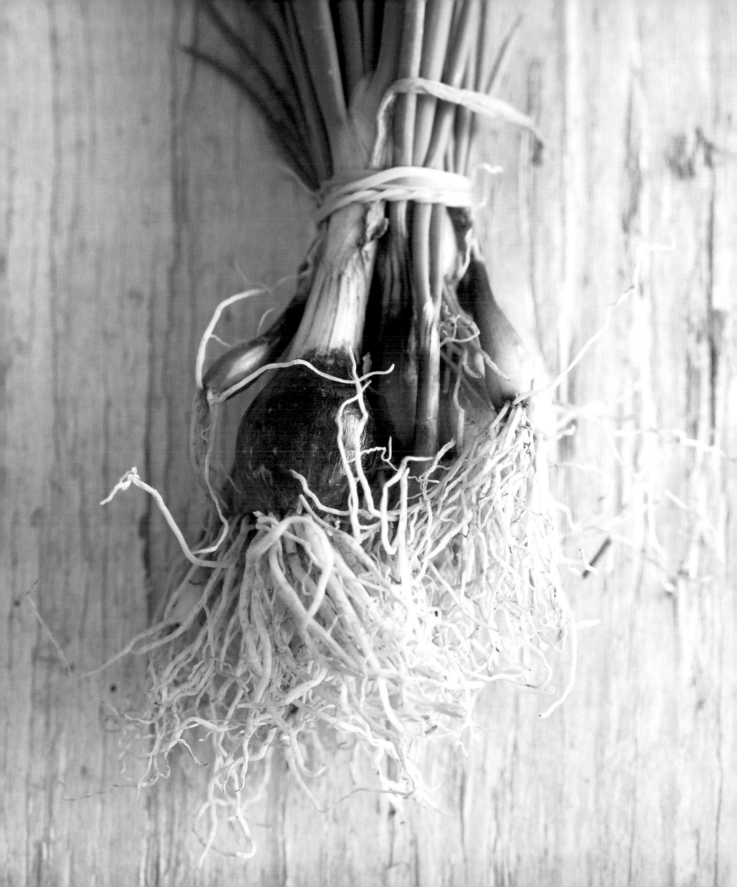

CHAPTER TWO *Nourishing yourself throughout the day is one of the smartest things you can do for your body: If you never get too hungry, you're unlikely to overeat. With these recipes, staying nourished and hydrated is a pleasure.*

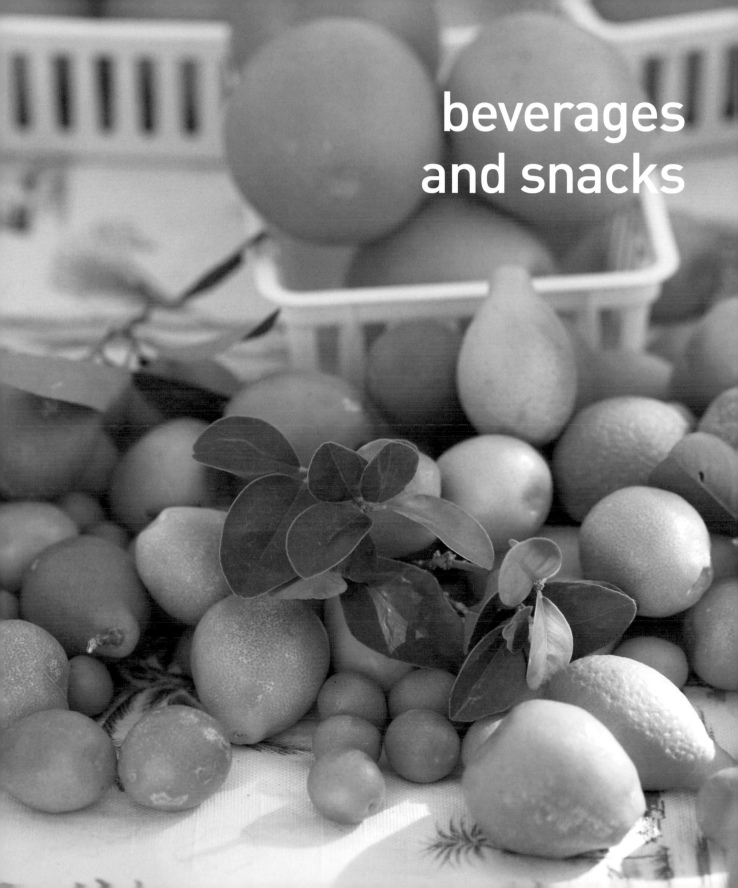

beverages
and snacks

beverages

ALMOSJITO

MAKES 1 SERVING (SEE PHOTO PAGE 38.)

1 tablespoon fresh
lime juice

¼ cup white grape juice

2 tablespoons fresh
orange juice

¼ cup sparkling water

1 tablespoon pure
maple syrup

4 fresh mint sprigs

1 cup ice cubes
(You need extra ice to
fill a 15-ounce glass.)

Combine the lime juice, white grape juice, orange juice, sparkling water, maple syrup, mint, and ice in a cocktail shaker. Shake and pour the mixture into a 15-ounce glass.

NUTRITION NOTE: *We have replaced the sugar in the original Cuban cocktail with a combo of white grape juice, fresh orange juice, and a splash of maple syrup for more flavor and nutrients.*

EACH SERVING CONTAINS

95 calories

24 g carbohydrate

0 g fat

0 mg cholesterol

1 g protein

5 mg sodium

1 g fiber

POMATINI

Gorgeous and refreshing.

MAKES 1 SERVING

½ cup white grape juice

2 tablespoons
pomegranate juice

1 tablespoon fresh
lime juice

Pinch sea salt

2 fresh mint leaves

1 cup ice cubes
(You need extra ice to
fill a 15-ounce glass.)

Combine the white grape juice, pomegranate juice, lime juice, salt, mint, and ice in a cocktail shaker. Shake and strain the mixture into an 8-ounce martini glass.

n **NUTRITION NOTE:** *Pomegranate juice has a wide spectrum of nutrients, from vitamin C to antioxidant polyphenols, with benefits in the areas of both cardiovascular disease and cancer.*

EACH SERVING CONTAINS

100 calories

25 g carbohydrate

0 g fat

0 mg cholesterol

1 g protein

27 mg sodium

1 g fiber

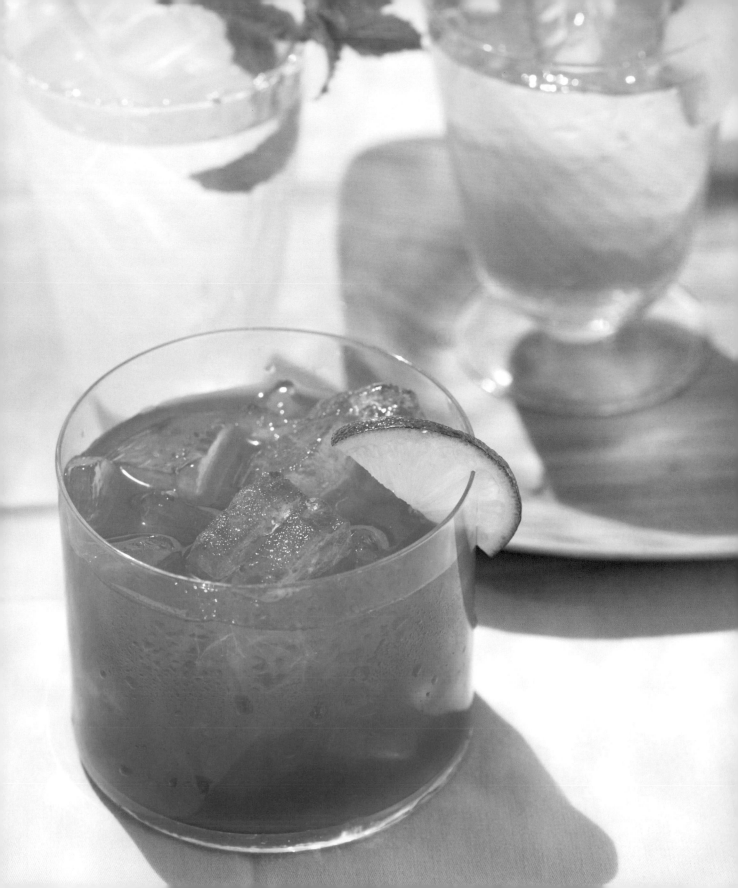

H$_2$-TINI

This sweet, delicious sipper is powered by the nutritional benefits of watermelon, which is a good low-calorie source of vitamins A, B$_6$, and C, plus fiber, potassium, and lycopene, a phytochemical that appears to protect against age-related health issues and prostate cancer. Look for a pale or buttery yellow spot on the bottom of the melon—it's one sign of ripeness—and choose a seedless melon to simplify the prep for this incomparable refresher.

MAKES 1 SERVING

1 cup fresh seedless watermelon in 1-inch cubes, plus 1 thin slice

1 lime wedge

¼ cup sparkling pear or apple juice

4 sprigs cilantro

1 cup ice cubes (You need extra ice to fill a 15-ounce glass.)

1. Whirl the watermelon chunks in a blender to make ½ cup watermelon juice.

2. Squeeze the lime wedge into a cocktail shaker. Add the squeezed lime wedge, pear juice, cilantro, and ice. Shake and strain the mixture into an 8-ounce martini glass. Garnish with a thin slice of watermelon.

EACH SERVING CONTAINS

70 calories

17 g carbohydrate

Trace fat

0 mg cholesterol

2 g protein

18 mg sodium

2 g fiber

DIRTY APPLE CHINI

Look for chai concentrate in the tea section of good grocery stores.

MAKES 1 SERVING

⅔ cup apple cider

2 tablespoons
sparkling water

1 tablespoon minced
fresh ginger

2 tablespoons Tazo
Chai Concentrate

1 cup ice cubes
(You need extra ice to
fill a 15-ounce glass.)

Combine the apple cider, sparkling water, ginger, chai, and ice cubes in a cocktail shaker. Shake and strain the mixture into an 8-ounce martini glass.

n NUTRITION NOTE: *Unfiltered apple cider that is cloudy in appearance has more nutritional benefit than cider that is clear.*

EACH SERVING CONTAINS

105 calories

26 g carbohydrate

Trace fat

0 mg cholesterol

1 g protein

9 mg sodium

Trace fiber

SPARKLING FRUIT SODA

An old-fashioned, fresh-tasting treat that's a healthy alternative to mass-marketed soft drinks.

MAKES EIGHT SERVINGS

FOR THE FRUIT PUREE

1¼ cups fresh fruit, such as mangoes, berries, or papayas

¼ cup cane sugarr

FOR THE SWEET AND SOUR MIX

2 tablespoons fresh lime juice

3 tablespoons fresh lemon juice

6 tablespoons water

3 tablespoons Simple Syrup

2 tablespoons fresh orange juice

½ cup Simple Syrup

6 cups club soda

1. Place the fruit and cane sugar in a blender and puree until smooth.

2. Combine the lime juice, lemon juice, water, Simple Syrup, and orange juice in a small bowl and mix well.

3. In each 15-ounce glass, place 3 tablespoons fruit puree, 2 tablespoons sweet and sour mix, 1 tablespoon Simple Syrup, and ¾ cup club soda and stir until well combined. Add ice and serve.

See the Simple Syrup recipe on page 42.

n NUTRITION NOTE: *Soft drinks, sweetened either with high-fructose corn syrup or artificial sweeteners, have become the beverage of choice for many adults and children alike. The health benefits of switching to green tea or a real fruit-based treat like this are huge.*

EACH SERVING CONTAINS

80 calories

21 g carbohydrate

Trace fat

0 mg cholesterol

Trace protein

26 mg sodium

2 g fiber

CHOCOLATE ESPRESSO SODA

MAKES FOUR SERVINGS

FOR THE CHOCOLATE
ESPRESSO SYRUP

½ cup brewed espresso

1 teaspoon pure
vanilla extract

1 tablespoon
Simple Syrup

¼ cup fruit juice
sweetened, low-fat
chocolate sauce

─────

¼ cup Simple Syrup

3 cups club soda

1. For Chocolate Espresso Syrup, combine the espresso, vanilla, Simple Syrup, and chocolate sauce in a small bowl and mix well.

2. Place 2 tablespoons chocolate espresso syrup, 1 tablespoon Simple Syrup and ¾ cup club soda in a 15-ounce glass and stir until well combined. Add ice and serve.

SIMPLE SYRUP

½ cup cane sugar

½ cup water

Mix the cane sugar and water in a small saucepan. Heat until the sugar dissolves.

n NUTRITION NOTE: *Making this chocolatey treat saves hundreds of calories over a blended mocha from your local coffee shop.*

EACH SERVING CONTAINS

80 calories

19 g carbohydrate

0 g fat

0 mg cholesterol

1 g protein

58 mg sodium

1 g fiber

LIMEADE

Cane sugar is a type of raw, less-refined sugar made from fresh cane juice that is simply evaporated and crystallized. It is straw colored with a richer, cleaner flavor than refined sugar. It also has a few more trace minerals than regular sugar. We have found that it can be equally substituted for regular sugar in desserts and as a sweetener.

MAKES EIGHT SERVINGS   (SEE PHOTO PAGE 38.)

¾ cup cane sugar

1 cup fresh lime juice

4 cups water

Combine the cane sugar and lime juice in a 2-quart pitcher. Add the water and mix well. Add ice and serve.

EACH SERVING CONTAINS

100 calories

27 g carbohydrate

0 g fat

0 mg cholesterol

Trace protein

3 mg sodium

Trace fiber

snacks

TRAIL MIX WITH ALMONDS AND CHOCOLATE CHIPS

Our guests who hike love to munch on this energy-rich, carbohydrate- and protein-balanced trail mix. It's packed with nutrients, including those in the chocolate.

MAKES ABOUT THIRTY-EIGHT ¼-CUP SERVINGS (SEE PHOTO PAGE 48.)

3½ cups whole almonds, blanched or unblanched

1 teaspoon sea salt

2 cups dried cranberries

2 cups dried tart cherries

1 cup dark raisins

2 cups semisweet chocolate chips

1. Preheat the oven to 350°F.

2. Spread the almonds evenly on a baking sheet, lightly spray with canola oil, and sprinkle with the salt. Roast for 10 to 15 minutes. Cool completely.

3. Combine the almonds, cranberries, cherries, raisins, and chocolate chips in a large bowl and mix well.

EACH SERVING CONTAINS

200 calories

26 g carbohydrate

10 g fat

2 mg cholesterol

4 g protein

52 mg sodium

3 g fiber

CRISPY ROASTED GARBANZO BEANS

A great "nosh." We serve these as a bar snack.

MAKES EIGHT ¼-CUP SERVINGS

1 tablespoon extra
virgin olive oil

¼ cup freshly grated
Parmesan

2 teaspoons garlic powder

½ teaspoon sea salt

1 tablespoon
onion powder

¼ teaspoon dried basil

½ teaspoon dried oregano

¼ teaspoon cayenne

½ teaspoon freshly
ground black pepper

Two 15-ounce cans
garbanzo beans

1. Preheat the oven to 325°F. Lightly spray a baking sheet with canola oil spray.

2. Combine the olive oil, Parmesan, garlic powder, salt, onion powder, basil, oregano, cayenne, and pepper in a large bowl.

3. Rinse and drain the garbanzo beans well and pat dry. Add the beans to Parmesan mixture and toss together until well coated.

4. Spread the beans evenly on the baking sheet and roast for 1¼ to 1½ hours, stirring every 15 minutes, or until golden brown and crunchy.

> **n** NUTRITION NOTE: *Snack well on garbanzo beans, which contain a perfect natural combination of complex carbohydrates and fiber. Garbanzos are also rich in folate, a vitamin that's important for heart health and for creating healthy babies.*

EACH SERVING CONTAINS

150 calories

21 g carbohydrate

4 g fat

3 mg cholesterol

8 g protein

175 mg sodium

5 g fiber

CANYON RANCH GRANOLA

There are lots of good commercial granolas out there: Look for organic ingredients, thus minimizing additives and preservatives. When you make your own, you can adjust the proportions and add-ins exactly to your taste, and you'll know it's good for you.

MAKES TWELVE ½-CUP SERVINGS

1½ cup rolled oats

½ cup oat flour

¼ cup cashews, halves or pieces

½ cup whole almonds, blanched or unblanched

Pinch ground cinnamon

Pinch sea salt

2 tablespoons apple juice concentrate

1 tablespoon pineapple or orange juice concentrate

¼ cup light coconut milk

1 tablespoon packed light brown sugar

1 tablespoon pure vanilla extract

1 teaspoon cashew butter

1 tablespoon pure maple syrup

¼ cup dried cranberries

¾ cup dried tart cherries

2 tablespoons honey, warmed

1. Preheat the oven to 275°F. Lightly spray a baking sheet with canola oil spray.

2. Combine the oats, oat flour, cashews, almonds, cinnamon, and salt in a medium bowl and mix well.

3. Combine the apple juice concentrate, pineapple juice concentrate, coconut milk, brown sugar, vanilla, cashew butter, and maple syrup in a small bowl and mix well. Stir into the oat mixture and mix until moistened.

4. Crumble the mixture onto the baking sheet and bake for 45 minutes to 1 hour, stirring after 25 minutes to allow for even cooking. Remove the granola from the oven, break it apart while it is still slightly warm, and stir in the cranberries, cherries, and honey. Cool on the baking sheet for about 1 hour. Store in a tightly sealed container.

n **NUTRITION NOTE:** *Although granola is a whole grain and filled with good fruit and nuts, our nutritionists have long cautioned our guests about the calorie level. This recipe is lower in calories than most because it has no oil, but a ½-cup serving still provides 200 calories. Portion carefully.*

c **COOK'S NOTE:** *You can make oat flour in the food processor from regular or quick rolled oats. Feel free to substitute almond butter or peanut butter for cashew butter.*

EACH SERVING CONTAINS

200 calories

32 g carbohydrate

6 g fat

0 mg cholesterol

5 g protein

53 mg sodium

4 g fiber

ROASTED EDAMAME

This is a great protein-packed to-go snack. You'll find shelled edamame (green soybeans) in the frozen foods section of most supermarkets.

MAKES SIX ¼-CUP SERVINGS

1 pound frozen shelled edamame (green soybeans)

½ teaspoon sea salt

½ teaspoon freshly ground black pepper

1½ teaspoons extra virgin olive oil

EACH SERVING CONTAINS

120 calories

9 g carbohydrate

6 g fat

0 mg cholesterol

9 g protein

144 mg sodium

3 g fiber

1. Preheat the oven to 400°F. Lightly spray a baking sheet with canola oil spray.

2. Thaw and drain the edamame in a colander. Pat dry.

3. Toss the edamame, salt, pepper, and olive oil in a large bowl. Spread the edamame evenly on the baking sheet and roast for 50 to 60 minutes, or until golden.

n NUTRITION NOTE: *We recommend real soy foods, such as edamame or tofu, rather than isolated soy protein in bars or powder as the best sources of soy isoflavones.*

c COOK'S NOTE: *Use only organic edamame because so many soybeans are genetically modified.*

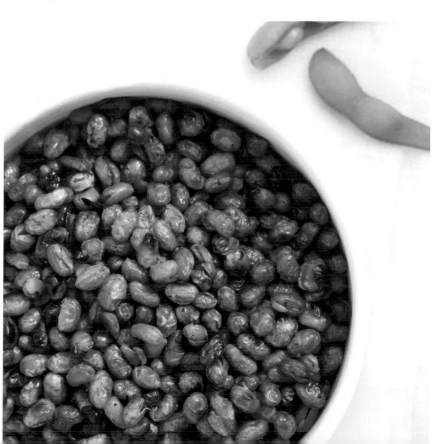

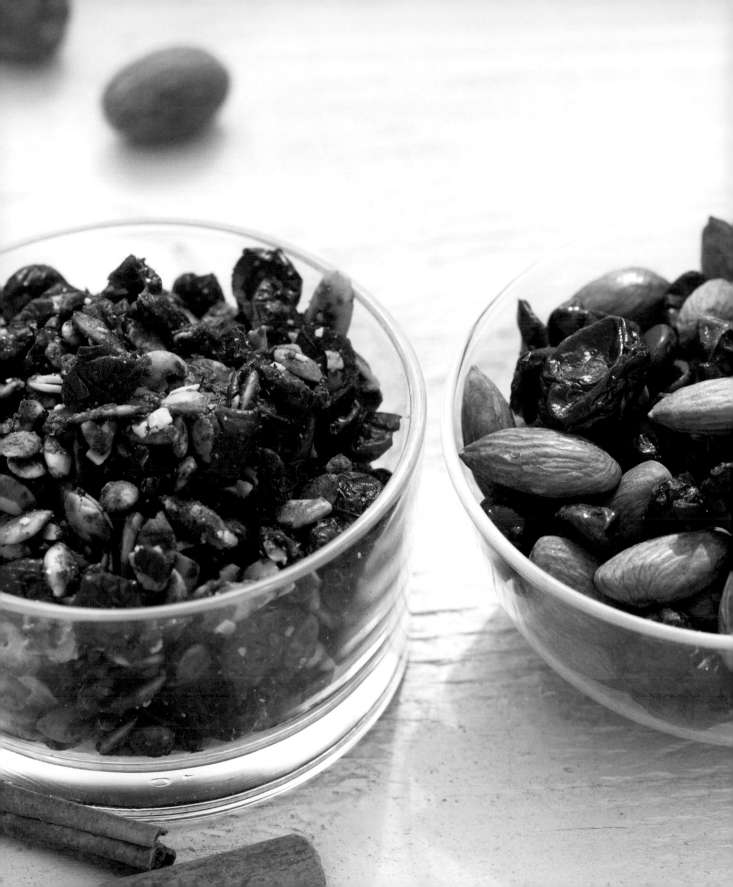

PUMPKIN CRUNCH

A favorite of Canyon Ranch guests.

MAKES TEN ¼-CUP SERVINGS

1 cup pumpkin seeds

1½ teaspoons canola oil

2 tablespoons pure
maple syrup

½ teaspoon ground
cinnamon

½ teaspoon ground
nutmeg

¼ teaspoon ground
allspice

½ teaspoon sea salt

1¼ cups dried cranberries

1. Preheat the oven to 300°F. Lightly spray a baking sheet with canola oil spray.

2. Toss the pumpkin seeds and canola oil in a small bowl. Spread the coated seeds evenly on the baking sheet. Roast for 20 minutes, or until almost dry.

3. Place the pumpkin seeds in a medium bowl and stir in the maple syrup until coated.

4. Combine the cinnamon, nutmeg, allspice, and salt in a small bowl. Add the spice mixture to the pumpkin seeds. Stir to combine.

5. Return the pumpkin seeds to the baking sheet and roast for 15 minutes, or until dry, stirring occasionally. Turn the pan several times to ensure even roasting, checking frequently—seeds burn easily. Set aside until completely cool, about 30 minutes.

6. Combine the seeds and dried cranberries in a large bowl. Store in a tightly sealed container.

n **NUTRITION NOTE:** *Pumpkin seeds are a rich source of healthy mono- and poly-unsaturated oils, besides being a good source of fiber, iron, magnesium, and phosphorus.*

EACH SERVING CONTAINS

125 calories

13 g carbohydrate

7 g fat

0 mg cholesterol

4 g protein

123 mg sodium

1 g fiber

CHAPTER THREE *Yes, it is the most important meal. Eating soon after you awake tells your body that you aren't starving, which means that your metabolism will be higher for the rest of the day. Study after study has found that people who eat breakfast are, on average, leaner than those who skip it.*

A word about eggs. Because the yolks contain cholesterol, eggs often get a bad rap. But cholesterol in foods does not have as much effect on blood cholesterol as we once thought—other factors in the diet are more significant—and eggs are a great source of high-quality protein, iron, choline, and other nutrients, and they combine beautifully with other foods in so many ways. Look for organic, locally raised eggs—try your local farmers' market.

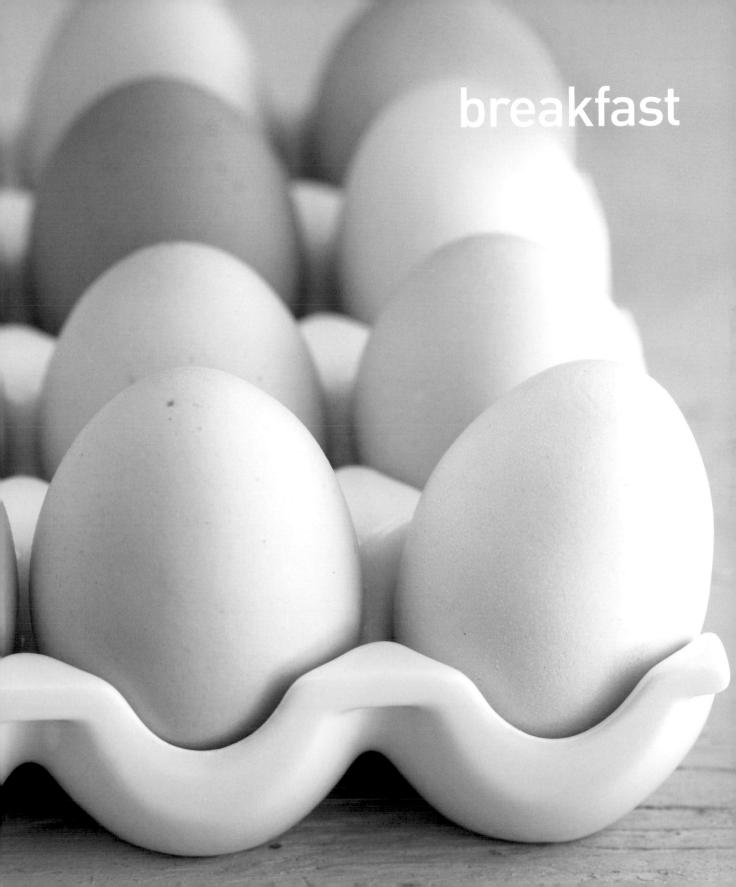

breakfast

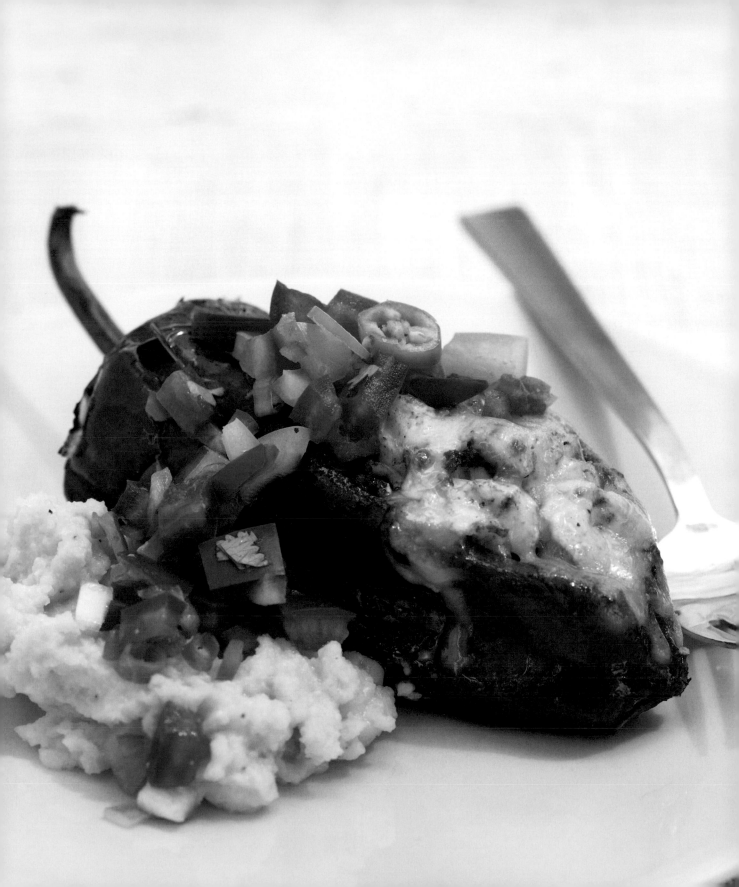

BREAKFAST RELLENOS

This is our hearty and healthy interpretation of a Mexican classic. Look for low-fat, nitrite- and nitrate-free sausage and the darkest green poblano peppers.

MAKES 4 SERVINGS

4 medium whole poblano peppers

½ pound low-fat, nitrite- and nitrate-free chicken chorizo or spicy chicken sausage

4 large eggs

4 large egg whites (about ½ cup)

½ cup shredded Monterey Jack

1 cup Soft Corn Polenta (page 115)

½ cup Pico de Gallo (page 189)

1. Preheat the broiler.

2. Roast the poblanos under the broiler until charred on all sides and the chiles begin to soften. Remove the skin and cut a slit lengthwise through the peppers. Remove the seeds and ribs and set aside. Poblanos are not considered hot chili peppers.

3. Sauté the chicken chorizo in a large sauté pan over medium heat until fully cooked and crumbly. Add the eggs and egg whites and cook to a soft scramble.

4. Stuff each pepper with ½ cup chorizo mixture so the filling is overflowing. Place on a baking sheet. Top each pepper with 2 tablespoons Monterey Jack and broil on high for 5 to 7 minutes, or until the cheese starts to melt.

5. Place ¼ cup soft corn polenta on a plate and top with one stuffed pepper. Serve with 2 tablespoons pico de gallo.

EACH SERVING CONTAINS

340 calories

17 g carbohydrate

16 g fat

268 mg cholesterol

33 g protein

758 mg sodium

3 g fiber

SAUSAGE AND EGG BREAKFAST BURRITOS

A good way to start your day right with some vegetables. Add whatever vegetable you find in your refrigerator.

MAKES 4 SERVINGS

Four 1-ounce low-fat, nitrate- and nitrite-free chicken sausage links

4 large eggs

Four 10-inch whole wheat tortillas

½ cup broccoli, chopped and steamed

cup shredded Cheddar

2 cups fresh seasonal fruit

1.   Brown the sausages in a medium sauté pan over medium heat. Let cool, then slice into ¼-inch pieces. Set aside.

2.   Lightly coat the same pan with canola oil spray. Beat the eggs with a fork or whisk in a medium bowl. Pour the eggs into the pan and scramble over medium heat until cooked through.

3.   Lay the tortillas on a flat surface. Top each with a quarter of the scrambled eggs, a quarter of the broccoli, one sliced sausage, and 2 tablespoons Cheddar. Roll up burrito style. Serve each burrito with ½ cup fresh fruit.

n **NUTRITION NOTE:** *Whole wheat or whole grain flour should be the first ingredient listed on the tortillas' ingredients label. Look for tortillas made with canola or other vegetable oil.*

EACH SERVING CONTAINS

380 calories

42 g carbohydrate

15 g fat

232 mg cholesterol

21 g protein

554 mg sodium

6 g fiber

SOUTHWEST SCRAMBLED EGGS

Pico de Gallo steps up the flavor of plain old scrambled eggs.

MAKES 4 SERVINGS

2 teaspoons canola oil

½ cup diced tomatoes

⅓ cup diced red onions

⅓ cup diced canned green chiles

¼ teaspoon sea salt

6 large eggs

¼ cup shredded low-fat mozzarella

½ cup Pico de Gallo (page 189)

1. Heat the canola oil in a large sauté pan over medium heat. Sauté the tomatoes, onions, and chiles until the onions are translucent. Season with the salt.

2. Beat the eggs in a medium mixing bowl with a fork or whisk. Add the eggs to the tomato mixture and scramble until the eggs are cooked through.

3. Evenly divide the eggs among four plates and top each serving with 1 tablespoon mozzarella and 2 tablespoons pico de gallo.

n **NUTRITION NOTE:** *This breakfast dish is actually more vegetables than eggs—the trick to a healthy meal.*

EACH SERVING CONTAINS

190 calories

7 g carbohydrate

12 g fat

326 mg cholesterol

14 g protein

332 mg sodium

1 g fiber

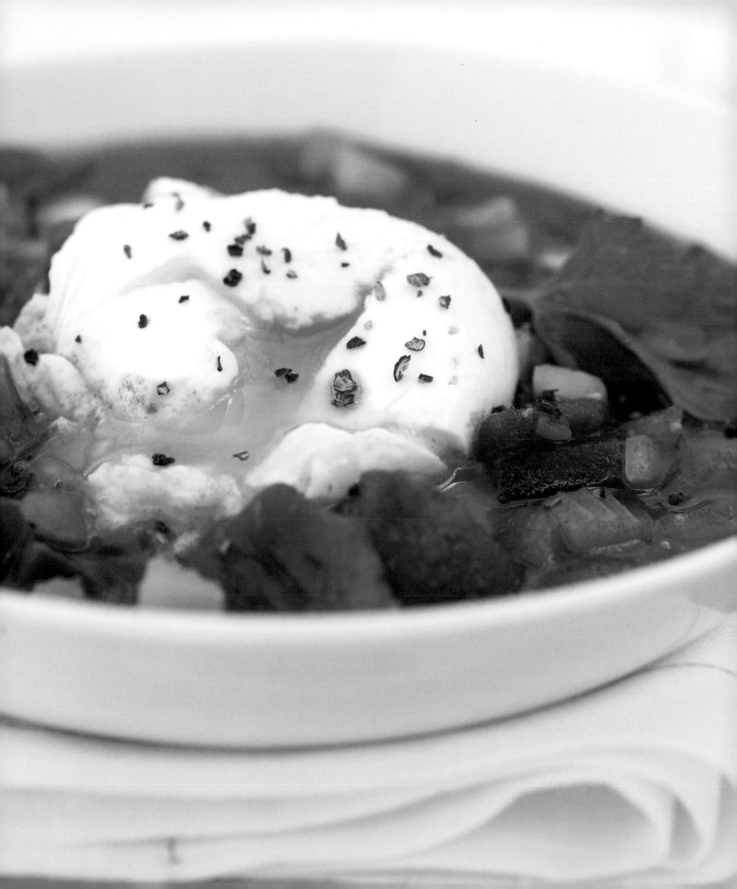

EGGS ZYDECO

Bring a taste of New Orleans to your breakfast table.

MAKES 8 SERVINGS

2 teaspoons extra
virgin olive oil

2 ounces fully cooked
andouille sausage or
spicy low-fat, nitrite-
and nitrate-free
chicken sausage

¼ cup diced yellow
bell peppers

¼ cup diced celery

½ cup diced yellow onions

1 tablespoon
minced garlic

1 tablespoon Blackening
Spice (page 193)

1 teaspoon sea salt

¼ teaspoon cayenne

1 cup diced tomatoes

2 cups low-sodium
tomato juice

½ cup water

1 tablespoon fresh
lemon juice

¼ teaspoon grated
lemon zest

2 teaspoons distilled
white vinegar

8 large eggs

1.   Heat the olive oil in a large sauté pan over medium heat. Sauté the sausage until it begins to crisp. Add the bell peppers, celery, onion, garlic, blackening spice, salt, and cayenne and sauté until the onions are translucent. Add the tomatoes, tomato juice, water, lemon juice, and lemon zest and bring to a simmer for 10 to 15 minutes, or until slightly thickened.

2.   Bring a large pot of water to a boil. The water should be at least 5 or 6 inches deep (the deeper the better). When the water boils, add the vinegar. Lower the heat to a slow simmer: The surface of the water should be moving, but not bubbling. Carefully crack the eggs one at a time into a teacup or large ladle. Lower the teacup into the water and pour the eggs out as gently as possible. The whites will coagulate and become firm and white. Most eggs will take between 2 and 3 minutes for the white to cook completely; the yolk should still be runny. Remove the eggs with a slotted spoon. Jiggle the spoon to shake off excess water.

3.   Pour ⅓ cup sausage-tomato sauce into a bowl and top with a poached egg.

n   NUTRITION NOTE: *If you can't find organic or truly farm-gathered eggs, choose those high in omega-3 fatty acids. They are laid by hens fed a diet rich in flaxseed.*

EACH SERVING CONTAINS

125 calories

7 g carbohydrate

7 g fat

216 mg cholesterol

8 g protein

449 mg sodium

1 g fiber

FRITTATA
WITH BELL PEPPERS AND ONIONS

Not just for breakfast: Frittatas makes great quick dinners. We substitute egg whites for some of the whole eggs in traditional recipes to reduce the saturated fat. Look for packaged egg whites in the egg section of most grocery stores.

MAKES 8 SERVINGS

8 large eggs

16 large egg whites (about 2 cups)

¼ cup 2% milk

½ teaspoon fresh lemon juice

⅛ teaspoon extra virgin olive oil

1 cup chopped red onions

½ cup chopped red bell peppers

½ cup chopped yellow bell peppers

¼ teaspoon sea salt

⅛ teaspoon freshly ground black pepper

1 cup shredded Cheddar

1. Preheat the oven to 375ºF. Lightly spray a 9-inch round cake pan or 8-inch cast iron skillet with canola oil spray.

2. Whisk together the eggs, egg whites, milk, and lemon juice in a large mixing bowl.

3. Heat the olive oil in a large sauté pan over medium-high heat. Sauté the onions, red bell peppers, and yellow bell peppers until tender. Season with the salt and pepper.

4. Add the onion mixture and Cheddar to the egg mixture and stir until combined. Pour the mixture into the prepared cake pan.

5. Bake for 20 to 30 minutes, or until the eggs are cooked and the cheese is melted. Let cool briefly. Cut into 8 pieces.

C COOK'S NOTE: *Substitute your favorite vegetables for the ones here—a cup each of spinach and sliced leeks, for example.*

EACH SERVING CONTAINS

175 calories

6 g carbohydrate

7 g fat

219 mg cholesterol

20 g protein

395 mg sodium

1 g fiber

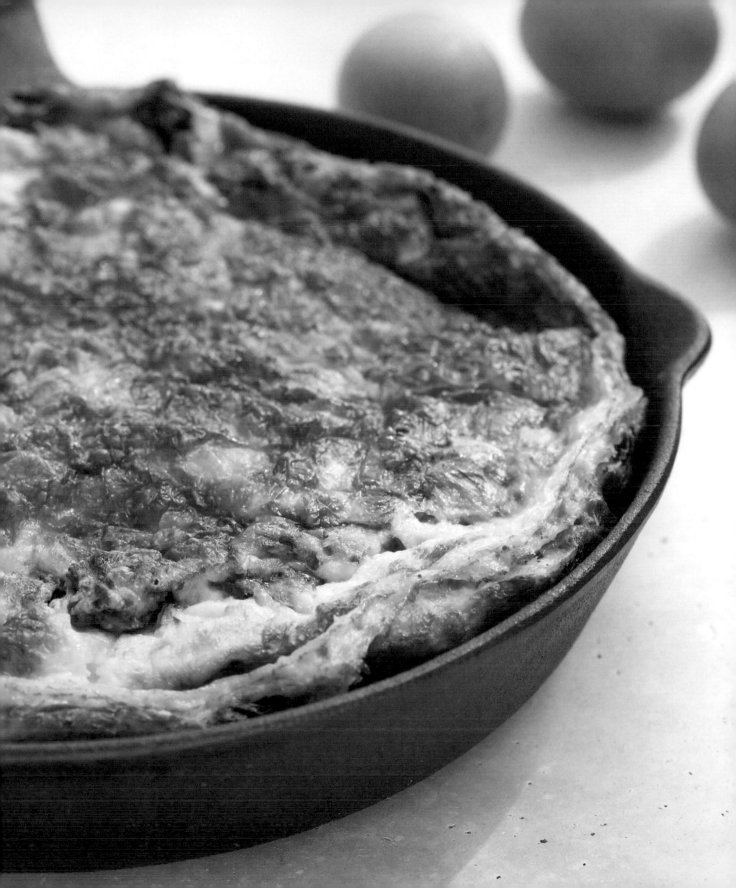

THAI FRENCH TOAST
WITH ORANGE GINGER SYRUP

A weekend treat that kids love.

MAKES 4 SERVINGS

1 large egg

4 large egg whites
(about ¼ cup)

3 tablespoons light
coconut milk

½ cup nonfat milk

¼ teaspoon ground nutmeg

½ teaspoon ground
cinnamon

½ teaspoon pure
vanilla extract

8 slices multigrain bread

FOR THE ORANGE
GINGER SYRUP

1 tablespoon orange
marmalade

1 teaspoon minced
fresh ginger

½ cup pure maple syrup

1 teaspoon fresh lime juice

315 calories
60 g carbohydrate
4 g fat
53 mg cholesterol
11 g protein
341 mg sodium
2 g fiber

EACH SERVING CONTAINS

1. Combine the egg, egg whites, coconut milk, nonfat milk, nutmeg, cinnamon, and vanilla in a shallow bowl and mix well.

2. Heat a sauté or grill pan and spray it with canola oil spray. Dip both sides of each bread slice in the egg mixture. Cook the bread over medium heat until golden brown, about 1 minute on each side.

3. For the Orange Ginger Syrup, combine the orange marmalade, ginger, maple syrup, and lime juice in a small bowl and whisk to blend well.

4. Serve 2 toast slices with 2 tablespoons of the orange ginger syrup.

n NUTRITION NOTE: *Ginger has antiinflammatory properties and cinnamon has been found to help stabilize blood sugar. So much good medicine and so much flavor!*

c COOK'S NOTE: *Light coconut milk is lower in fat than regular coconut milk. It adds a subtle yet flavorful note to this breakfast treat.*

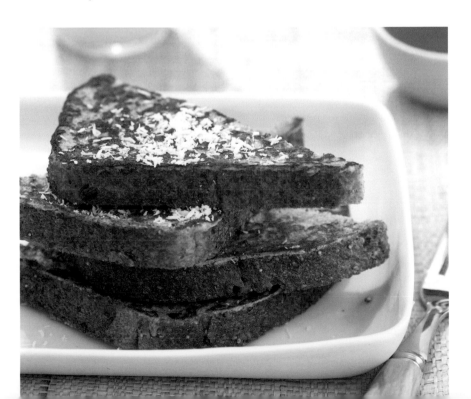

PECAN WAFFLES

Top with your favorite seasonal fruits.

MAKES 8 WAFFLES

1 cup unbleached all-purpose flour

⅓ cup whole wheat flour

½ teaspoon baking soda

3 tablespoons cane sugar

1⅓ cups buttermilk

1 large egg

½ teaspoon pure vanilla extract

2 tablespoons unsalted butter, melted

3 tablespoons chopped pecans

1 cup pure maple syrup

1. Preheat a waffle iron.

2. Combine the all-purpose flour, whole wheat flour, baking soda, and cane sugar in a medium bowl. Set aside.

3. Combine the buttermilk, egg, vanilla, and butter in a large bowl and mix well. Gradually add the dry ingredients and stir until just combined. Fold in the pecans.

4. Lightly spray the waffle iron with canola oil spray. Pour ½ cup batter on the iron. Cook for 4 to 5 minutes, or until the waffle is golden brown and begins to pull away from the iron.

5. Serve each waffle with 2 tablespoons maple syrup.

n **NUTRITION NOTE:** *Pecans have been rated fourteenth among the fifteen foods with the highest antioxidant capacity. No other nut rated as high.*

EACH SERVING CONTAINS

190 calories

25 g carbohydrate

9 g fat

32 mg cholesterol

5 g protein

110 mg sodium

2 g fiber

CREAM CHEESE–STUFFED FRENCH TOAST

A great summer brunch item.

MAKES 4 SERVINGS

¼ cup low-fat cream cheese

8 slices multigrain bread

1 cup sliced fresh strawberries

½ cup nonfat milk

2 large eggs

⅛ teaspoon ground cinnamon

¼ teaspoon pure vanilla extract

1 tablespoon canola oil

½ cup pure maple syrup

1. With a handheld mixer, beat the cream cheese in a small bowl until softened. Evenly spread 1 tablespoon cream cheese on 1 slice of bread. Top the cream cheese with ¼ cup of the sliced strawberries. Top with a second slice of bread to form a sandwich. Repeat with the remaining ingredients.

2. Beat together the milk, eggs, cinnamon, and vanilla in a wide, shallow bowl. Dip each sandwich into the egg mixture, coating both sides.

3. Heat a large sauté pan over medium heat and lightly coat with canola oil spray. Cook each sandwich until golden brown on both sides.

4. Serve each French toast sandwich with 2 tablespoons maple syrup.

n **NUTRITION NOTE:** *To make this special breakfast particularly healthy, use a whole grain bread with a good amount of fiber and a generous amount of fresh fruit.*

EACH SERVING CONTAINS

445 calories

72 g carbohydrate

12 g fat

114 mg cholesterol

14 g protein

544 mg sodium

5 g fiber

CARIBBEAN FRENCH TOAST

An exotic variation on traditional French toast.

MAKES 4 SERVINGS

½ cup 2% milk

2 tablespoons rum or
pure rum extract

1 large egg

½ teaspoon ground
cinnamon

Pinch ground nutmeg

Pinch ground allspice

8 slices multigrain bread

2 medium bananas, sliced

½ cup small diced
fresh pineapple

½ cup pure maple syrup

1. Combine the milk, rum, egg, cinnamon, nutmeg, and allspice in a wide shallow bowl. Mix well.

2. Heat a sauté or grill pan over medium heat and lightly coat with canola oil spray. Dip both sides of the bread slices in the egg mixture. Cook until golden brown, about 1 minute on each side.

3. Serve 2 slices of French toast, topped with a quarter of the sliced bananas, and 2 tablespoons of the diced pineapple with 2 tablespoons of the maple syrup.

EACH SERVING CONTAINS

340 calories

66 g carbohydrate

5 g fat

55 mg cholesterol

9 g protein

311 mg sodium

4 g fiber

GRILLED PEANUT BUTTER AND BANANA SANDWICH

Kids really go for this portable, nutrition-packed breakfast.

MAKES 4 SERVINGS

FOR THE BANANA
PEANUT BUTTER

3 tablespoons low-fat cream cheese

3 tablespoons natural peanut butter

½ banana, mashed

2 tablespoons honey

⅛ teaspoon sea salt

———————

8 slices multigrain bread

4 medium bananas

1. Combine the cream cheese, peanut butter, banana, honey, and salt in a small mixing bowl. With an electric mixer on low speed, mix to combine, then increase speed and mix until well blended, about 30 seconds. Spread 2 heaping tablespoons banana peanut butter on each of 4 slices of bread.

2. Lightly spray a large sauté pan with canola oil spray and heat to medium high. Slice the whole bananas in half crosswise and then in half again lengthwise. Place the sliced bananas in the sauté pan and sauté until caramelized, about 3 to 4 minutes.

3. Divide the cooked bananas evenly and place on top of the peanut butter bread slices. Place the 4 remaining slices of bread on top to make sandwiches.

4. Wipe the sauté pan.

5. Place the sandwiches in the sauté pan and cook over medium heat until golden brown on each side.

6. Slice each sandwich in half on the diagonal and serve.

n NUTRITION NOTE: *Look at the fiber in this imaginative breakfast sandwich. The protein and potassium are impressive also.*

EACH SERVING CONTAINS

430 calories

78 g carbohydrate

11 g fat

7 mg cholesterol

11 g protein

501 mg sodium

8 g fiber

BREAKFAST FRUIT TART

*This makes a lovely centerpiece for brunch or, with
a cup of yogurt, a great quick breakfast.*

MAKES 8 SERVINGS

4 tablespoons
unsalted butter

¼ cup low-fat
cream cheese

½ cup plus 1 tablespoon
cane sugar

¼ teaspoon sea salt

¾ cup whole wheat
pastry flour

¾ cup unbleached
all-purpose flour

3 medium plums,
pitted and sliced

1 cup fresh blueberries

1 large egg

1. Preheat the oven to 325°F. Lightly spray a 10-inch tart pan with canola oil spray and dust with all-purpose flour.

2. Combine the butter, cream cheese, ½ cup of the cane sugar, and salt in a food processor and process until mixed. Add the pastry flour and all-purpose flour and process until a dough is formed.

3. Press the dough into the bottom of the tart pan to form a crust. Arrange the plum slices around outer rim of the tart pan and spread the blueberries in the center.

4. Combine the egg and the remaining 1 tablespoon cane sugar in a small bowl. Beat with a wire whisk until mixed. Pour over the blueberries.

5. Bake for 40 minutes. Cool until the tart comes away from the sides of the pan. Cut into 8 slices to serve.

n NUTRITION NOTE: *We often recommend eating the rainbow in vegetables and fruits. There are just a few ways to eat purple, plums and blueberries being two of the finest.*

c COOK'S NOTE: *If plums and blueberries are not available, try other seasonal fruits.*

EACH SERVING CONTAINS

160 calories

26 g carbohydrate

5 g fat

31 mg cholesterol

3 g protein

73 mg sodium

2 g fiber

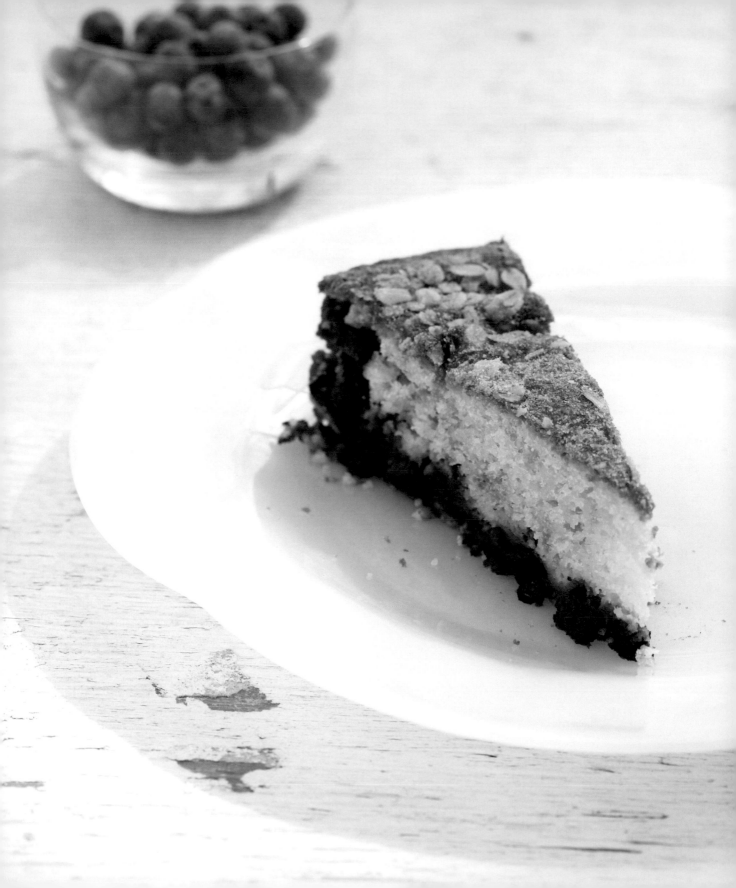

COFFEE CRUMB CAKE

A yummy breakfast cake that can double as a healthy dessert.

MAKES 16 SLICES

FOR THE CRUMB TOPPING

⅓ cup steel-cut oats

3 tablespoons whole wheat flour

3 tablespoons firmly packed light brown sugar

¼ teaspoon ground cinnamon

Pinch sea salt

1 tablespoon canola oil

———

5 tablespoons plus 1 teaspoon unsalted butter

¼ cup low-fat cream cheese

1⅓ cups cane sugar

3 large egg yolks

1 teaspoon pure vanilla extract

2 cups unbleached all-purpose flour

2½ teaspoons aluminum-free baking powder

½ teaspoon baking soda

½ teaspoon sea salt

1¼ cups buttermilk

1 pound fresh blueberries, raspberries, or cranberries

2 cups chopped pecans

1. Preheat the oven to 325°F. Lightly spray a 10-inch round cake pan with canola oil spray and dust with all-purpose flour.

2. Combine the oats, flour, brown sugar, cinnamon, salt, and canola oil in a medium bowl and mix well. Set aside.

3. With an electric mixer, cream the butter, cream cheese, and cane sugar in a large mixing bowl. Add the egg yolks and vanilla and beat until just combined.

4. Sift together the flour, baking powder, baking soda, and salt in another large bowl.

5. Add half the flour mixture to the butter mixture and mix briefly. Add ¾ cup of the buttermilk and mix briefly. Add the remaining flour mixture and mix until just combined. Add the remaining buttermilk and mix until just combined. Do not overmix.

6. Pour the batter into the prepared pan and top with the blueberries. Sprinkle the crumb topping and pecans evenly over the top of the batter.

7. Bake for 30 minutes. Rotate the cake 180 degrees and bake for an additional 20 minutes, or until a toothpick inserted in the center comes out clean. Cool on a wire rack until the cake pulls away from the pan. Cut into 16 slices to serve.

n NUTRITION NOTE: *This cake is loaded with blueberries, a rich source of anthocyanins, the antioxidant pigments linked to protection against heart disease.*

c COOK'S NOTE: *The blueberries will naturally sink to the bottom of the pan during baking because they are denser than the batter.*

EACH SERVING CONTAINS

310 calories

45 g carbohydrate

13 g fat

70 mg cholesterol

5 g protein

229 mg sodium

2 g fiber

BISCUITS AND SAUSAGE GRAVY

Spa food? You bet! Make extra biscuits and enjoy strawberry shortcake (see page 346) tonight.

MAKES 12 SERVINGS

1¼ cups unbleached all-purpose flour

¾ cup whole wheat flour

1¼ teaspoons sea salt

1 tablespoon plus 1 teaspoon aluminum-free baking powder

3 tablespoons chilled unsalted butter

⅓ cup low-fat cream cheese

¾ cup buttermilk

FOR THE SAUSAGE GRAVY

1½ teaspoons extra virgin olive oil

½ cup chopped yellow onions

1 tablespoon chopped garlic

1 pound raw low-fat, nitrite- and nitrate-free chicken or turkey breakfast sausage

2 teaspoons dried sage

(continued)

1. Preheat the oven to 400°F. Lightly spray a large baking sheet with canola oil spray.

2. Sift together the all-purpose flour, whole wheat flour, salt, and baking powder in a large mixing bowl.

3. Cut the butter and cream cheese into the flour mixture, using a pastry cutter. Stir in the buttermilk until just combined.

4. Transfer the mixture to a lightly floured work surface and knead gently just until a dough forms. Roll out the dough to ½-inch thick. Using a 2½-inch round cutter, form 12 biscuits and arrange them about 1 inch apart on the prepared baking sheet.

5. Lightly spray the tops of the biscuits with canola oil spray and bake for 10 minutes, or until golden in color and cooked through.

6. Heat the olive oil over medium-high heat in a large saucepan. Sauté the onions and garlic until the onions are translucent. Add the sausage, sage, bay leaves, and pepper and sauté, breaking up the sausage into smaller pieces. Cook until the sausage is just about cooked through.

7. Stir in the béchamel sauce and chicken stock and bring to a simmer for 20 to 25 minutes. Stir in the hot sauce, Worcestershire, and vinegar. Remove the bay leaves.

8. Serve ½ cup sausage gravy over each biscuit.

3 bay leaves

1 teaspoon freshly
ground black pepper

4 cups Béchamel
Sauce (page 175)

½ cup chicken stock

1 teaspoon hot sauce,
such as Tabasco

1½ teaspoons
Worcestershire sauce

2 teaspoons distilled
white vinegar

NUTRITION NOTE: *These biscuits are a bit healthier than those your grandmother made. We have reduced the fat by substituting the low-fat cream cheese for some of the butter and mixed some whole wheat flour into the all-purpose flour.*

EACH SERVING CONTAINS

250 calories

26 g carbohydrate

11 g fat

40 mg cholesterol

12 g protein

721 mg sodium

2 g fiber

APPLE CINNAMON-CRUSTED OATMEAL

So much better—and better for you—than flavored instant oatmeal.

MAKES 8 SERVINGS

2 cups uncooked steel-cut oats

¼ cup cane sugar

¼ cup wheat germ

1 teaspoon ground cinnamon

1 cup minced apple, about one small apple

1. Cook the oats according to the package directions. In a small bowl, combine the cane juice, wheat germ, and cinnamon. Set aside.

2. Divide the cooked oatmeal among 8 serving bowls.

3. Layer 2 tablespoons of the minced apple and top with 1 tablespoon of the cane sugar, wheat germ, and cinnamon mixture on top of the oatmeal and serve.

n **NUTRITION NOTE:** *Steel-cut oats are a great source of soluble fiber called beta-glucon, which lowers blood cholesterol.*

EACH SERVING CONTAINS

190 calories

36 g carbohydrate

3 g fat

0 mg cholesterol

7 g protein

4 mg sodium

5 g fiber

HOMEMADE FRUIT PRESERVES

MAKES TWENTY 2-TABLESPOON SERVINGS

1¼ pounds fresh
or frozen fruit, such as
strawberries, blueberries,
or peach slices

1 tablespoon fresh
lemon juice

¾ cup frozen white
grape juice concentrate

3 tablespoons dry pectin
(Sure Jell, found in
most grocery stores)

1 tablespoon cornstarch

4 tablespoons water

1. Bring the fruit, lemon juice, and grape juice concentrate to a boil in a large saucepan over medium heat. Reduce the heat to a simmer and cook for 45 minutes, or until slightly thickened and bubbles begin forming very low in the fruit mixture; you will hear popping or splattering sounds.

2. Stir together the pectin, cornstarch, and water in a small bowl until well combined.

3. Add the pectin mixture to the fruit and bring it back up to a boil. Boil for 1 minute, then remove from the heat immediately. Cool completely and store in the refrigerator in a tightly sealed container for a week.

n NUTRITION NOTE: *We are encouraging local and seasonal eating for vegetables and fruits. This is a fine way to deal with the abundance of fruit available only in season.*

c COOK'S NOTE: *1¼ pounds blueberries equal about 4 cups; 1¼ pounds strawberries or sliced peaches equal about 5 cups.*

EACH SERVING CONTAINS

50 calories

12 g carbohydrate

0 g fat

0 mg cholesterol

0 g protein

6 mg sodium

1 g fiber

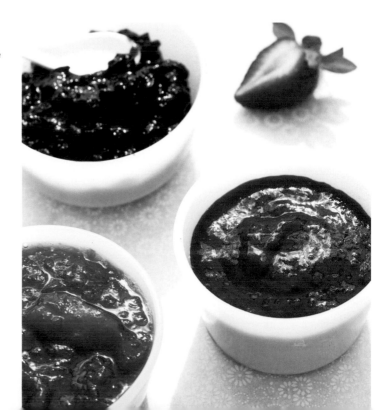

CHAPTER FOUR | *Everything Canyon Ranch does advances wellness: That's true right down to our appetizers and side dishes, which are designed to stimulate the appetite and round out the nutritional profile of our entrées while creating a balance of color, texture, and flavor. We provide our chef's suggestions for pairing main dishes and sides in the entrée recipes, but feel free to combine your own favorites. Any meal you create using this cookbook will be a healthy one—great nutrition is built into every dish.*

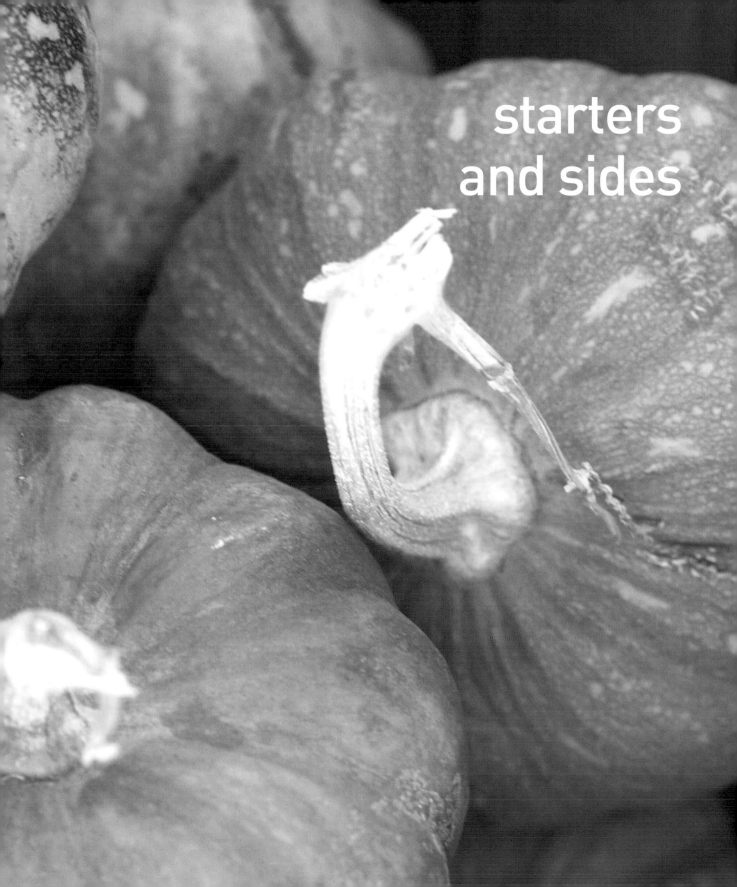

starters
and sides

FLATBREADS

Wholesome, tasty, and infinitely versatile, this multigrain flatbread recipe is the starting point for as many light, nourishing meals as you can imagine. Look for three of our favorite combinations on pages 77 to 80.

MAKES 12 FLATBREAD CRUSTS

¾ cup warm water (90° to 105°F)

1 teaspoon instant active dry yeast

1 teaspoon honey

1 tablespoon blackstrap molasses

1 cup whole wheat bread flour

½ cup cooked seven-grain cereal

½ cup oat flour

1 cup unbleached all-purpose flour

1 teaspoon sea salt

1 tablespoon minced fresh oregano

2 tablespoons grated Parmesan

1. Mix together the water, yeast, honey, and molasses in a large bowl. Add ½ cup of the bread flour, the seven-grain cereal, oat flour, all-purpose flour, and salt. Mix by hand until combined. Add the remaining bread flour and mix by hand until the dough is no longer sticky. If necessary, add extra bread flour 1 tablespoon at a time.

2. Gather the dough into a ball. Place in a medium bowl lightly sprayed with canola oil spray and cover the bowl with plastic wrap. Let sit in a warm place until doubled in size, about 1 hour.

3. Turn out the dough onto a lightly floured work surface. Divide it into 12 portions and roll into balls. Cover with plastic wrap and let rest for about 1 hour.

4. Preheat the oven to 350°F. Lightly coat a baking sheet with canola oil spray.

5. Working in batches suited to the size of your oven, roll out balls of dough with a rolling pin until very thin, about $\frac{1}{16}$ inch thick and 9 or 10 inches in diameter, and place on the baking sheet.

6. Parbake for 3 to 4 minutes. Remove from the oven and spray each flatbread crust lightly with canola oil spray and dust with a pinch of the oregano and ½ teaspoon of the Parmesan. Return to the oven and bake for an additional 5 minutes. (If you wish to use the flatbreads later, let cool on wire racks, wrap tightly in plastic wrap, and freeze.)

7. Arrange your favorite toppings on the crusts, return them to the oven, and bake for 10 to 15 minutes, or until the toppings are heated through.

n NUTRITION NOTE: *It's hard to find a prebaked product like this that is free of pre-servatives, additives, or dough conditioners. This is clean as well as healthy.*

c COOK'S NOTE: *To make oat flour, whir uncooked steel-cut oats in a blender until finely ground. To make cracker bread, parbake the dough as above. After spraying the crusts with olive oil and dusting them with oregano and Parmesan, return them to the oven for about 10 minutes, or until crisp.*

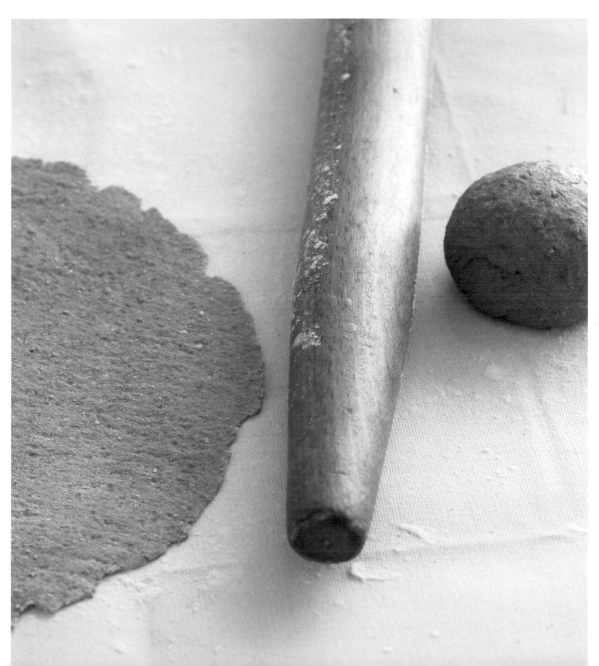

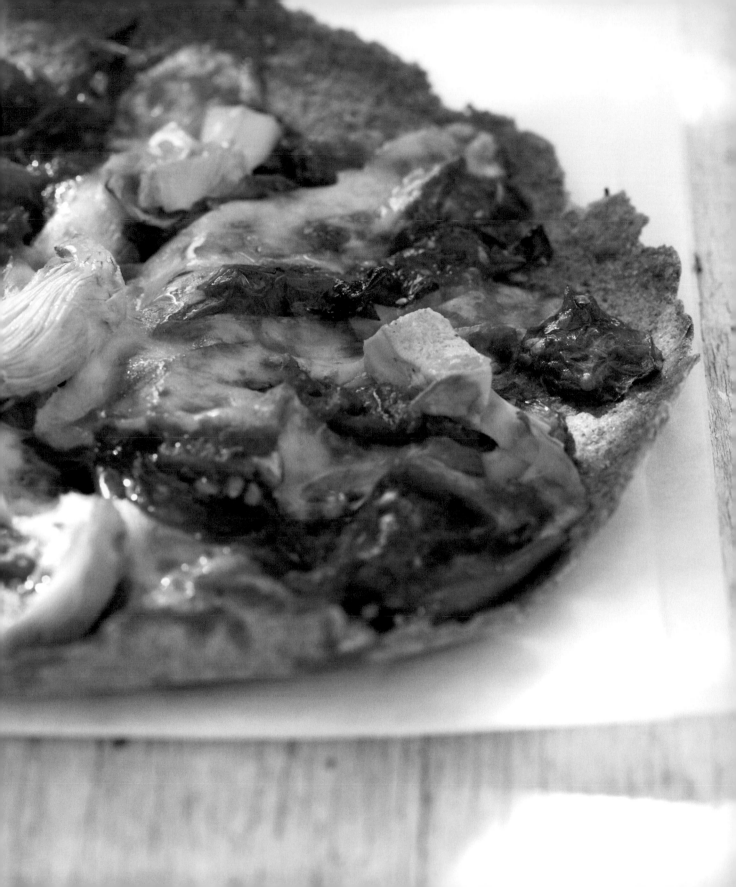

ARTICHOKE TOMATO FLATBREADS

MAKES 4 INDIVIDUAL FLATBREADS

4 parbaked Flatbreads
(page 74)

¾ pound Roma
tomatoes (about 4)

¾ teaspoon sea salt

½ pound frozen artichoke
bottoms (about 6 to 8)

1 tablespoon extra
virgin olive oil

1 tablespoon fresh
lemon juice

Pinch freshly ground
black pepper

½ cup shredded
mozzarella

1. Preheat the oven to 400°F.

2. Slice the tomatoes in half. Roast sliced side up on a baking sheet sprayed with canola spray for 15 minutes. Cool slightly and halve. Slice crosswise into ¼-inch slices. Place the tomatoes in a colander to drain off any excess liquid. Season with ½ teaspoon of the salt.

3. Place the frozen artichoke bottoms in a shallow baking dish. Pour in 1 cup of water and cover with aluminum foil. Roast for 25 to 30 minutes, until tender. Uncover, drain, and cool slightly before julienning. Toss the julienned artichokes with the olive oil, lemon juice, the remaining ¼ teaspoon of salt, and the pepper in a medium bowl.

4. Lower the oven temperature to 350°F.

5. Spread ⅓ cup roasted tomatoes to within ½ inch of a flatbread's edges. Distribute ¼ cup artichokes evenly across the flatbread and sprinkle 2 tablespoons mozzarella over the top. Repeat with the remaining flatbreads.

6. Bake until the crusts become golden and the cheese melts, about 5 minutes.

C COOK'S NOTE: *You can also use leftover cooked artichoke bottoms from the Artichoke Salad (page 144) or the Artichoke Fritters (page 91) for this.*

EACH SERVING CONTAINS

275 calories

35 g carbohydrate

10 g fat

15 mg cholesterol

14 g protein

592 mg sodium

5 g fiber

MEDITERRANEAN FLATBREADS

Look for unsulfured sun-dried tomatoes. Reconstitute them in a little hot water to make them plumper and more juicy before using. Drain before using.

MAKES 4 INDIVIDUAL FLATBREADS

4 parbaked Flatbreads (page 74)

¾ pound Roma tomatoes (about 4)

½ teaspoon sea salt

1 cup diced yellow bell peppers

½ cup sun-dried tomatoes, julienned

2 tablespoons kalamata olives

½ cup feta

1. Preheat the oven to 400°F.

2. Slice the Roma tomatoes in half. Roast sliced side up on a baking sheet sprayed with canola oil spray for 15 minutes. Cool slightly and halve. Place the tomatoes in a colander to drain off any excess liquid. Season with the salt.

3. Toss together the Roma tomatoes, bell peppers, sun-dried tomatoes, and olives in a medium bowl.

4. Lower the oven temperature to 350°F.

5. Spread ⅓ cup tomato-olive mixture to within ½ inch of a flatbread's edges. Sprinkle 2 tablespoons of the feta over the top. Repeat with the remaining flatbreads.

6. Bake until the crusts become golden and the cheese melts, about 5 minutes.

EACH SERVING CONTAINS

285 calories

45 g carbohydrate

8 g fat

25 mg cholesterol

12 g protein

674 mg sodium

6 g fiber

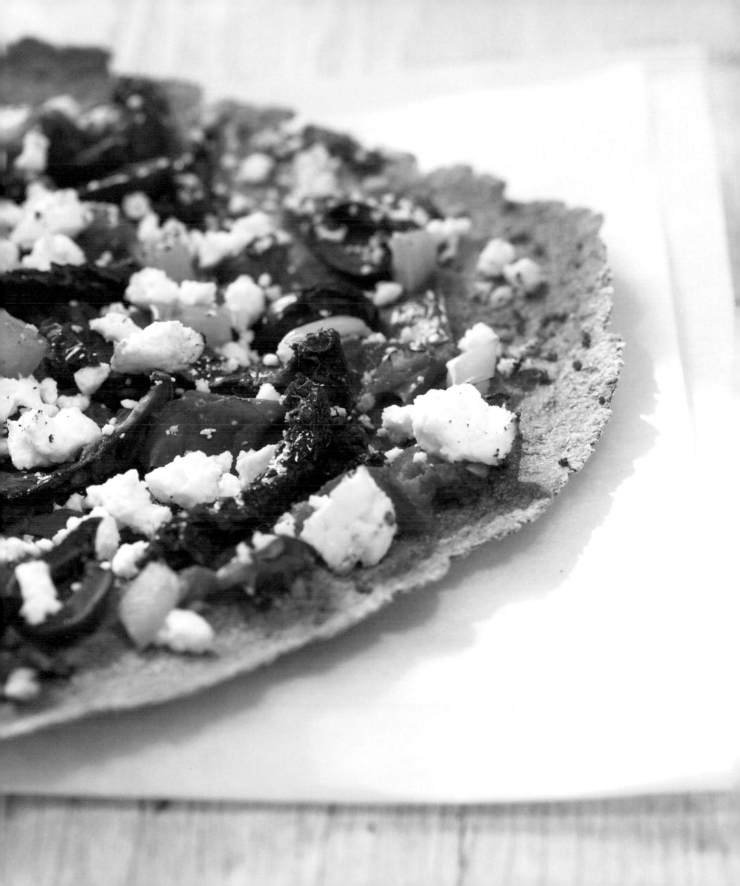

PEAR AND BLUE CHEESE FLATBREADS

MAKES 4 INDIVIDUAL FLATBREADS

4 parbaked Flatbreads
(page 74)

FOR THE BLUE
CHEESE SAUCE

½ cup crumbled
blue cheese

3 tablespoons plain
low-fat yogurt

½ cup half-and-half

———————

2 medium Bartlett
pears, cored and
cut into 24 slices

1 teaspoon fresh tarragon

1 teaspoon fresh rosemary

4 heaping tablespoons
grated Parmesan

1. Preheat the oven to 350°F.

2. Combine the blue cheese, yogurt, and half-and-half in a blender and puree until smooth.

3. Spread ¼ cup blue cheese sauce to within ½ inch of a flatbread's edges. Arrange 6 pear slices on top of the sauce and sprinkle with ¼ teaspoon tarragon and ¼ teaspoon rosemary. Top with 1 heaping tablespoon Parmesan. Repeat with the remaining flatbreads.

4. Bake until the crusts become golden and the cheese melts, about 5 minutes.

EACH SERVING CONTAINS

315 calories

37 g carbohydrate

13 g fat

34 mg cholesterol

15 g protein

636 mg sodium

4 g fiber

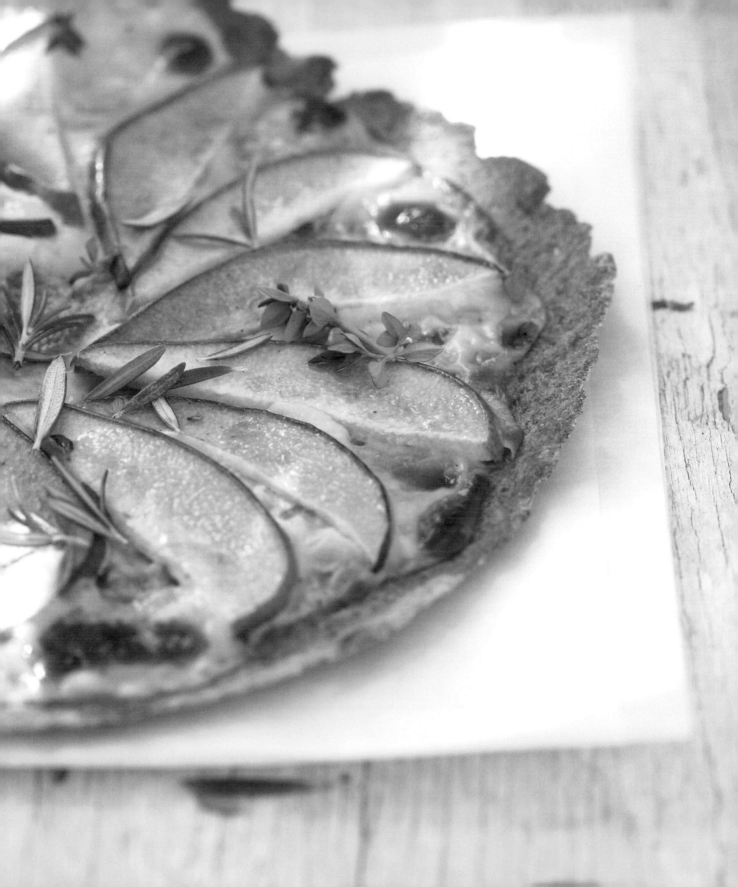

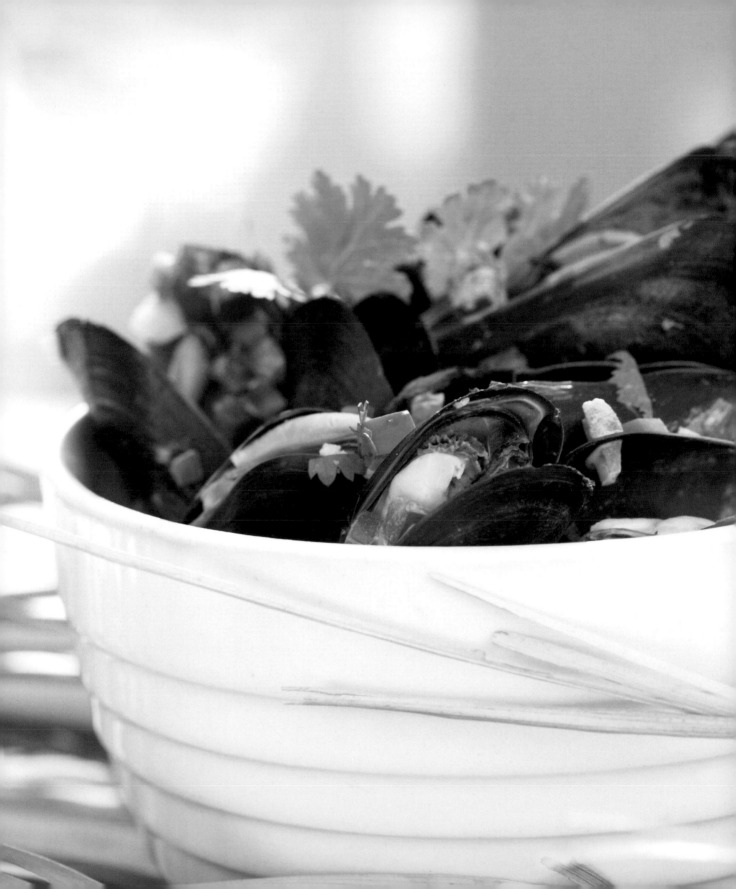

CURRIED MUSSELS

MAKES 5 SERVINGS

1 tablespoon extra virgin olive oil

½ cup diced yellow onions

1 tablespoon curry powder

1½ teaspoons minced garlic

1 tablespoon minced jalapeño peppers

1 cup light coconut milk

1 teaspoon sea salt

½ teaspoon freshly ground black pepper

2½ pounds fresh black mussels in the shell, washed and debearded

¼ cup diced tomatoes

1 tablespoon minced fresh cilantro

1. Heat the olive oil in a large stockpot over medium heat. Sauté the onions and curry powder until the onions are translucent. Add the garlic and sauté until golden. Stir in the jalapeños, coconut milk, salt, and pepper. (Wear gloves while handling hot chile peppers or wash your hands thoroughly before touching your eyes, nose, or mouth.)

2. Add the mussels and cover the pot. Steam the mussels until fully open. Add the tomatoes and cilantro. Evenly divide the mussels and sauce among five bowls.

n NUTRITION NOTE: *The turmeric in curry powder is a source of curcumin, an anti-inflammatory component of several spices.*

c COOK'S NOTE: *Clean mussels thoroughly. Discard any that are slightly open and don't close when you squeeze the shell together.*

EACH SERVING CONTAINS

120 calories

6 g carbohydrate

6 g fat

16 mg cholesterol

8 g protein

547 mg sodium

1 g fiber

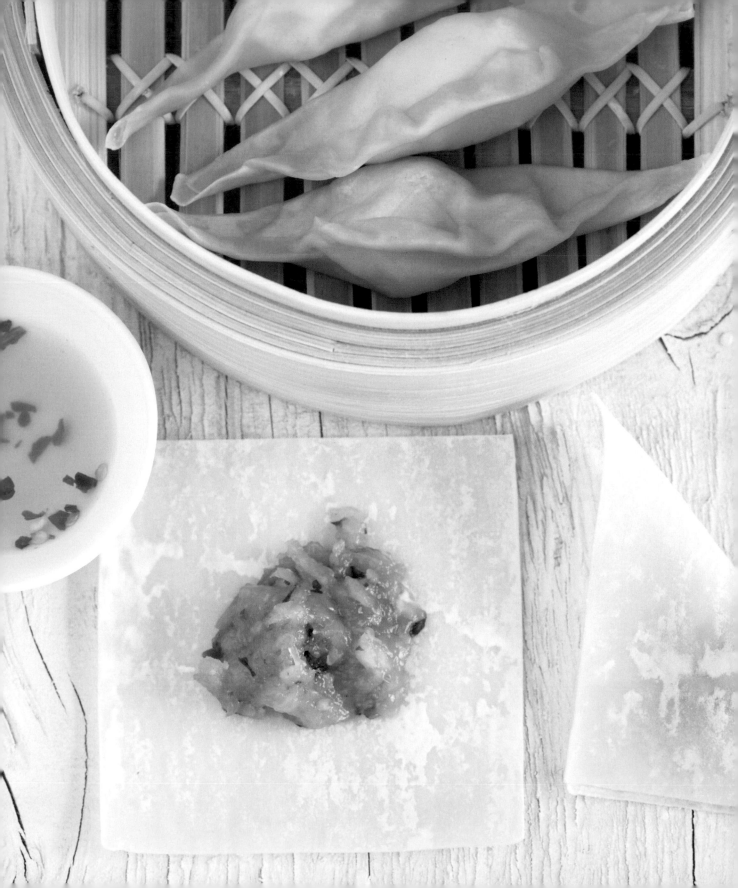

CHICKEN POT STICKERS

Double the size of the portions for a great casual main dish. Children love these with a milder version of this dipping sauce. (You can store extra sauce tightly covered in the refrigerator for up to a week.)

MAKES EIGHT 3-POT STICKER SERVINGS

FOR THE RED CHILE DIPPING SAUCE

½ teaspoon crushed red pepper flakes, or to taste

½ cup rice vinegar

1 teaspoon sea salt

2 teaspoons ground coriander

2 tablespoons minced garlic

2 tablespoons cane sugar

———

5 ounces boneless, skinless chicken breast

1 teaspoon minced fresh ginger

½ teaspoon minced garlic

¼ cup chopped scallions

Dash Tabasco

1 tablespoon low-sodium tamari sauce

1 teaspoon minced fresh basil

1 teaspoon minced fresh cilantro

1 tablespoon large egg white (about ½ large white)

24 wonton wrappers (Look for wonton wrappers in the produce section of most supermarkets.)

2 teaspoons canola oil

1. Combine the pepper flakes, rice vinegar, salt, coriander, garlic, and cane sugar in a small bowl. Set aside.

2. Place the chicken, ginger, garlic, scallions, Tabasco, tamari, basil, and cilantro in a food processor and process until a ball forms. Add the egg white and mix until combined.

3. Place 1½ teaspoons of the chicken mixture in the center of each wonton wrapper, wet the edges with water, and fold over and press lightly to seal.

4. Lightly spray the pot stickers with canola oil spray and place them in a large sauté pan over medium heat. Add ¼ cup of water. Cover the pan and steam for 5 to 6 minutes, or until the internal temperature of the pot stickers reaches 165°F. Uncover and allow the water to boil off. Add the canola oil and cook for 1 to 2 more minutes, or until the bottoms are browned.

5. Serve 3 pot stickers with 1 tablespoon red chile dipping sauce.

EACH SERVING CONTAINS

120 calories

19 g carbohydrate

2 g fat

12 mg cholesterol

7 g protein

338 mg sodium

1 g fiber

VEGETABLE NORI ROLLS

Canyon Ranch does sushi!

MAKES EIGHT 2-PIECE SERVINGS

1¼ cups cooked long-grain brown rice

2 tablespoons rice vinegar

4 nori sheets (dried seaweed sheets)

1 small carrot, julienne

1 small cucumber, julienned

1 red bell pepper, julienned

1 avocado, sliced

2 tablespoons plus 1 teaspoon pickled ginger

2 tablespoons plus 2 teaspoons low-sodium tamari sauce

1 tablespoon plus 1 teaspoon wasabi paste

EACH SERVING CONTAINS

65 calories
—
10 g carbohydrate
—
2 g fat
—
0 mg cholesterol
—
2 g protein
—
188 mg sodium
—
2 g fiber

1   When preparing the rice, cook it a little longer with a little extra water to make it sticky. Let cool slightly. Sprinkle with the rice vinegar and toss gently. Set aside until cool enough to handle.

2.   Place 1 nori sheet on top of a bamboo rolling mat (available in most cookware stores or at Target) and lightly brush with water. Moisten your fingers with water and distribute ⅓ cup of the cooked rice over the nori to within 1 inch of the edges. Divide the carrots, cucumbers, bell peppers, and avocados into four equal piles. Lay each pile lengthwise across the rice.

3.   Roll tightly, away from you, using the bamboo rolling mat to grip the nori. Place the roll seam side down on a tray and let rest. Repeat with the remaining nori sheets.

4.   Cut each roll into quarters. Serve each roll with 1 teaspoon pickled ginger, 1 teaspoon tamari, and ½ teaspoon wasabi paste.

n   NUTRITION NOTE: *Sushi made with brown rice is a little sweeter, chewier, and higher in fiber than that made with white rice.*

c   COOK'S NOTES: *You'll find pickled ginger in the Asian section of most specialty food stores or online at gingerpeople.com. We prefer ginger without artificial coloring and artificial sweeteners. Wasabi paste and nori sheets can be purchased in the Asian foods section of most supermarkets.*

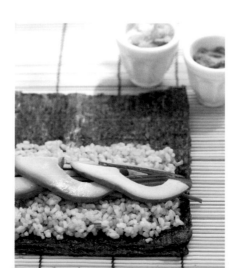
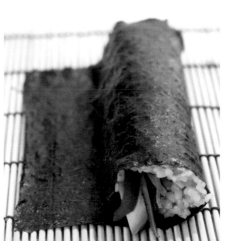

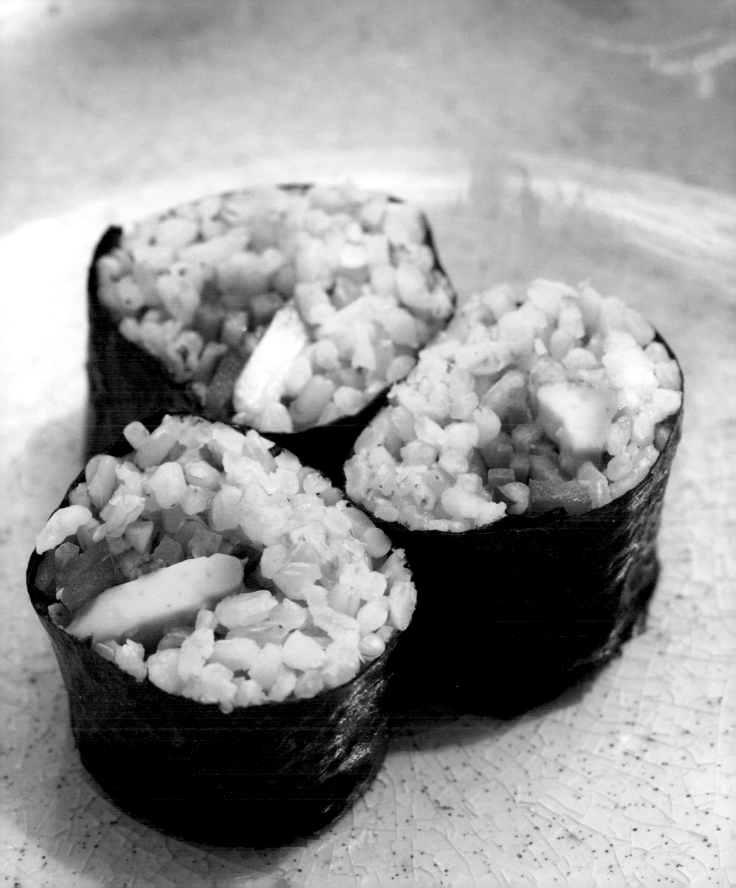

ROASTED TOMATOES WITH RADICCHIO

*The sweetness of roasted tomatoes really works
with the slight bitterness of radicchio.*

MAKES 6 SERVINGS

6 Roma tomatoes

1 tablespoon plus 1
teaspoon minced shallots

2 teaspoons minced garlic

¾ teaspoon sea salt

¾ teaspoon freshly
ground black pepper

1 small head radicchio

18 cloves roasted
garlic (see page 20)

¾ cup fat-free ricotta

1. Preheat the oven to 350°F.

2. Cut the tomatoes in half and core them. Place in a roasting pan cut side up. Mix together the shallots, garlic, ½ teaspoon of the salt, and ½ teaspoon of the pepper in a small bowl. Sprinkle shallot mixture over the tomatoes. Roast for 15 minutes. Set aside.

3. Preheat the grill. Do not turn off the oven.

4. Stand the radicchio upright on its stem and cut it lengthwise into 3 or 4 slices roughly ¾ inch thick. (Leave the stem on to prevent the slices from falling apart while grilling.) Season with the remaining ¼ teaspoon salt and the remaining ¼ teaspoon pepper. Grill and slightly caramelize the outside. Remove the radicchio from the grill and cut out the stem. Julienne.

5. Place ¼ cup radicchio and 2 tomato halves topped with 3 cloves roasted garlic and 2 tablespoons ricotta in each of six 4-ounce ramekins. Bake for 5 minutes.

> *n*   NUTRITION NOTE: *In addition to its other benefits, garlic has antiviral, antibacterial, and antifungal properties.*

EACH SERVING CONTAINS

60 calories

10 g carbohydrate

1 g fat

3 mg cholesterol

6 g protein

170 mg sodium

1 g fiber

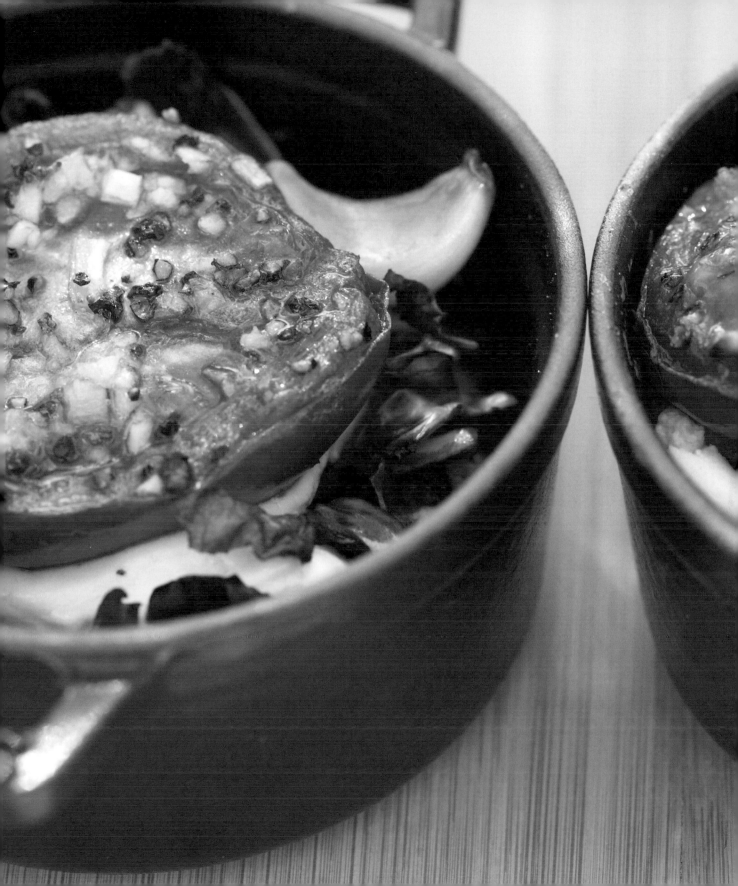

BAKED MOZZARELLA
WITH CHUNKY TOMATO SAUCE

Our light, tasty adaptation of a popular restaurant starter.
Fresh mozzarella makes a tremendous difference.

MAKES 6 SERVINGS

FOR THE COATING

½ cup unbleached all-purpose flour

½ teaspoon sea salt

¼ teaspoon freshly ground black pepper

---

2 large egg whites (about ¼ cup)

1½ cups whole wheat bread crumbs

6 ounces fresh mozzarella, sliced into 6 pieces

Chunky Tomato Sauce (page 174)

1. Preheat the oven to 400°F.

2. Combine the flour, salt, and pepper in a medium bowl

3. Beat/whip the egg whites in a medium bowl.

4. Put the bread crumbs in a bowl.

5. Dredge the mozzarella slices in the coating and shake off any excess. Dip in the egg whites, and then roll them in the bread crumbs until coated. Dip the mozzarella in the egg whites again, then roll once more in the bread crumbs.

6. Sear each side of the mozzarella in a sauté pan over medium heat for 1 minute.

7. Lightly spray a baking sheet with canola oil spray. Lightly spray the mozzarella slices and place them on the sheet.

8. Bake for 2 to 3 minutes. Turn over the pieces and bake for another 2 to 3 minutes, or until browned and crisp.

9. Serve each piece of mozzarella topped with ¼ cup of the chunky tomato sauce.

EACH SERVING CONTAINS

120 calories

10 g carbohydrate

5 g fat

18 mg cholesterol

9 g protein

289 mg sodium

1 g fiber

ARTICHOKE FRITTERS

Frozen artichoke hearts or bottoms are available at most major supermarkets, which makes this delicious vegetable a snap to include in your diet. We love these scrumptious fritters alongside Cod with Olive Salsa (page 226).

MAKES 4 SERVINGS

½ pound frozen artichoke hearts or bottoms

2 large egg whites (about ¼ cup)

3 tablespoons freshly grated Parmesan

½ teaspoon minced garlic

1 tablespoon minced shallots

1 teaspoon minced fresh flat-leaf parsley

Pinch freshly ground black pepper

3 tablespoons unbleached all-purpose flour

½ teaspoon aluminum-free baking powder

1. Boil the artichokes in salted water (¼ cup salt per 1 gallon water) in a large saucepan for 7 to 10 minutes, or until tender. Drain and chop the artichokes.

2. Fold together the artichokes, egg whites, Parmesan, garlic, shallots, parsley, and pepper in a large bowl.

3. Mix the flour and baking powder in a small bowl or cup.

4. Slowly mix into the artichoke mixture.

5. Lightly spray a large sauté pan with canola oil. Pour ⅓ cup artichoke mixture into the pan and flatten it with a spatula. Repeat with the remaining batter. Sauté the fritters on each side over medium heat until cooked through.

EACH SERVING CONTAINS

75 calories

10 g carbohydrate

2 g fat

5 mg cholesterol

6 g protein

180 mg sodium

2 g fiber

BRAISED RED CABBAGE

Wonderful with duck or chicken or our Beef Short Ribs (page 202).

MAKES FOUR ½-CUP SERVINGS

1 tablespoon extra
virgin olive oil

½ cup julienned
yellow onions

4 cups shredded
red cabbage

2 bay leaves

Pinch ground cloves

1 teaspoon sea salt

½ teaspoon freshly
ground black pepper

½ teaspoon caraway seed

¼ cup red wine

2 tablespoons red
wine vinegar

¼ cup water

1 cup julienned Red
Delicious apples

2 tablespoons honey

1. Preheat the oven to 350°F.

2. Heat the olive oil in a medium ovenproof sauté pan over medium heat. Sauté the onions in olive oil until golden. Add the red cabbage. Cover and cook for about 2 minutes. Add the bay leaves, cloves, salt, pepper, caraway seed, wine, vinegar, and water. Mix well and cover tightly.

3. Transfer the sauté pan to the oven and braise for 25 minutes, or until the cabbage is wilted. Add the apples and honey and mix well. Cover and braise for an additional 10 minutes. Remove and discard the bay leaves.

n **NUTRITION NOTE:** *Purple cabbage joins the list of vegetables and fruits rich in anthocyanins, the purple and dark red pigments that protect against cancer and heart disease.*

EACH SERVING CONTAINS

120 calories

21 g carbohydrate

4 g fat

0 mg cholesterol

2 g protein

252 mg sodium

3 g fiber

CHILLED GREEN BEAN SALAD

A great use for leftover green beans.

MAKES 4 SERVINGS

1 pound green
beans, trimmed

1 tablespoon extra
virgin olive oil

1½ teaspoons
minced garlic

1 teaspoon grated
lemon zest

1 tablespoon minced
fresh flat-leaf parsley

½ teaspoon sea salt

⅛ teaspoon freshly
ground black pepper

1. Boil the green beans in water in a large saucepan over medium heat until tender. Drain the green beans and shock in ice water to stop the cooking process. Drain well.

2. Transfer the green beans to a large serving bowl and toss with the olive oil, garlic, lemon zest, parsley, salt, and pepper. Divide the green beans evenly among four plates.

EACH SERVING CONTAINS

65 calories

9 g carbohydrate

4 g fat

0 mg cholesterol

2 g protein

241 mg sodium

4 g fiber

BROCCOLINI WITH GARLIC AND OLIVE OIL

Broccolini, which is sometimes called baby broccoli in markets, is a trademarked cross between broccoli and Chinese kale. It has long slender stalks and tiny heads that look like miniature broccoli heads. It's crunchy, with a sweet, subtly peppery flavor.

MAKES 4 SERVINGS

1 tablespoon extra virgin olive oil

1½ pounds fresh Broccolini

1½ teaspoons minced garlic

¼ teaspoon sea salt

¼ teaspoon freshly ground black pepper

Heat the olive oil in a large sauté pan over medium heat. Sauté the Broccolini and garlic until the Broccolini is cooked and still slightly crisp. Season with the salt and pepper. Divide evenly among four plates.

EACH SERVING CONTAINS

60 calories

8 g carbohydrate

3 g fat

0 mg cholesterol

3 g protein

94 mg sodium

3 g fiber

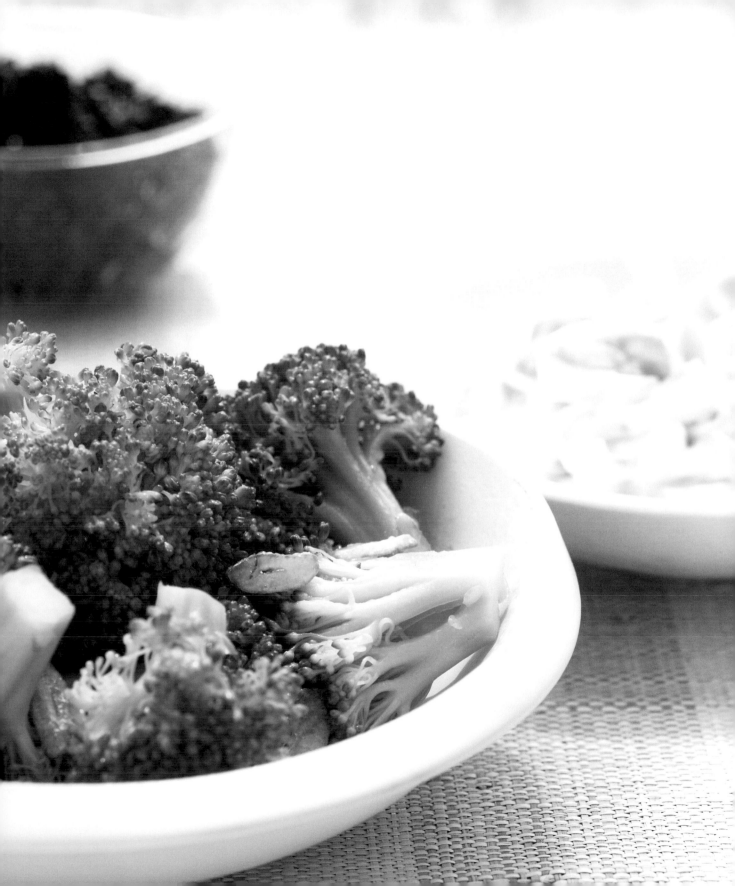

CREAMED LEEKS

Old-fashioned comfort food.

MAKES FOUR ½-CUP SERVINGS   [SEE PHOTO ON PAGE 95.]

1½ tablespoons
unsalted butter

½ pound chopped
leeks, white part only

1⅓ tablespoons
unbleached all-
purpose flour

⅔ cup 1% milk

½ teaspoon sea salt

⅛ teaspoon freshly
ground black pepper

2 teaspoons fresh
lemon juice

1. Melt the butter in a small saucepan over medium heat. Sauté the leeks until translucent. Add the flour and cook for 5 minutes, stirring constantly.

2. Keeping the heat on medium, add the milk and continue stirring until the milk thickens and coats the leeks, about 8 to 10 minutes.

3. Remove from the heat and add the salt, pepper, and lemon juice.

EACH SERVING CONTAINS

100 calories

12 g carbohydrate

5 g fat

14 mg cholesterol

2 g protein

261 mg sodium

1 g fiber

PARSNIP CARROT PUREE

This puree is a great alternative to mashed potatoes that's rich in vitamins A and C and antioxidants.

MAKES EIGHT ⅓-CUP SERVINGS

¾ pound parsnips (about 3 medium), peeled

¾ pound carrots (about 3 medium), peeled

2 tablespoons unsalted butter

1 tablespoon chopped scallions

1 teaspoon sea salt

1 tablespoon cane sugar

1. Bring 2 quarts of water to boil in a large saucepan.

2. Chop the parsnips and carrots into 1-inch cubes. Place in the boiling water and cook until soft, about 10 minutes. Drain.

3. Place the vegetables in a blender and add the butter, scallions, salt, and cane sugar. Puree until smooth.

EACH SERVING CONTAINS

85 calories

12 g carbohydrate

4 g fat

10 mg cholesterol

1 g protein

342 mg sodium

3 g fiber

RAINBOW VEGETABLE SALAD

All the colors of health.

MAKES 4 SERVINGS

½ cup julienned red bell peppers

⅓ cup julienned carrots

⅓ cup diced celery

¼ cup julienned red onions

¼ cup julienned fennel

1 tablespoon chopped fresh flat-leaf parsley

FOR THE DRESSING

2 teaspoons minced shallots

2 tablespoons prepared horseradish

½ teaspoon minced garlic

3 tablespoons fresh lemon juice

2 tablespoons water

Pinch sea salt

1 teaspoon Dijon mustard

1. Toss together the bell peppers, carrots, celery, onions, fennel, and parsley in a large bowl. Set aside.

2. Combine the shallots, horseradish, garlic, lemon juice, water, salt, and mustard in a small bowl. Whisk until well mixed.

3. Pour the dressing over the vegetable mixture and toss until well combined. Divide evenly among four plates.

EACH SERVING CONTAINS

25 calories

6 g carbohydrate

Trace fat

0 mg cholesterol

1 g protein

105 mg sodium

1 g fiber

ROASTED FENNEL

The fennel bulb is a vegetable. Its seed is a spice: You can't make Italian sausage without it. If you've never tasted the bulb, which has a mild licorice flavor, try this recipe.

MAKES 4 SERVINGS

1 fennel bulb, top removed

¼ teaspoon sea salt

¼ teaspoon freshly ground black pepper

1. Preheat the oven to 400°.

2. Cut the fennel bulb into quarters. Lightly coat with canola oil spray and season with the salt and pepper.

3. Place the quarters on a baking sheet and roast for about 20 minutes, or until the fennel just begins to brown.

4. Add ½ cup water to the pan and cover with aluminum foil. Continue to roast until soft, about another 20 minutes. Divide evenly among four plates.

EACH SERVING CONTAINS

20 calories

4 g carbohydrate

Trace fat

0 mg cholesterol

1 g protein

146 mg sodium

2 g fiber

SAUTÉED KALE

This simple preparation works for any type of green—chard, mustard, or dandelion greens, what have you.

MAKES 4 SERVINGS

1 teaspoon extra virgin olive oil

2 tablespoons sliced shallots

1 bunch kale, thick stems removed

½ teaspoon sea salt

¼ teaspoon freshly ground black pepper

2 tablespoons water

2 tablespoons apple cider vinegar

1. Heat the olive oil in a large sauté pan over medium heat. Sauté the shallots until translucent.

2. Add the kale, salt, and pepper. Add the water to steam and soften the vegetables. Cook uncovered, stirring occasionally, until the liquid is almost gone. Add the vinegar and cook until the pan is almost dry.

n **NUTRITION NOTE:** *Not only is kale rich in beta-carotene and lutein (the carotenoid linked to protection against macular degeneration), but it is also an excellent source of calcium, which is better absorbed than the calcium in milk.*

EACH SERVING CONTAINS

35 calories

5 g carbohydrate

1 g fat

0 mg cholesterol

2 g protein

243 mg sodium

1 g fiber

SAUTÉED SPINACH AND GARLIC

To remove every speck of grit from fresh spinach, float it in a clean sink with plenty of cold water. Swish and drain. With very muddy spinach, do this twice. Don't forget to wash bagged spinach, too.

MAKES 4 SERVINGS

1 tablespoon extra virgin olive oil

2 teaspoons minced garlic

1 pound spinach, washed and torn into large pieces

¼ teaspoon sea salt

¼ teaspoon freshly ground pepper

1. Heat the olive oil in a large sauté pan over medium-low heat. Sauté the garlic until just beginning to turn golden brown.

2. Add the spinach and cook briefly until wilted. Season with the salt and pepper. Divide evenly among four plates.

n **NUTRITION NOTE:** *Although a nutritional analysis of spinach shows it is a good source of calcium, it isn't well absorbed because it is bound to oxalic acid. There are several other reasons to eat spinach, though, including beta-carotene, lutein, folic acid, vitamin C, and fiber.*

EACH SERVING CONTAINS

60 calories

5 g carbohydrate

4 g fat

0 mg cholesterol

3 g protein

207 mg sodium

3 g fiber

SOUTHWEST GREEN CABBAGE SALAD

This type of tangy, clean-flavored raw cabbage salad is traditionally served with fish tacos and other classic Mexican dishes.

MAKES FOUR SERVINGS

2 cups shredded
green cabbage

1 tablespoon fresh
lime juice

1 tablespoon chopped
fresh cilantro

½ teaspoon sea salt

1. Bruise the cabbage with a meat mallet until it becomes a bit juicy.

2. Combine the cabbage, lime juice, cilantro, and salt in a medium bowl and toss together. Drain the liquid before serving. Divide evenly among four plates.

n NUTRITION NOTE: *Fresh cabbage is loaded with vitamin C as well as indoles, which help with metabolism of hormones.*

EACH SERVING CONTAINS

15 calories

4 g carbohydrate

Trace fat

0 mg cholesterol

1 g protein

240 mg sodium

1 g fiber

MASHED BUTTERNUT SQUASH WITH MAPLE SYRUP

A cold-weather favorite at Canyon Ranch in Lenox, Massachusetts.

MAKES SIX ½-CUP SERVINGS

3 pounds butternut squash

1 tablespoon pure maple syrup

Pinch sea salt

Pinch freshly ground black pepper

2 teaspoons unsalted butter

1. Preheat the oven to 350°F.

2. Cut the squash in half, scoop out the seeds, and place the halves in a large baking pan cut side down. Add enough water to barely cover the bottom of the pan.

3. Bake for 40 to 60 minutes, or until the squash is very tender.

4. Scoop out the cooked squash and transfer it to a medum mixing bowl. Add the maple syrup, salt, pepper, and butter. With an electric mixer at medium speed, beat until smooth.

n NUTRITION NOTE: *Butternut squash provides as much beta-carotene, potassium, and fiber as sweet potatoes but with fewer calories because of its higher water content.*

EACH SERVING CONTAINS

90 calories

19 g carbohydrate

2 g fat

5 mg cholesterol

2 g protein

125 mg sodium

5 g fiber

MASHED LIMA BEANS

A fiber-rich alternative to mashed potatoes.

MAKES 4 SERVINGS

1 pound frozen lima
beans, thawed

2 tablespoons extra
virgin olive oil

½ cup buttermilk

¾ teaspoon sea salt

¼ teaspoon freshly
ground black pepper

1. Steam the lima beans in a large saucepan fitted with a steamer basket for 20 minutes, or until tender. Transfer to a medium bowl.

2. Add the olive oil, buttermilk, salt, and pepper to the lima beans. Mash the mixture with a potato masher until smooth. Divide evenly among four plates.

n NUTRITION NOTE: *Beans of all types are rich in protein, fiber, magnesium, and folic acid. They make an extremely healthy alternative to mashed potatoes.*

c COOK'S NOTE: *For a smoother consistency, process in a food processor.*

EACH SERVING CONTAINS

135 calories

16 g carbohydrate

5 g fat

1 mg cholesterol

6 g protein

261 mg sodium

4 g fiber

MASHED POTATOES

So good, and so easily varied.

MAKES 4 SERVINGS

1 pound Yukon golds
or other creamy type
of potatoes, peeled and
cut into large dice

2 teaspoons
unsalted butter

½ teaspoon sea salt

¼ teaspoon freshly
ground black pepper

¼ to ½ cup 2% milk

1. Combine 1 quart water and the potatoes in a medium saucepan. Bring to a boil and cook for 15 to 20 minutes, or until the potatoes are tender. Drain.

2. Place the potatoes in a medium mixing bowl and add the butter, salt, and pepper. With an electric mixer on medium speed, slowly beat in the milk until the potatoes are fluffy. Divide evenly among four plates.

n NUTRITION NOTE: *These are lean mashed potatoes and full of flavor, but watch your serving size. Weigh your raw potato carefully. Our recommended portion is small, but satisfying.*

c COOK'S NOTE: *For Horseradish Mashed Potatoes, add 1 tablespoon prepared horseradish along with the butter, salt, and pepper.*
For Garlic Mashed Potatoes, add 1 teaspoon minced fresh garlic and 2 teaspoons minced fresh chives along with the butter, salt, and pepper.

EACH SERVING CONTAINS

110 calories

21 g carbohydrate

2 g fat

5 mg cholesterol

3 g protein

243 mg sodium

3 g fiber

MASHED SESAME SOYBEANS

Yes, you can mash soybeans, too.

MAKES 4 SERVINGS

2 tablespoons sesame seeds

1½ cups shelled edamame (green soybeans), steamed

½ cup vegetable stock

⅛ teaspoon freshly ground black pepper

1 tablespoon low-sodium tamari sauce

¼ teaspoon sea salt

1. Preheat the oven to 350°F.

2. Spread the sesame seeds evenly on a baking sheet and toast for a few minutes until golden. Cool.

3. Place the toasted sesame seeds in a spice grinder, and pulse until some oil is visible.

4. Add the edamame, vegetable stock, pepper, tamari sauce, salt, and sesame seeds to a food processor and puree until smooth.

5. Divide evenly among four plates.

n NUTRITION NOTE: *This is probably the highest protein mashed vegetable side dish you could serve. Soybeans are the superstars of the legume world. They are the only plant food that delivers complete protein, and are also a good source of folate, iron, and magnesium. Other phytonutrient compounds in soybeans may help to lower blood cholesterol and prevent cancer.*

EACH SERVING CONTAINS

130 calories

9 g carbohydrate

7 g fat

0 mg cholesterol

10 g protein

264 mg sodium

4 g fiber

COCONUT BLACK RICE

Many intriguing, exotic whole grains are now reaching Western markets. Look for Chinese black rice in Asian and gourmet specialty stores. It has a slightly sweet, nutty flavor and is a good source of iron and fiber.

MAKES 4 SERVINGS   (SEE PHOTO ON PAGE 95.)

1½ teaspoons
unsalted butter

2 tablespoons diced
yellow onions

2 tablespoons diced
yellow bell peppers

2 tablespoons diced
red bell peppers

½ cup Chinese black rice

½ cup chicken stock

½ cup water

½ cup light coconut milk

½ teaspoon sea salt

Pinch freshly ground
black pepper

1. Melt the butter over medium heat in a large saucepan. Sauté the onions, yellow bell peppers, and red bell peppers until the onions are translucent.

2. Add the rice, chicken stock, water, and coconut milk, and bring to a boil, stirring occasionally. Cover and reduce the heat to medium low for 20 minutes, or until all the liquid is absorbed. Season with the salt and pepper and fluff with a fork. Divide evenly among four plates.

n NUTRITION NOTE: *Notice the serving size for this recipe. We recommend modest portions of starchy side dishes even when they are studded with vegetables and whole grains like this one. It's a matter of calories.*

EACH SERVING CONTAINS

110 calories

19 g carbohydrate

2 g fat

2 mg cholesterol

2 g protein

286 mg sodium

1 g fiber

COLD NOODLE SALAD

Look for udon noodles, sesame oil, and black sesame seeds in Asian specialty stores or in the Asian foods section of well-stocked supermarkets. Whole grain udon noodles deliver more fiber.

MAKES SIX ½-CUP SERVINGS

½ cup julienned cucumber

½ cup chopped scallions

½ cup julienned red bell peppers

½ cup julienned carrots

¾ cup sliced shiitake mushrooms (about 6 medium caps, stems removed)

2 tablespoons black sesame seeds

¼ cup water

FOR THE DRESSING

2 tablespoons fresh lemon juice

1 tablespoon fresh ginger juice

1 tablespoon sesame oil

¼ teaspoon crushed red pepper flakes (optional)

1 tablespoon cane sugar

1 teaspoon sea salt

Pinch freshly ground black pepper

———

2 cups cooked udon noodles (about 6 ounces dry noodles)

1. Combine the cucumber, scallions, and bell peppers in a medium bowl and refrigerate while cooking the other ingredients.

2. Preheat the wok or sauté pan on high heat and lightly spray with canola oil spray.

3. Sauté or stir-fry the carrots, mushrooms, and sesame seeds in a medium sauté pan. Add the water a tablespoon at a time, continuing to cook until the carrots and mushrooms are just tender. Cool.

4. Add the carrot mixture to the cucumber mixture and refrigerate.

5. Combine the lemon juice, ginger juice, sesame oil, red pepper flakes, if using, cane sugar, salt, and pepper in a small bowl and mix well.

6. When ready to serve, toss the dressing and noodles with the vegetable mixture.

C COOK'S NOTE: *To make fresh ginger juice, grate fresh ginger using a cheese grater, collect the grated ginger in the palm of your hand, and squeeze out the juice.*

EACH SERVING CONTAINS

130 calories

19 g carbohydrate

5 g fat

0 mg cholesterol

4 g protein

343 mg sodium

3 g fiber

GRITS CAKE

Hominy grits are ground white or yellow corn kernels.

MAKES TWELVE 2.75 X 2-INCH SERVINGS

½ cup minced red onions

¼ cup minced leeks, white part only

1 teaspoon minced garlic

3¼ cups 2% milk

5 tablespoons plus 1 teaspoon unsalted butter

¼ cup heavy cream

¾ teaspoon sea salt

½ teaspoon freshly ground black pepper

1¼ cups quick-cooking grits

2 tablespoons minced scallions

2 tablespoons minced fresh chives

1. Lightly spray a large saucepan with canola oil spray. Sauté the onions, leeks, and garlic over medium heat until translucent. Stir in the milk, butter, cream, salt, and pepper. Whisk in the grits and bring to a boil. Cook for 5 minutes. Remove from the heat and mix in the scallions and chives.

2. Lightly spray an 8-inch square baking pan with canola oil spray. Pour in the grits mixture and let set. Place in the refrigerator until cold. Unmold and cut into 12 cakes.

3. Lightly spray a large sauté pan with canola oil spray. Sauté the cakes lightly on both sides until golden brown.

n NUTRITION NOTE: Allium *vegetables, the family of onion and garlic, are known for their health properties, especially protection against cardiovascular disease and cancer. This Southern version of polenta has four varieties of* allium *vegetables.*

EACH SERVING CONTAINS

130 calories

15 g carbohydrate

7 g fat

20 mg cholesterol

3 g protein

140 mg sodium

1 g fiber

MACARONI AND CHEESE

The new multigrain elbow macaroni makes this classic even more satisfying and nutritious.

MAKES 18 SERVINGS

3 cups elbow macaroni

½ cup diced yellow onions

1 tablespoon canola oil

Pinch ground cloves

¼ teaspoon freshly ground black pepper

1 bay leaf

¼ cup cornstarch

1 quart 2% milk

1 teaspoon Worcestershire sauce

½ teaspoon garlic powder

1½ teaspoons sea salt

½ teaspoon distilled white vinegar

2 cups shredded Cheddar (about 8 ounces)

¼ cup freshly grated Parmesan

½ cup whole wheat bread crumbs

1. Cook the elbow macaroni according to the package instructions. Rinse, drain, and cool.

2. Preheat the oven to 375ºF. Lightly coat a 9 x 13-inch baking pan with canola oil.

3. Sauté the onions over medium heat in the canola oil in a large saucepan, until translucent. Add the cloves, black pepper, and bay leaf.

4. Mix the cornstarch with the milk in a large bowl.

5. Add the milk mixture to the onion mixture and bring to a simmer over low heat. Cook for 2 to 3 minutes, or until thickened. Add the Worcestershire, garlic powder, salt, and vinegar. Stir in the Cheddar and Parmesan until melted. Remove and discard the bay leaf. Stir in the macaroni and mix gently. Pour the macaroni mixture into the baking pan and top with the bread crumbs.

6. Bake for 25 to 20 minutes, or until the bread crumbs are golden brown. Cut into eighteen 2.5 x 3-inch squares.

n NUTRITION NOTE: *We have saved calories in this dish by using cornstarch instead of butter and flour to thicken the sauce.*

EACH SERVING CONTAINS

165 calories

19 g carbohydrate

6 g fat

17 mg cholesterol

8 g protein

286 mg sodium

1 g fiber

OAT CAKES

Substitute vegetable stock for the milk to create a vegan oat cake.

MAKES 12 2.75 X 2-INCH SERVINGS

2 teaspoons extra
virgin olive oil

1 cup diced yellow onions

½ teaspoon minced garlic

1½ cups steel-cut oats

1½ cups 2% milk

1½ cups nonfat milk

¾ teaspoon sea salt

½ teaspoon freshly
ground black pepper

2 tablespoons minced
fresh chives

2 tablespoons
minced scallions

1.   Heat the olive oil in a saucepan. Sauté the onions and garlic over medium heat until the onions are translucent. Add the oats, 2% milk, and nonfat milk and cook until thick enough for a spoon to stand up in. Stir in the salt, pepper, chives, and scallions.

2.   Lightly coat an 8-inch square baking pan with canola oil spray. Pour in the oat mixture and refrigerate, covered, for at least 8 hours or overnight. Cut into 12 servings.

3.   Lightly spray a large sauté pan with canola oil spray. Sauté the cakes lightly on both sides until golden brown.

n   NUTRITION NOTE: *Oats, especially steel-cut oats, are a great source of the viscous fiber that lowers cholesterol and blood sugar levels. Now they're not just for breakfast anymore.*

EACH SERVING CONTAINS

110 calories

17 g carbohydrate

3 g fat

3 mg cholesterol

5 g protein

142 mg sodium

2 g fiber

POMEGRANATE COUSCOUS

Whole wheat couscous adds a subtle nutty flavor, plus an extra dose of fiber. Natural food stores often stock it.

MAKES 4 SERVINGS

1 teaspoon extra
virgin olive oil

3 tablespoons
minced shallots

¾ cup water

¼ cup pomegranate juice

¼ teaspoon sea salt

Pinch freshly ground
black pepper

⅔ cup couscous

2 teaspoons minced
fresh mint

1. Heat the olive oil in a medium saucepan over medium heat. Sauté the shallots until softened.

2. Increase the heat to medium high. Add the water, pomegranate juice, salt, and pepper and bring to a boil. Add the couscous and bring back to a boil. Cover, turn off the heat, and let sit for 10 minutes. Fluff with a fork. Stir in the mint.

EACH SERVING CONTAINS

125 calories

26 g carbohydrate

1 g fat

0 mg cholesterol

4 g protein

123 mg sodium

1 g fiber

POTATO MEDLEY

Prettier and better for you than plain white potatoes.

MAKES 4 SERVINGS

2 teaspoons extra virgin olive oil

¼ teaspoon sea salt

¼ teaspoon freshly ground black pepper

½ teaspoon garlic granules

2 cups (1 large) peeled and diced sweet potatoes

1½ cups (2 to 3 medium) peeled, diced Yukon gold potatoes

1. Preheat the oven to 400°F.

2. Combine the olive oil, salt, pepper, and garlic granules in a large bowl. Add the sweet potatoes and Yukon gold potatoes and toss to coat.

3. Spread the potatoes evenly on a large baking sheet and roast for 10 minutes, or until tender. Divide evenly among four plates.

EACH SERVING CONTAINS

120 calories

23 g carbohydrate

2 g fat

0 mg cholesterol

2 g protein

124 mg sodium

3 g fiber

ROASTED ACORN SQUASH

Sweet and simple to prepare, this is a fall favorite.

MAKES 8 SERVINGS

2 large acorn squash, cleaned and cut into 8 wedges

6 tablespoons evaporated cane juice

1 teaspoon sea salt

1 teaspoon ground cinnamon

Pinch freshly ground black pepper

1. Preheat the oven to 375°F.

2. Steam the squash in a large saucepan with a steamer basket for 15 minutes.

3. Combine the cane juice, salt, cinnamon, and pepper in a small bowl.

4. Arrange the squash skin side down on a baking sheet. Season each wedge with a scant tablespoon of the cane juice mixture.

5. Bake for 15 minutes, or until the sugar caramelizes.

n NUTRITION NOTE: *The fiber, potassium, and beta-carotene in the squash and the cinnamon in the topping make this a sweet side dish that's healthy even for diabetics.*

EACH SERVING CONTAINS

75 calories

20 g carbohydrate

Trace fat

0 mg cholesterol

1 g protein

190 mg sodium

2 g fiber

SOFT CORN POLENTA

Double the portion size and serve the polenta with a side of Broccolini with Garlic and Olive Oil (page 94) for a satisfying vegetarian meal. Polenta is a tasty cornmeal mush, a staple in Italian cooking. Look for quick-cooking dry polenta in Italian specialty grocery stores.

MAKES 4 SERVINGS

1 tablespoon unsalted butter

3 tablespoons finely minced onions

3 tablespoons white corn kernels, cut from the cob or frozen

1¼ cups 2% milk

¼ cup quick-cooking polenta

Pinch sea salt

Pinch freshly ground black pepper

1 teaspoon cane sugar

2 tablespoons freshly grated Parmesan

1. Heat the butter in a medium saucepan over medium heat. Sauté the onions until translucent. Add the corn and sauté briefly, about 30 seconds. Add the milk and bring to a boil.

2. Lightly whisk in the polenta, salt, pepper, and cane sugar. Cook until thickened, about 3 minutes. Stir in the Parmesan until melted. Divide evenly among four plates.

n NUTRITION NOTE: *This recipe provides a good example of the sweetness of some whole foods. Let foods such as fresh corn help satisfy your sweet tooth rather than relying on the intensity of concentrated sweets or artificial sweeteners.*

c COOK'S NOTE: *For a creamier consistency, add more milk, ¼ cup at a time.*

EACH SERVING CONTAINS

120 calories

13 g carbohydrate

5 g fat

16 mg cholesterol

5 g protein

100 mg sodium

1 g fiber

CRANBERRY ORZO

Orzo is a tiny rice-shaped pasta that's often used in soups.

MAKES 4 SERVINGS

¾ teaspoon
unsalted butter

2 tablespoons diced
yellow onions

½ teaspoon minced garlic

⅔ cup dry orzo pasta

¾ cup plus 2 tablespoons
chicken stock

¼ teaspoon sea salt

Pinch freshly ground
black pepper

3 tablespoons dried
cranberries

1. Heat the butter in a large saucepan over medium heat. Sauté the onions and garlic until the onions are translucent. Add the orzo and sauté for 3 to 4 minutes, or until golden brown.

2. Add the chicken stock and simmer, stirring frequently, until the liquid is almost absorbed. Remove from the heat and stir in the salt, pepper, and cranberries. Divide evenly among four plates.

EACH SERVING CONTAINS

125 calories

24 g carbohydrate

1 g fat

3 mg cholesterol

4 g protein

106 mg sodium

1 g fiber

WHOLE WHEAT CROUTONS

So much tastier than packaged croutons.

MAKES EIGHT ¼-CUP SERVINGS

4 slices (about 2 cups) whole grain bread, cut into cubes

1 teaspoon extra virgin olive oil

⅓ teaspoon sea salt

¼ teaspoon freshly ground black pepper

1 teaspoon herbs de Provence (basil, fennel seed, lavender, rosemary, sage, and thyme)

1. Preheat the oven to 400°F.

2. Lightly spray the bread cubes with extra virgin olive oil. Sprinkle with the salt, pepper, and herbs de Provence. Spread the bread cubes evenly on a baking sheet.

3. Bake until crispy, about 8 minutes. Allow to cool.

EACH SERVING CONTAINS

55 calories

10 g carbohydrate

1 g fat

0 mg cholesterol

2 g protein

151 mg sodium

1 g fiber

CHAPTER FIVE | *Homemade soup is one of the good things in life, and so satisfying and easy to make that we simply don't see a reason to eat canned soup, which is never as tasty as homemade and often has too much sodium to be healthy. The portion sizes we give are for first courses; we understand, though, that the occasions when you'll have time to prepare and serve a three-course feast are probably rare. These soups make wonderful meals—just double the portion size and serve with crusty multigrain bread or a sandwich or salad.*

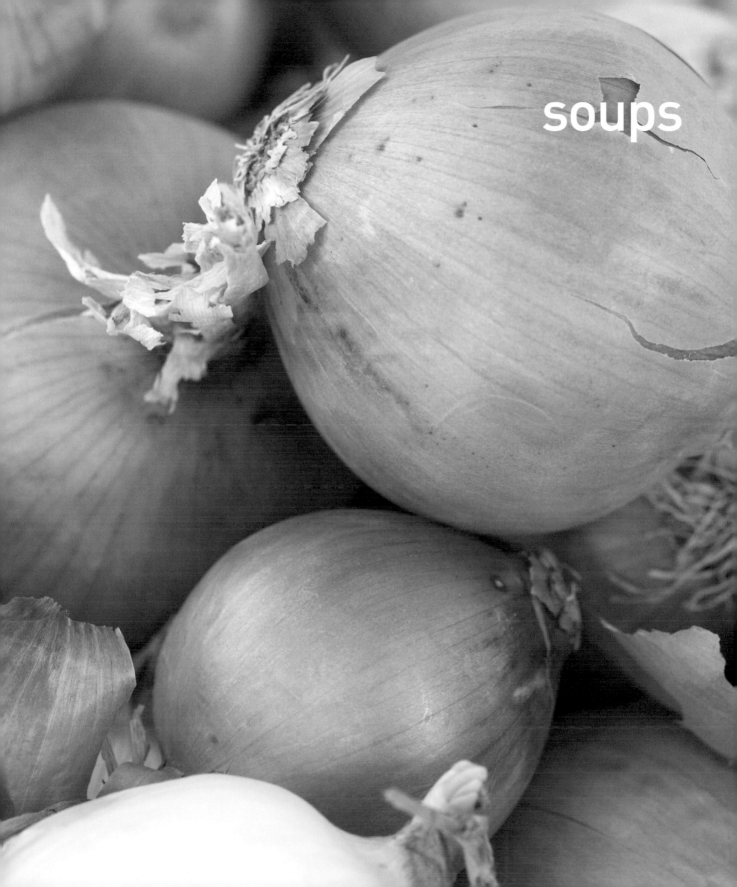

soups

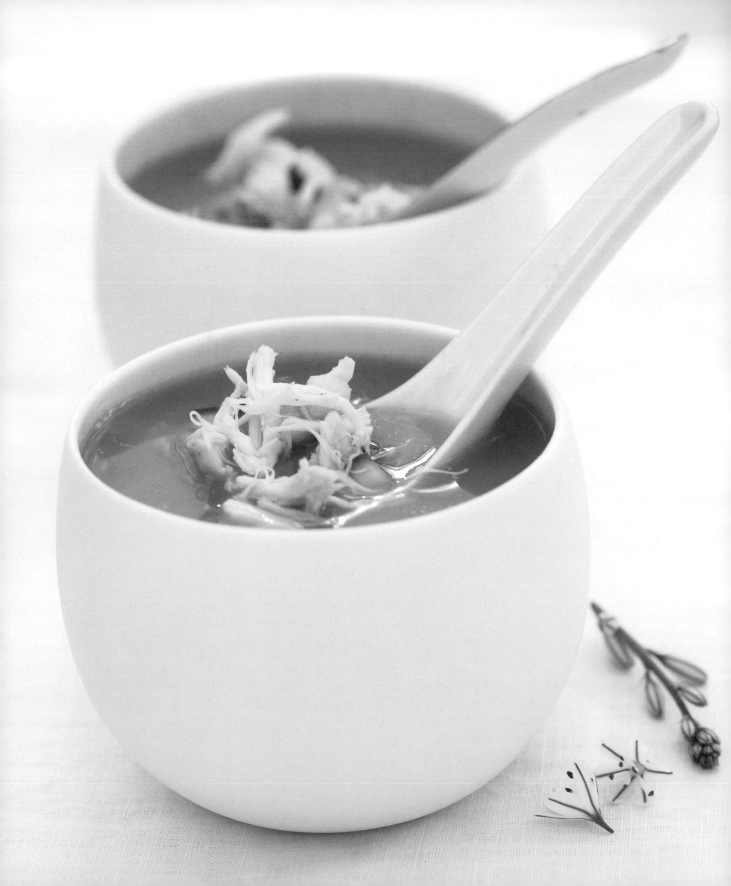

YELLOW GAZPACHO

For the best flavor and spectacular color, use yellow tomatoes in season.

MAKES SIX ¾-CUP SERVINGS

2¼ pounds diced yellow tomatoes

⅓ cup diced yellow bell peppers

2 teaspoons chopped shallots

2 teaspoons champagne vinegar

1 teaspoon extra virgin olive oil

½ teaspoon sea salt

Pinch freshly ground black pepper

⅓ cup peeled, diced cucumbers

¾ cup lump crabmeat

1½ teaspoons fresh lime juice

1. Combine the tomatoes, bell peppers, shallots, vinegar, olive oil, salt, and pepper in a blender and puree until smooth. Pour through a fine-mesh strainer into a medium bowl.

2. Combine the cucumbers, crabmeat, and lime juice in another medium bowl and marinate for about 10 minutes.

3. Serve ¾ cup gazpacho topped with 3 tablespoons crabmeat mixture.

C COOK'S NOTE: *If the gazpacho is not served immediately, it may separate, so be sure to stir or shake well before serving.*

EACH SERVING CONTAINS

60 calories

6 g carbohydrates

2 g fat

22 mg cholesterol

7 g protein

236 mg sodium

1 g fiber

CHILLED CUCUMBER SOUP
WITH ARUGULA

Peppery arugula gives this cool summer soup a savory finish.

MAKES SIX ¾-CUP SERVINGS

3 medium cucumbers, peeled and diced

1 cup water

¼ cup diced onions (white or sweet onions are best)

2 tablespoons fresh lemon juice

1 teaspoon minced garlic

1½ teaspoons sea salt

¼ teaspoon freshly ground black pepper

2 tablespoons heavy cream

¼ cup julienned arugula

1. Combine the cucumbers, water, onions, lemon juice, garlic, salt, and pepper in a blender and puree until very smooth. Refrigerate in a covered bowl for at least 30 minutes, or until well chilled.

2. Serve ¾ cup cucumber soup with 1 teaspoon cream and a sprinkle of arugula.

EACH SERVING CONTAINS

35 calories

4 g carbohydrate

2 g fat

6 mg cholesterol

1 g protein

319 mg sodium

1 g fiber

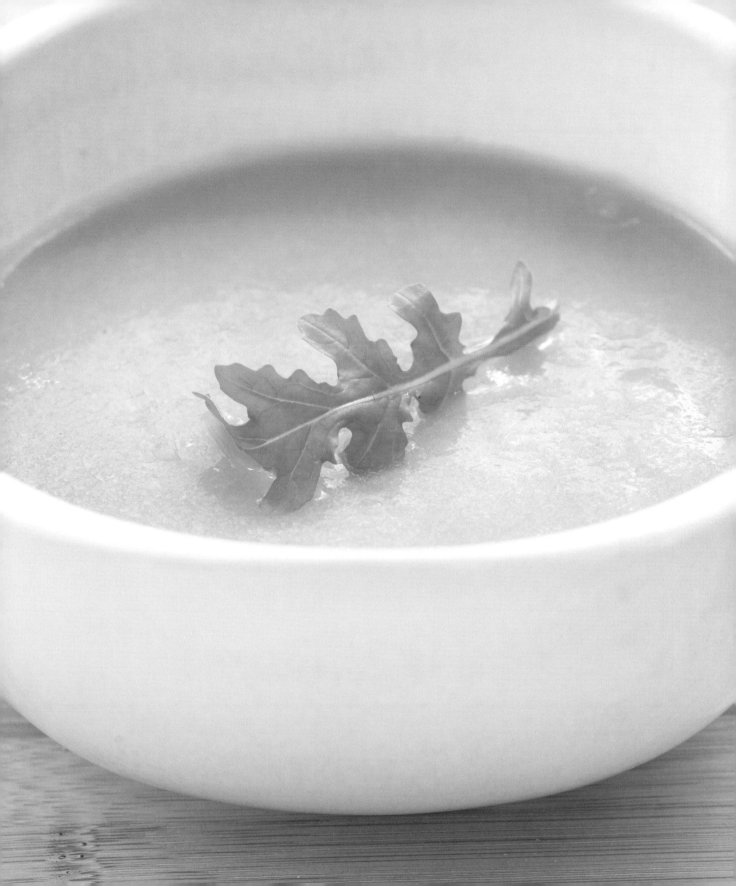

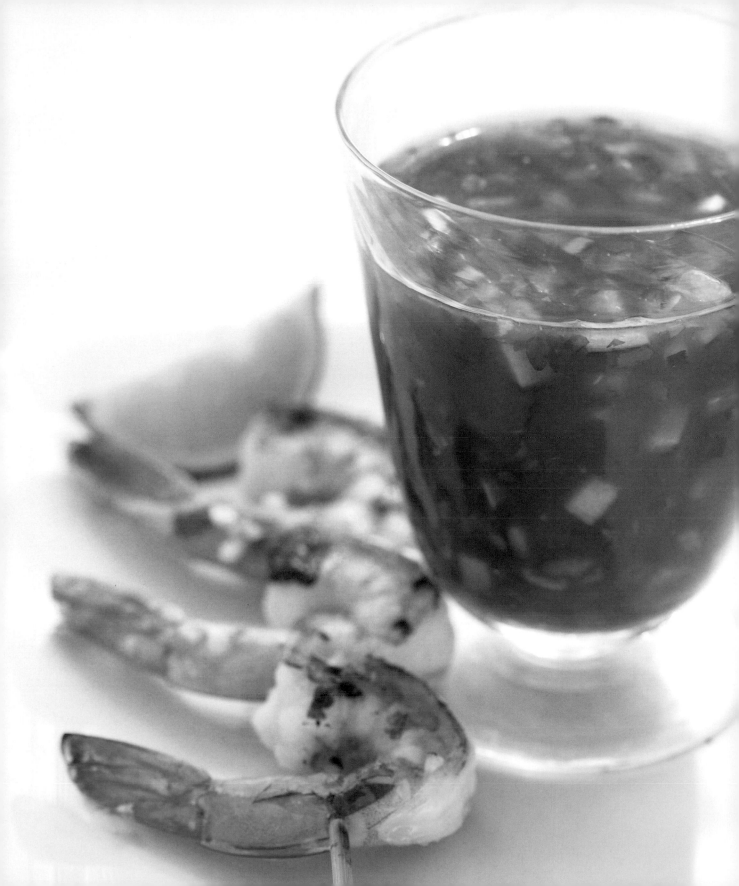

SPELT BERRY GAZPACHO
WITH CILANTRO LIME SHRIMP

Spelt, a type of wheat dating back to the time of Moses, is a good source of riboflavin, niacin, dietary fiber, and zinc. These chewy whole grain berries are also higher in protein than regular wheat.

MAKES SIX ½-CUP SERVINGS

¾ cup spelt

½ cup peeled, diced tomatoes

¼ cup diced red onions

¼ cup peeled, diced cucumbers

⅛ cup diced celery

1 tablespoon minced fresh cilantro

1 tablespoon fresh lime juice

½ teaspoon sea salt

1 cup low-sodium tomato juice

1½ teaspoons minced serrano peppers

FOR THE CILANTRO LIME SHRIMP

⅓ cup fresh lime juice

2 tablespoons minced fresh cilantro

2 teaspoons minced garlic

½ pound (18 shrimp) medium shrimp, peeled and deveined

1. Preheat the grill or broiler.

2. Place the spelt in a large saucepan with 2 quarts of water and bring to a boil. Lower to simmer and cook for 1 to 1½ hours, or until the spelt berries begin to split open but are still somewhat chewy. Drain in a colander.

3. Combine the spelt, tomatoes, onions, cucumbers, celery, cilantro, lime juice, salt, tomato juice, and serranos in a large bowl. (Wear gloves when handling hot chile peppers or wash your hands thoroughly before touching your eyes, nose, or mouth.) Refrigerate for 4 hours or overnight.

4. In a shallow glass baking dish, combine the lime juice, cilantro, and garlic.

5. For ease of grilling, skewer the 18 shrimp on three 6-inch bamboo skewers, and place in the marinade for 10 minutes.

6. Grill or broil the shrimp until cooked through, about 2 minutes on each side. Allow the shrimp to cool slightly.

7. Serve ½ cup spelt berry gazpacho in a martini glass with 3 shrimp.

EACH SERVING CONTAINS

150 calories

25 g carbohydrate

1 g fat

53 mg cholesterol

11 g protein

251 mg sodium

4 g fiber

CREAM OF TOMATO TARRAGON SOUP

Tarragon makes this soup considerably more interesting than plain old tomato.

MAKES SIX ¾-CUP SERVINGS

1 teaspoon extra
virgin olive oil

¼ cup diced yellow onions

1 tablespoon
minced garlic

⅓ cup canned
pureed tomatoes

½ cup white wine

1½ cups chopped
fresh tomatoes

2⅓ cups vegetable stock

2 tablespoons
heavy cream

¾ teaspoon sea salt

⅛ teaspoon freshly
ground black pepper

½ teaspoon minced
fresh tarragon

1. Heat the olive oil over medium heat in a large saucepan. Sauté the onions and garlic until soft. Add the pureed tomato and cook until tawny in color, 4 to 5 minutes. Add the white wine and reduce by half.

2. Add the chopped tomatoes and the vegetable stock, bring to a boil, reduce the heat to low, and simmer for 30 minutes. Add the heavy cream and remove from the heat. Cool slightly.

3. Pour the tomato mixture into a blender and puree until smooth. Pour the puree through a fine-mesh strainer into a medium bowl and reserve the liquid. Stir in the salt, pepper, and tarragon.

n NUTRITION NOTE: *This fragrant soup is made creamy by only two tablespoons of cream. It's loaded with lycopene from the tomatoes.*

60 calories

5 g carbohydrate

3 g fat

6 mg cholesterol

1 g protein

247 mg sodium

1 g fiber

EACH SERVING CONTAINS

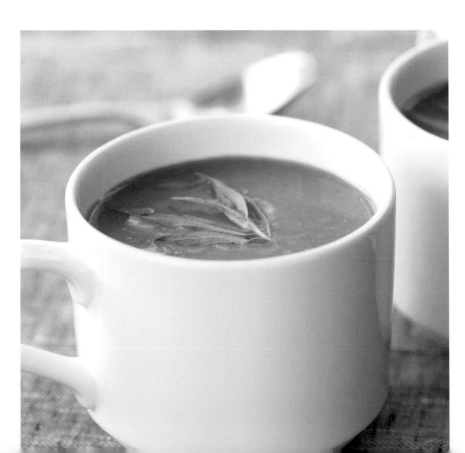

FRENCH ONION SOUP

Our light, elegant take on a sometimes overly rich classic.

MAKES SIX ¾-CUP SERVINGS

2 teaspoons extra virgin olive oil

1 pound yellow onions, halved and thinly sliced

1 tablespoon minced garlic

⅓ cup white wine

¼ teaspoon minced fresh thyme

1 tablespoon chopped fresh flat-leaf parsley

1 bay leaf

Pinch freshly ground black pepper

2¼ cups chicken stock

⅓ cup beef stock

1 teaspoon sea salt

¼ teaspoon Worcestershire sauce

Six ½-inch-thick slices whole wheat French baguette

3 tablespoons shredded Swiss

1. Heat the olive oil in a heavy-bottomed medium saucepan over low heat. Sauté the onions and garlic until caramelized, stirring often so they don't burn.

2. Add the white wine and bring to a boil over medium heat. Cook until almost dry.

3. Add the thyme, parsley, bay leaf, pepper, chicken stock, and beef stock. Bring to a boil and simmer for 20 minutes. Add the salt and Worcestershire.

4. Preheat the broiler.

5. Arrange the bread slices on a small baking sheet. Sprinkle each with ½ teaspoon of the Swiss. Broil until the cheese is melted and the crust is brown, 30 to 60 seconds.

6. Divide the soup among six bowls, top each with 1 cheese crouton, and sprinkle over another ½ teaspoon Swiss.

EACH SERVING CONTAINS

150 calories

23 g carbohydrate

3 g fat

6 mg cholesterol

5 g protein

393 mg sodium

3 g fiber

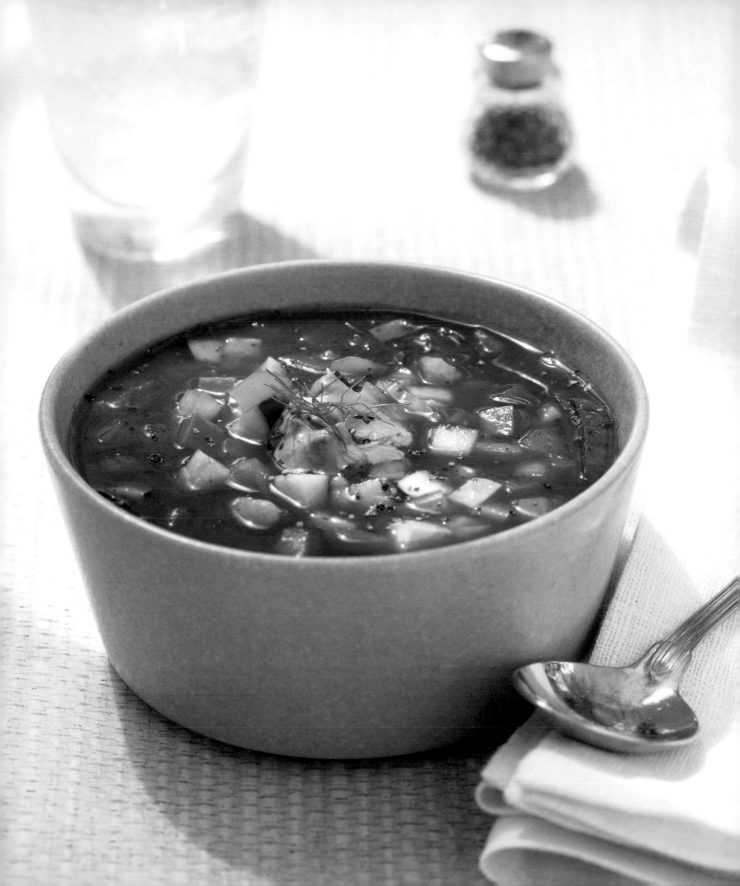

ITALIAN VEGETABLE SOUP
WITH CANNELLINI BEANS

Fantastic nutrition and a complete meal in a bowl.

MAKES SIX ¾-CUP SERVINGS

2 teaspoons extra
virgin olive oil

½ cup diced yellow onions

¼ cup diced fennel

¼ cup diced celery

¼ cup diced carrots

1 cup unpeeled,
diced tomatoes

½ cup diced zucchini

½ cup diced yellow squash

3½ cups vegetable stock

½ teaspoon minced
fresh oregano

½ teaspoon minced
fresh thyme

1 teaspoon minced
fresh parsley

1 small bay leaf

2 cups chiffonade
of spinach

1 cup cooked or canned
cannellini beans

1 tablespoon red
wine vinegar

1 tablespoon freshly
grated Parmesan

¾ teaspoon sea salt

⅛ teaspoon freshly
ground black pepper

1. Heat the olive oil in a large saucepan over medium heat. Sauté the onions, fennel, celery, and carrots until the onions are translucent. Add the tomatoes and cook for 5 minutes. Add the zucchini and yellow squash and cook for 5 more minutes.

2. Add the vegetable stock, oregano, thyme, parsley, and bay leaf and simmer for 1 hour.

3. Add the spinach, cannellini beans, vinegar, Parmesan, salt, and pepper and mix well. Remove and discard the bay leaf.

n NUTRITION NOTE: *The addition of spinach and cannellini beans to this minestrone-like soup increases the folic acid while the entire spectrum of vegetables and beans results in a full 5 grams of fiber in each ¾-cup serving.*

EACH SERVING CONTAINS

100 calories

17 g carbohydrate

2 g fat

0 mg cholesterol

6 g protein

307 mg sodium

5 g fiber

AJIACO SOUP

Chicken soups called ajiaco *are traditional in Latin America. The name is likely a derivative of the word* aji, *which means "hot pepper." This delectable, warming soup is a unique blend of mildly spicy flavors in a creamy coconut milk base.*

MAKES SIX ¾-CUP SERVINGS

1 teaspoon canola oil

Two 4-ounce boneless, skinless chicken breast halves, small diced

1 cup diced yellow onions

½ teaspoon minced garlic

1 teaspoon paprika

Pinch cayenne

3½ cups chicken stock

¾ cup corn fresh or thawed frozen kernels

1 cup diced yucca root or potatoes

1 cup light coconut milk

½ teaspoon sea salt

2 tablespoons fresh lime juice

1. Heat the canola oil in a large sauté pan over medium heat. Sauté the chicken until golden brown and cooked through, 2 to 3 minutes. Add the onions and garlic and sauté until the onions are translucent. Add the paprika and cayenne and cook briefly.

2. Stir in the chicken stock, corn, yucca, coconut milk, and chicken. Simmer for 30 minutes, or until the yucca is cooked through. Season with the salt and lime juice.

> **C** COOK'S NOTE: *Adding yucca root (also known as manioc or cassava) to this hearty soup is a way to introduce you to a popular Latin American staple. Depending on where you live, look for it in a Latin American specialty grocery store or in a natural foods supermarket. It has a tough brown skin, which should be removed prior to cooking, with crisp white flesh when peeled. Cut out the tough center core as well. It deserves nutritional kudos since it is a good source of vitamin C, iron, magnesium, and potassium.*

EACH SERVING CONTAINS

175 calories

20 g carbohydrate

4 g fat

28 mg cholesterol

12 g protein

199 mg sodium

2 g fiber

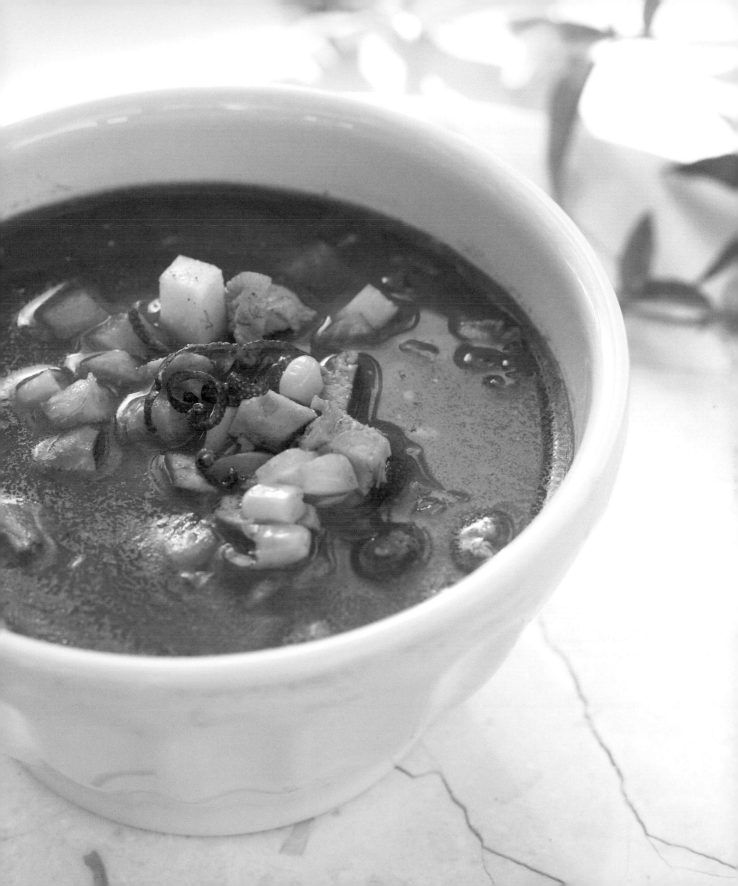

SWEET 100 TOMATO SOUP

This soup is all about the quality of the tomatoes.

MAKES FIVE ¾-CUP SERVINGS

1 pound Sweet 100 or other small sweet tomatoes

1 tablespoon extra virgin olive oil

½ cup diced yellow onions

1 tablespoon minced garlic

1 teaspoon grated lemon zest

2 cups vegetable stock

¾ teaspoon sea salt

¼ teaspoon freshly ground black pepper

1 tablespoon honey

⅔ cup Fennel and Garlic Salsa (page178)

2 tablespoons minced fresh basil

1. Stem the tomatoes and slice them in half.

2. Heat the olive oil over medium heat in a large saucepan. Sauté the onions and garlic until the onions are translucent. Add the tomatoes, lemon zest, and vegetable stock. Bring to a boil and simmer for 2 minutes. Remove from the heat.

3. Add the salt, pepper, and honey. Pour the tomato mixture into a blender and puree until smooth. Strain through a fine-mesh strainer into a bowl.

4. Serve ¾ cup tomato soup with 2 tablespoons fennel and garlic salsa and garnish with 1 heaping teaspoon basil.

EACH SERVING CONTAINS

90 calories

12 g carbohydrate

5 g fat

0 mg cholesterol

2 g protein

320 mg sodium

2 g fiber

CARAWAY CHICKEN SOUP WITH SPAETZLE

Comfort food with an Eastern European inflection.

MAKES EIGHT ¾-CUP SERVINGS

1½ quarts chicken stock

¼ cup beef stock

¾ teaspoon sea salt

1 teaspoon ground
caraway seed

3 tablespoons
unsalted butter

¼ cup unbleached
all-purpose flour

FOR THE SPAETZLE

3 tablespoons
all-purpose flour

1 large egg

Pinch salt

1. Combine the chicken stock, beef stock, salt, and caraway in a large saucepan. Bring to a boil, reduce to low, and simmer for 10 minutes.

2. Combine the butter and flour in a small bowl to make a paste. Add to the chicken stock mixture and stir well to combine.

3. Combine the flour, egg, and salt in a small bowl. Mix with a whisk until a very soft batter forms.

4. Position a colander over the saucepan and press the batter through the holes into the simmering soup. Cook for at least 5 more minutes, stirring occasionally to break up the spaetzle.

n NUTRITION NOTE: *We control the calories in this rich-tasting soup by serving only ¾ cup. Caraway seeds, in addition to adding wonderful flavor, are a source of terpenes, a category of phytochemicals being explored for protection against cancer.*

c COOK'S NOTE: *If you choose not to add beef stock, use more chicken stock. The size of the holes in your colander will determine the size of your spaetzle.*

EACH SERVING CONTAINS

100 calories

7 g carbohydrate

6 g fat

45 mg cholesterol

3 g protein

350 mg sodium

Trace fiber

TORTILLA SOUP

This is a light, easy version of a Sonoran classic.

MAKES FIVE ¾-CUP SERVINGS

FOR THE CHICKEN LIME BROTH

1 quart chicken stock

4 tablespoons fresh lime juice

———————

½ cup chopped avocado

5 ounces (about ¾ cup) cooked chicken thigh meat

⅓ cup chopped tomatoes

¼ cup minced red onions

¼ cup chopped fresh cilantro

¼ cup shredded sharp Cheddar

2 teaspoons minced fresh jalapeño peppers

¼ teaspoon sea salt

15 corn tortilla chips

1. Bring the chicken stock and 2 tablespoons of the lime juice to a boil over medium-high heat in a large saucepan.

2. Toss the avocado with the remaining 2 tablespoons of the lime juice in a medium bowl. Add the chicken, tomatoes, onions, cilantro, Cheddar, jalapeños, and salt. (Wear gloves when handling hot chile peppers, or wash your hands thoroughly before touching your eyes, nose, or mouth.)

3. Divide the chicken mixture among five bowls. Place 3 tortilla chips in each bowl and pour in ¾ cup chicken lime broth.

n **NUTRITION NOTE:** *Look for corn tortilla chips made with nonhydrogenated canola oil or high-oleic safflower oil. Baked tortilla chips are a good alternative, but they may be higher in sodium.*

EACH SERVING CONTAINS

140 calories

9 g carbohydrate

7 g fat

31 mg cholesterol

12 g protein

211 mg sodium

2 g fiber

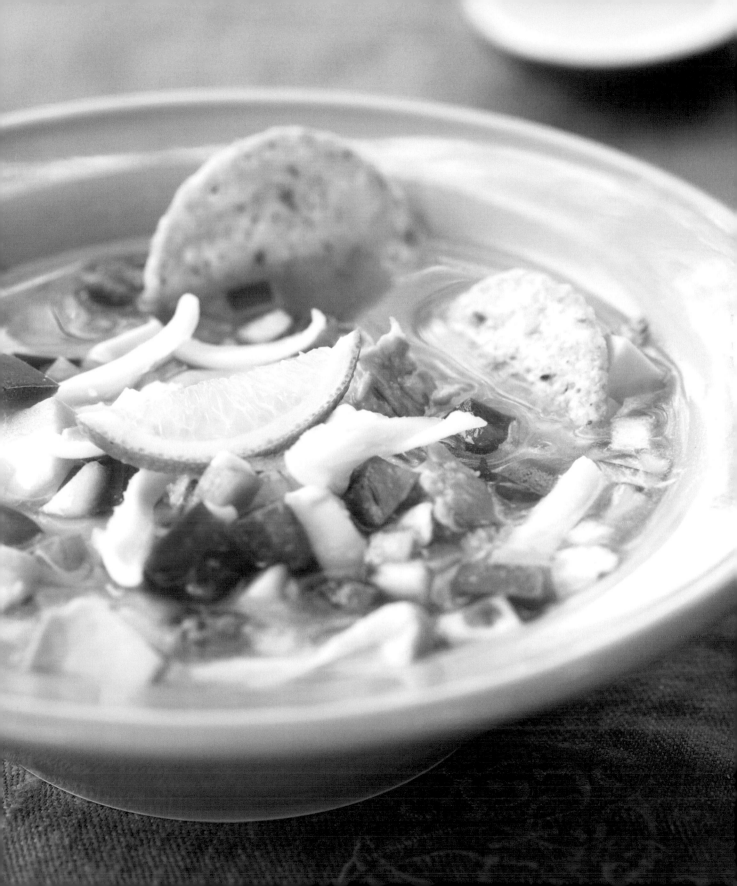

YELLOW SPLIT PEA AND POTATO SOUP

A satisfying, warming soup for a cold evening.
Double the portion for a hearty meal.

MAKES SIX ¾-CUP SERVINGS

1 teaspoon extra
virgin olive oil

½ cup diced yellow onions

¼ cup chopped celery

¼ cup diced carrots

½ teaspoon minced garlic

¼ teaspoon whole
fennel seed

½ teaspoon dried basil

1 bay leaf

¼ teaspoon dried thyme

Dash liquid smoke

2 cups peeled, diced
Yukon gold potatoes

½ cup yellow split peas

1 quart chicken or
vegetable stock

1½ teaspoons
Worcestershire sauce

1 teaspoon sea salt

⅛ teaspoon freshly
ground black pepper

1. Heat the olive oil over medium heat in a large saucepan. Sauté the onions, celery, carrots, and garlic for 5 minutes, or until the onions are translucent.

2. Add the fennel seed, basil, bay leaf, thyme, and liquid smoke and cook for 1 minute, stirring constantly.

3. Add the potatoes, split peas, and chicken stock and bring to a simmer, stirring occasionally, for about 45 minutes, or until the split peas and potatoes are soft.

4. Remove from the heat and stir in the Worcestershire, salt, and pepper. Ladle ¾ cup soup into serving bowls and serve hot.

n   NUTRITION NOTE: *This pleasing soup is quite high in fiber—7 grams in only ¾ cup. Split pea soup is traditionally made with bacon or ham, but here we impart that same smoky flavor by using a dash of liquid smoke, avoiding the sodium and nitrates found in those processed meats.*

EACH SERVING CONTAINS

130 calories

23 g carbohydrate

1 g fat

4 mg cholesterol

7 g protein

349 mg sodium

7 g fiber

PUREE OF WHITE BEAN
AND CELERY ROOT SOUP

Celery root and olive oil give a wonderful flavor to this simple, wholesome soup.

MAKES SIX ¾-CUP SERVINGS

¼ cup extra virgin olive oil

10 ounces celery root, peeled and chopped (about 2 cups)

1 cup dried white cannellini beans, soaked overnight in water to cover

1½ quarts water

1 teaspoon sea salt

½ teaspoon freshly ground black pepper

1. Heat the olive oil over medium heat in a large sauce pot. Add the celery root and sauté for 5 to 7 minutes, or until it starts to brown and caramelize.

2. Drain the beans and add them to the celery root sauté.

3. Add the water to the bean mixture and bring to a boil. Reduce the heat to low and simmer, uncovered, for 45 minutes, or until the beans are soft.

4. Pour into a blender (in batches if necessary) and puree until smooth. Season with the salt and pepper.

n NUTRITION NOTE: *Both beans and celery root are very rich in potassium, which can help normalize blood pressure. Potassium also protects against bone loss.*

EACH SERVING CONTAINS

210 calories

25 g carbohydrate

9 g fat

0 mg cholesterol

9 g protein

369 mg sodium

6 g fiber

CHIPOTLE BLACK BEAN SOUP

Hearty and nourishing, with chipotle chiles for a smoky Southwestern flavor.

MAKES FIVE ¾-CUP SERVINGS

¼ cup dried black beans

¼ cup diced carrots

½ cup diced yellow onions

¼ cup diced celery

5 cups chicken stock

¼ teaspoon ground cumin

1 bay leaf

⅛ teaspoon dried oregano

¼ cup canned
crushed tomatoes

½ teaspoon canned
chipotle chiles

1 teaspoon chopped
fresh cilantro

1 teaspoon
Worcestershire sauce

⅛ teaspoon liquid smoke

¾ teaspoon sea salt

⅓ cup nonfat sour cream

2 tablespoons
chopped scallions

1. Cover the black beans with at least 2 cups of water in a large saucepan and soak overnight. Pour off the bean soaking water, then rinse and drain the beans.

2. Lightly coat a large saucepan with canola oil spray. Sauté the carrots, onions, and celery over medium-high heat until soft, about 5 minutes.

3. Add the beans, chicken stock, cumin, bay leaf, oregano, tomatoes, and chipotle peppers. Bring to a boil and then reduce the heat to low, cover, and cook until the beans are very soft and the soup has thickened slightly, about 1 hour.

4. Stir in the cilantro, Worcestershire, liquid smoke, and salt. Remove from the heat. Remove and discard the bay leaf.

5. Serve ¾ cup soup and garnish each serving with 1 tablespoon sour cream and 1 teaspoon chopped scallions.

EACH SERVING CONTAINS

150 calories

24 g carbohydrate

1 g fat

14 mg cholesterol

12 g protein

329 mg sodium

7 g fiber

CREAM OF MUSHROOM SOUP

You'll never go back to canned.

MAKES SIX ¾-CUP SERVINGS

2 teaspoons
unsalted butter

1¼ cups chopped
yellow onions

2 teaspoons minced garlic

6 cups sliced button
mushrooms

¼ cup white wine

¼ cup dry sherry

2⅔ cups vegetable stock

⅔ cup half-and-half

¾ teaspoon sea salt

⅛ teaspoon freshly
ground black pepper

1. Melt the butter in a large saucepan over medium heat. Sauté the onions and garlic until the onions are translucent.

2. Add 5½ cups of the mushrooms (reserve ½ cup for later) and cook over medium-high heat until just starting to brown. Add the white wine and sherry and reduce by half.

3. Add the vegetable stock, bring to a simmer, and cook for 5 minutes.

4. Remove from the heat. Stir in the half-and-half. Pour the mushroom mixture into a blender (in batches, if necessary) and puree until smooth.

5. Pour the soup back into the saucepan and stir in the reserved mushroom slices, salt, and pepper. Simmer for 2 to 3 minutes, before serving.

n NUTRITION NOTE: *White mushrooms, the stars of this elegant soup, are rich sources of B vitamins, especially riboflavin, and the important electrolyte potassium.*

EACH SERVING CONTAINS

110 calories

9 g carbohydrate

5 g fat

13 mg cholesterol

3 g protein

287 mg sodium

2 g fiber

CREAM OF PARSNIP SOUP

A delicious use for a sweet, often-ignored vegetable.

MAKES EIGHT ¾-CUP SERVINGS

2 teaspoons
unsalted butter

1 cup diced shallots

¼ cup diced yellow onions

¾ cup white wine

3½ cups peeled,
chopped parsnips

5 cups chicken stock

¾ teaspoon sea salt

Pinch freshly ground
black pepper

1 teaspoon white balsamic
or white wine vinegar

¾ cup half-and-half

1. Heat the butter over medium heat in a large saucepan. Sauté the shallots and onions until translucent.

2. Add the white wine and bring to a boil. Reduce the heat to medium low and simmer until reduced by half.

3. Add the parsnips and chicken stock and bring to a boil. Add the salt, pepper, and vinegar. Reduce the heat and simmer for 40 minutes, or until creamy. Remove from the heat and stir in the half-and-half.

n **NUTRITION NOTE:** *Parsnips are related to carrots and are a good source of fiber. When they are cooked for this soup, they add a creaminess that is enhanced by just a little half-and-half.*

EACH SERVING CONTAINS

140 calories

20 g carbohydrate

4 g fat

15 mg cholesterol

4 g protein

203 mg sodium

4 g fiber

POTATO VEGETABLE BISQUE

MAKES THIRTEEN ¾-CUP SERVINGS

5 cups peeled, cubed potatoes

1 cup large diced zucchini

2 quarts chicken stock

½ cup frozen peas

1½ teaspoons sea salt

⅛ teaspoon freshly ground black pepper

½ teaspoon minced garlic

¾ teaspoon dried marjoram

40 to 50 Whole Wheat Croutons (page 117)

1. Combine the potatoes, zucchini, and chicken stock in a large saucepan over medium heat and cook until soft.

2. Place the potato mixture in a blender and puree until smooth.

3. Return the puree to the saucepan. Add the peas and cook over medium heat until the peas are thawed. Add the salt, pepper, garlic, and marjoram. Cook for 5 more minutes.

4. Serve ¾ cup bisque garnished with 3 to 4 croutons per serving.

n NUTRITION NOTE: *A bisque is a creamy soup usually made with milk or cream. This version has no dairy at all, but is made creamy by pureeing potatoes with zucchini that have been cooked in stock. For a vegetarian version of this soup, use vegetable stock instead.*

EACH SERVING CONTAINS

155 calories

31 g carbohydrate

1 g fat

4 mg cholesterol

7 g protein

406 mg sodium

4 g fiber

Just say no to boring salads. This fantastically good-for-you category can be as interesting and satisfying as it is virtuous. A note on washing vegetables: At the Ranch, we meticulously wash all the produce we serve, with particular care for fruits and vegetables that are served raw. We recommend that you do the same. And be sure to wash prewashed, bagged vegetables just as carefully as the ones you buy au naturel. As one of our demonstration chefs likes to tell guests, "No one is as careful as you."

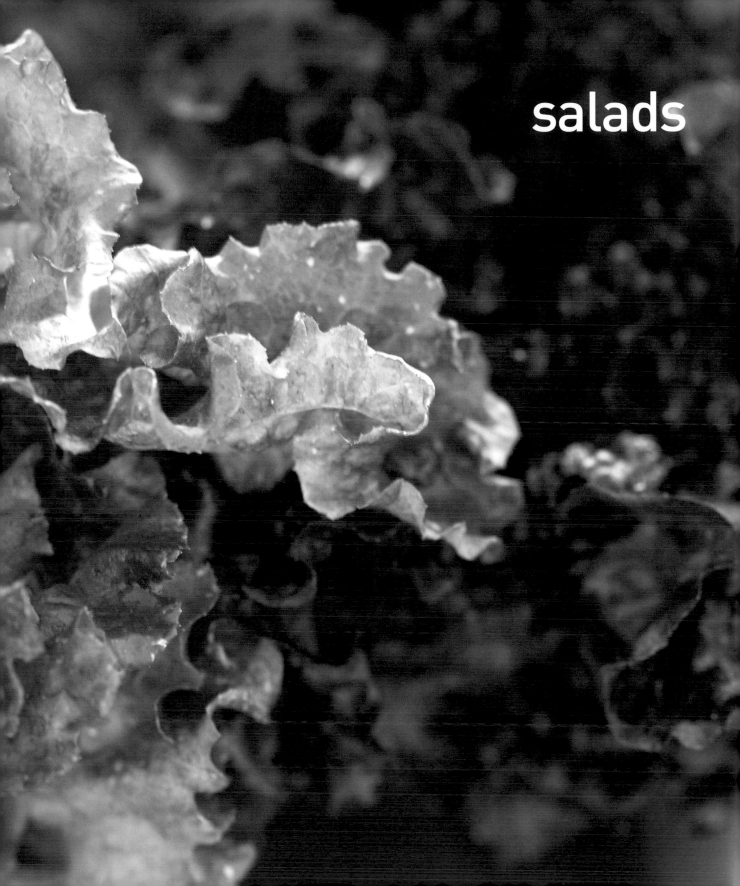

salads

ARTICHOKE SALAD

This makes a great side dish or appetizer.

MAKES TWELVE ½-CUP SERVINGS

2 pounds (about
four 9-ounce boxes)
frozen artichoke
hearts or bottoms

½ cup minced
yellow onions

1 tablespoon lemon zest

3 tablespoons fresh
lemon juice

1 tablespoon extra
virgin olive oil

1 tablespoon minced
fresh flat-leaf parsley

¼ teaspoon sea salt

¾ cup shaved
pecorino Romano

Freshly ground
black pepper

1. Boil the artichokes in heavily salted water (¼ cup salt per 1 gallon water) in a large saucepan for 7 to10 minutes, or until tender. Drain. Cut the artichokes into bite-size pieces.

2. Toss the artichokes with the onions, lemon zest, lemon juice, olive oil, parsley, and salt in large bowl. Keep the salad warm.

3. Serve each ½-cup portion of warm salad with 1 tablespoon pecorino Romano and a grinding of pepper.

n NUTRITION NOTE: *Use organic lemons for zesting to avoid pesticide residues in the peel.*

EACH SERVING CONTAINS

80 calories

8 g carbohydrate

7 mg cholesterol

4 g fat

5 g protein

230 mg sodium

4 g fiber

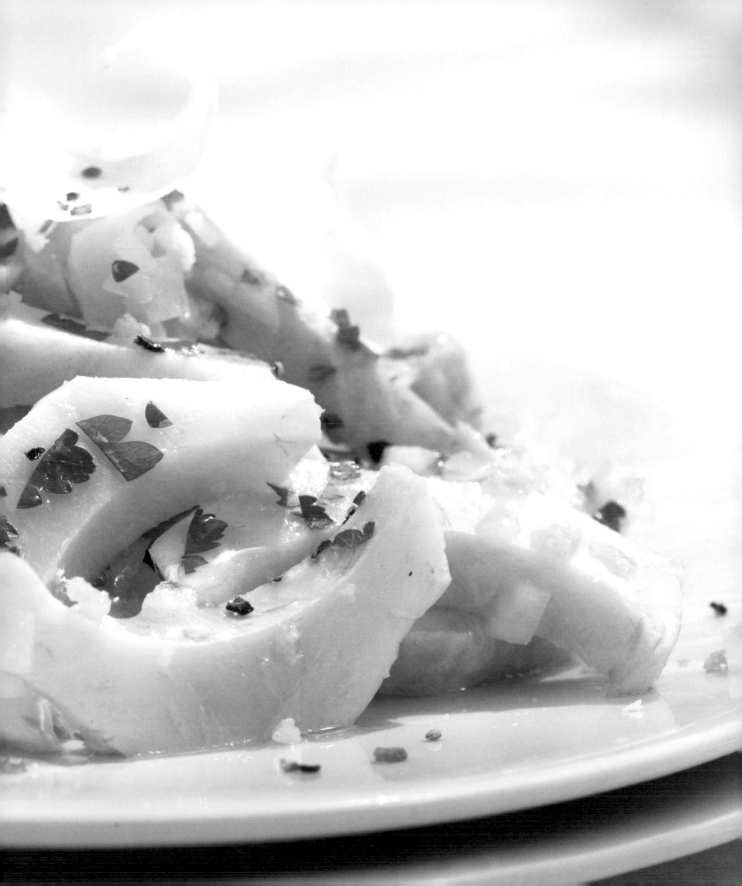

ARUGULA PEAR SALAD

*Store the extra dressing in a tightly covered jar
in the refrigerator for up to 2 weeks.*

MAKES 4 SERVINGS

⅔ cup red wine vinegar

⅔ cup champagne vinegar

½ cup vegetable stock

1 tablespoon
minced shallots

2 teaspoons freshly
ground black pepper

4 teaspoons white
miso paste

1 tablespoon chopped
fresh oregano

1 tablespoon chopped
fresh rosemary

2 firm Bartlett pears,
cored and cut in half

4 cups arugula, washed

1 tablespoon plus 1
teaspoon coarsely
chopped toasted pecans

1 ounce blue cheese,
crumbled

1. Combine the wine vinegar, champagne vinegar, vegetable stock, shallots, pepper, and miso paste in a blender and puree until smooth. Mix in the oregano and rosemary by hand.

2. Cut the pears in ½-inch slices. Place in a steamer basket over boiling water for about 3 minutes, or until soft.

3. Combine the arugula, pecans, and ½ cup rosemary vinaigrette.

4. Divide the salad into four equal portions and top each with one-quarter each crumbled blue cheese and sliced pears.

n NUTRITION NOTE: *With its peppery, mustard flavor, arugula makes a lively addition to this salad. It's also a good source of beta-carotene and vitamin C.*

c COOK'S NOTE: *Look for white miso paste in the refrigerated section of natural foods stores.*

EACH SERVING CONTAINS

80 calories

9 g carbohydrate

4 g fat

6 mg cholesterol

3 g protein

267 mg sodium

2 g fiber

FRISÉE SALAD
WITH SHERRY SHALLOT VINAIGRETTE

Frisée is a feathery, delicately bitter member of the chicory family. This dressing works well with any young greens.

MAKES 4 SERVINGS

FOR THE SHERRY
SHALLOT VINAIGRETTE

⅓ cup Dijon mustard

½ cup sherry vinegar

¼ cup red wine vinegar

¼ cup water

¼ cup diced shallots

¼ cup honey

¼ cup canola oil

½ cup chopped frisée

1½ cups fennel, very
thinly sliced and chopped

½ cup diced mangoes

3 tablespoons
roasted, unsalted
chopped cashews

½ cup crumbled feta

1. Combine the mustard, sherry vinegar, red wine vinegar, water, shallots, and honey in a blender and blend until well mixed. While blending, slowly drizzle in the canola oil.

2. Combine the frisée, fennel, mangoes, cashews, and feta in a medium bowl. Add ⅓ cup sherry shallot vinaigrette and toss. Divide the salad into four equal portions. Store the extra dressing in a tightly covered jar in the refrigerator for up to two weeks.

C COOK'S NOTE: *Fennel, which is used both as an herb and as a vegetable, is a good source of fiber and potassium. Use a mandoline to make thin, even slices.*

EACH SERVING CONTAINS

165 calories

18 g carbohydrate

9 g fat

8 mg cholesterol

3 g protein

301 mg sodium

3 g fiber

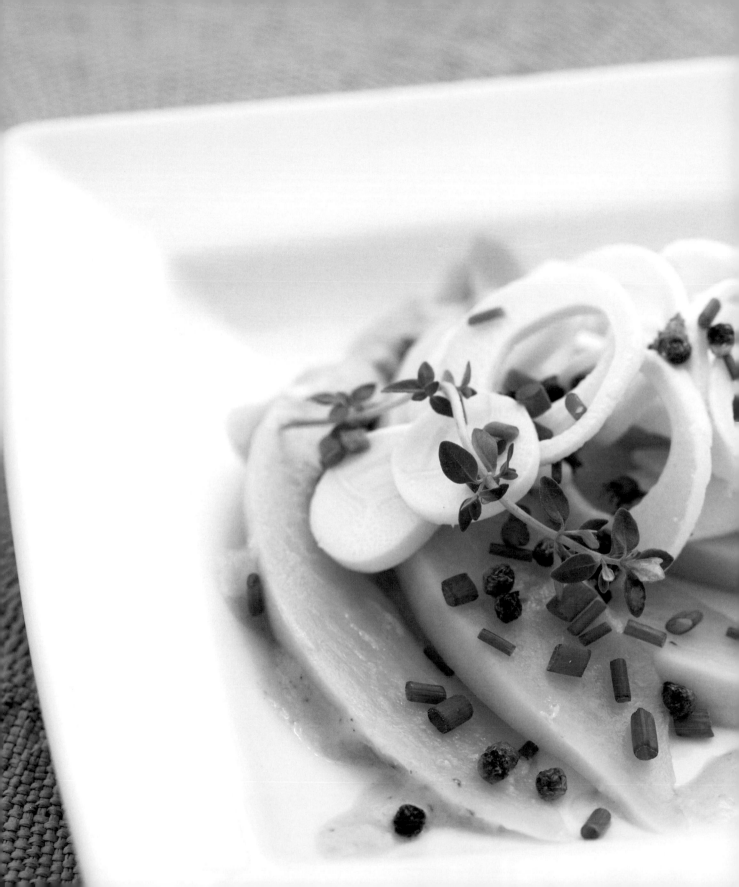

HEARTS OF PALM SALAD

Look for fresh hearts of palm in exceptionally well-stocked produce sections or order them online.

MAKES EIGHT ¼-CUP SERVINGS

1 pound fresh
hearts of palm

2 papayas or mangos

FOR THE DRESSING

1 tablespoon extra
virgin olive oil

½ teaspoon minced
fresh thyme

¼ cup chopped shallots

1 tablespoon
Dijon mustard

¼ teaspoon minced garlic

¼ cup champagne vinegar

2 tablespoons water

¼ teaspoon sea salt

¼ teaspoon cane sugar

1. Peel off the outer layer of the hearts of palm. Thinly slice the hearts and put in a bowl.

2. Peel and slice the papayas.

3. Combine the olive oil, thyme, shallots, mustard, garlic, vinegar, water, salt, and cane sugar in a blender and puree until smooth. Toss the hearts of palm with the dressing.

4. Serve ¼ cup hearts of palm with 3 to 4 papaya slices.

n NUTRITION NOTE: *Fresh hearts of palm bear only slight resemblance to their canned counterpart. They are the tender, young shoots of palm that are easy to peel and slice. They are not a source of palm oil.*

EACH SERVING CONTAINS

50 calories

8 g carbohydrate

2 g fat

0 mg cholesterol

1 g protein

204 mg sodium

2 g fiber

GRILLED CAESAR SALAD

Create a complete meal by adding grilled shrimp
or Spicy Lobster (see Cook's Note) to this revised classic.

MAKES 4 SERVINGS

FOR THE CAESAR SALAD DRESSING

1 teaspoon minced anchovy fillet

¼ cup roasted garlic (see page 20)

2 tablespoons freshly grated Parmesan

3 tablespoons fresh lemon juice

2 tablespoons water

2 teaspoons Worcestershire sauce

¼ teaspoon freshly ground black pepper

1 tablespoon extra virgin olive oil

---

2 romaine lettuce hearts

¼ teaspoon sea salt

¼ teaspoon freshly ground black pepper

4 whole wheat lavash crackers

1. Combine the anchovy, garlic, Parmesan, lemon juice, water, Worcestershire, pepper, and olive oil in a blender and puree until smooth.

2. Preheat the grill.

3. Cut the romaine hearts in half. Lightly spray with canola oil spray and sprinkle with the salt and pepper. Place on the grill to mark and cook slightly, 1 minute on each side.

4. Place one romaine half on each of four plates and top with 1 tablespoon dressing. Serve with a lavash cracker.

n **NUTRITION NOTE:** *Pick romaine hearts with as much green in the leaves as you can find. With salad greens, more color means more nutritional value.*

c **COOK'S NOTE:** *For Spicy Lobster, simply rub 4 lobster tails with a mixture of:*
½ teaspoon paprika
½ teaspoon ground turmeric
½ teaspoon chili powder
½ teaspoon ground cumin
¼ teaspoon sea salt
¼ teaspoon freshly ground black pepper

Place the lobster tails under the broiler for 5 to 10 minutes, or until the lobster is pink. Remove the shells and chop the tails into 1-inch pieces. Top each serving of Caesar salad with the lobster.

EACH SERVING CONTAINS

125 calories

16 g carbohydrate

6 g fat

3 mg cholesterol

5 g protein

241 mg sodium

5 g fiber

MIXED GREENS
WITH PINEAPPLE VINAIGRETTE

The sweetness and acidity of pineapple really complements mixed greens.

MAKES 4 SERVINGS

FOR THE PINEAPPLE VINAIGRETTE

¼ cup frozen pineapple juice concentrate

3 tablespoons champagne vinegar

1 tablespoon extra virgin olive oil

¼ teaspoon sea salt

Pinch freshly ground black pepper

1½ teaspoons minced fresh mint

---

4 cups organic mixed greens

1 tablespoon plus 1 teaspoon coarsely chopped toasted walnuts

¼ cup crumbled goat cheese

1. Combine the pineapple concentrate, vinegar, olive oil, salt, pepper, and mint in a blender and blend until well mixed.

2. Serve 1 cup mixed greens tossed with 1 teaspoon walnuts, 1 tablespoon goat cheese, and 2 tablespoons pineapple vinaigrette.

n **NUTRITION NOTE:** *Many salad greens have a pleasant bitterness, the result of the healthful phytochemicals found in them. In Chinese medicine, bitter is a desired flavor that helps control cravings for sweets.*

EACH SERVING CONTAINS

120 calories

9 g carbohydrate

8 g fat

7 mg cholesterol

4 g protein

128 mg sodium

1 g fiber

QUINOA WALNUT SALAD

Nutty, delicate-flavored, nourishing quinoa (pronounced KEEN-wah) was a cornerstone of the Inca diet: It deserves to be more prominent in ours. Quinoa is higher in protein than any other grain, and it is a good source of fiber, B complex vitamins, iron, magnesium, manganese, and phosphorus. Rinse it very well to remove its protective soapy, natural coating, then cook it as you would white rice.

MAKES 8 SERVINGS

1 cup quinoa

¼ cup chopped walnuts

FOR THE DRESSING

½ tablespoon champagne vinegar

½ teaspoon sea salt

¼ teaspoon freshly ground black pepper

⅛ teaspoon ground nutmeg

½ teaspoon walnut oil

⅓ cup fresh chopped scallions

2 tablespoons fresh chervil

1 pint water

1. Preheat the oven to 350°F. Lightly coat two baking sheets with canola oil spray.

2. Rinse the quinoa thoroughly: Cover it with cool water, swirl, and pour off the water. Repeat at least twice.

3. Spread the walnuts evenly on one baking sheet and the quinoa evenly on the other. Toast both for 5 to 10 minutes, redistributing after 2 to 3 minutes for even toasting. Cool completely.

4. Combine the vinegar, salt, pepper, and nutmeg in a small bowl. Whisk in the walnut oil. Add the scallions, chervil, and walnuts. Mix and let sit for 5 to 10 minutes to allow the flavors to develop.

5. Boil the water and add the quinoa. Cook covered over medium-low heat until the grains begin to pop open, 15 to 20 minutes. Drain and cool.

6. Combine the quinoa with the dressing. Divide into ⅓-cup portions.

n NUTRITION NOTE: *Quinoa is an ancient grain that is particularly high in protein and is also gluten-free. It cooks quickly and complements the nuts in this chewy, fragrant salad.*

c COOK'S NOTE: *Store walnut oil in the refrigerator to increase its shelf life. Chervil has a slight flavor of anise. You can substitute fennel leaves or 1 tablespoon chopped fresh tarragon and 1 tablespoon chopped flat-leaf parsley.*

110 calories

16 g carbohydrate

4 g fat

0 mg cholesterol

3 g protein

123 mg sodium

2 g fiber

EACH SERVING CONTAINS

SPINACH AND CANDIED PECAN SALAD

A contemporary classic made even more nourishing (and interesting) by the addition of colorful vegetables and berries.

MAKES FIVE 1-CUP SERVINGS

FOR THE DRESSING

¾ cup fresh or thawed frozen raspberries

2 tablespoons cane sugar

¼ cup honey

2 tablespoons champagne vinegar

1 tablespoon minced fresh chives

Pinch sea salt

Pinch freshly ground black pepper

FOR THE CANDIED PECANS

¼ cup chopped pecans

1 tablespoon cane sugar

─────

3 cups chiffonade of spinach

½ cup chopped button mushrooms

¼ cup shredded carrots

2 tablespoons minced red bell peppers

2 tablespoons minced yellow bell peppers

2 tablespoons finely sliced red onions

¼ cup sliced apples

½ cup fresh raspberries

1. Preheat the oven to 400°F.

2. Combine the raspberries and cane sugar in a blender and puree until smooth. Strain to remove the seeds, if desired.

3. Add the honey, vinegar, chives, salt, and pepper and puree until well blended. Set aside.

4. Spread the pecans evenly on a baking sheet. Lightly spray with canola oil spray and sprinkle with cane sugar. Toast for 5 minutes, shaking the pan once for even toasting. Cool completely.

5. Combine the spinach, mushrooms, carrots, red peppers, yellow peppers, onions, apples, and raspberries in a large bowl. Stir in the pecans and add the dressing. Toss together until well combined. Evenly divide the salad among five plates.

n   NUTRITION NOTE: *Spinach may be the most nutritious of all the salad greens. It is rich in beta-carotene, vitamin C, magnesium, folic acid, and fiber.*

EACH SERVING CONTAINS

135 calories

24 g carbohydrate

5 g fat

0 mg cholesterol

2 g protein

38 mg sodium

3 g fiber

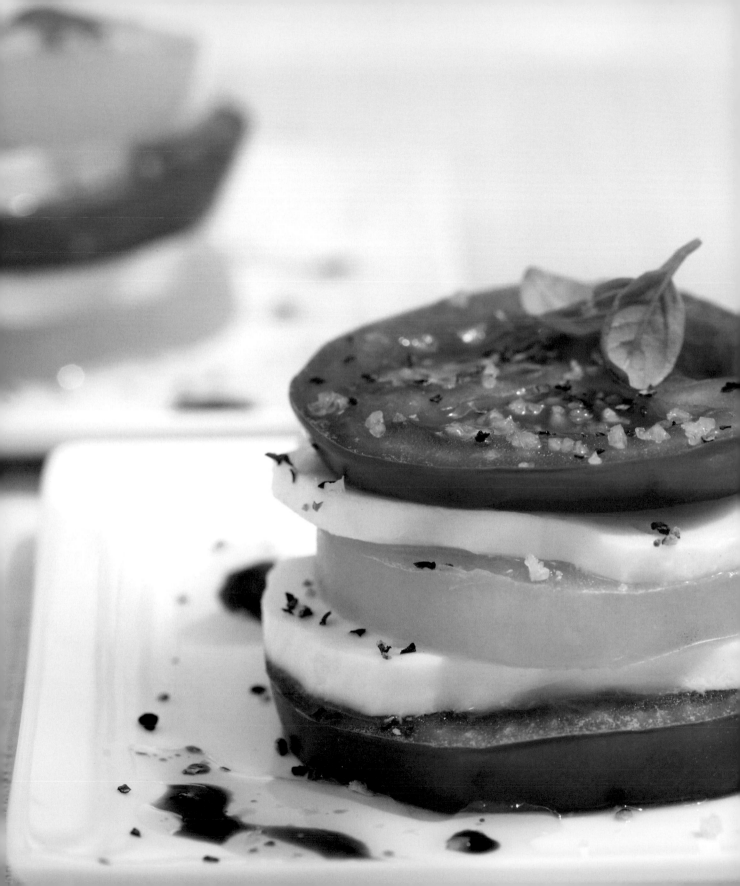

NAPOLEON OF HEIRLOOM TOMATOES AND MOZZARELLA

Gorgeous. Heirloom tomatoes are generally nonhybridized plants that produce full and richly flavored fruit. They come in many shapes, sizes, and colors, so pick your favorite and enjoy!

MAKES 4 SERVINGS

1 medium red tomato

1 medium yellow tomato

4 ounces fresh mozzarella

1 cup chopped fresh basil

1 tablespoon balsamic vinegar

½ teaspoon sea salt

¼ teaspoon freshly ground black pepper

1. Slice each tomato into 4 equal slices.

2. Cut the mozzarella into 8 thin slices, each weighing ½ ounce.

3. Combine the basil, vinegar, salt, and pepper in a small bowl and toss together.

4. To build a napoleon, place 1 red tomato slice on a plate and top with 1 mozzarella slice. Place a yellow tomato slice on the mozzarella and top the tomato with another slice of mozzarella. Repeat for each serving.

5. Top each napoleon with ¼ cup basil-vinegar mixture.

n **NUTRITION NOTE:** *The intense color and sweetness of vine-ripened tomatoes signal greater nutritional value. Shop a local farmers' market in the summer for heirloom varieties.*

c **COOK'S NOTE:** *Fresh mozzarella is generally purchased in an 8-ounce ball. To prepare ½-ounce slices, cut the ball in half lengthwise, then cut each half into 8 even slices.*

EACH SERVING CONTAINS

95 calories

6 g carbohydrate

5 g fat

18 mg cholesterol

8 g protein

393 mg sodium

2 g fiber

FATOOSH SALAD

This vegan salad is truly special. Sumac—look for it in Middle Eastern grocery stores—gives the dressing a beautiful pink color and an elusive astringency that brings all the other flavors together. Make this salad heartier by adding chopped cooked chicken or salmon.

MAKES 4 SERVINGS

FOR THE DRESSING

2 teaspoons sesame tahini

2 tablespoons fresh
lemon juice

1 teaspoon ground sumac

2 tablespoons water

1¼ teaspoons extra
virgin olive oil

½ teaspoon sea salt

¼ teaspoon freshly
ground black pepper

---

1 cup canned garbanzo beans,
rinsed well and drained

1 cup chopped romaine lettuce

½ cup chopped tomatoes

½ cup peeled and
diced cucumbers

¼ cup diced red onions

FOR THE PITA CHIPS

1 whole wheat pita

1 tablespoon Za'atar
Spice Mix (page 214)

---

1 tablespoon plus 1 teaspoon
toasted pine nuts

2 teaspoons minced
fresh mint

1. Preheat the oven to 375°F.

2. Whisk together the tahini, lemon juice, sumac, water, olive oil, salt, and pepper in a small bowl.

3. Combine the garbanzo beans, romaine, tomatoes, cucumbers, and onions in a large bowl. Add the dressing and toss well.

4. Separate the pita pocket into two halves. Cut each half into 8 triangles. Place the pita triangles evenly on a baking sheet and generously spray with canola oil. Sprinkle the spice mix over the triangles and toss to coat.

5. Bake for 5 minutes, or until brown and crisp.

6. Divide the salad into four equal portions. Top each portion with 4 pita chips, 1 teaspoon pine nuts, and ½ teaspoon mint.

EACH SERVING CONTAINS

255 calories

39 g carbohydrate

8 g fat

0 mg cholesterol

10 g protein

577 mg sodium

8 g fiber

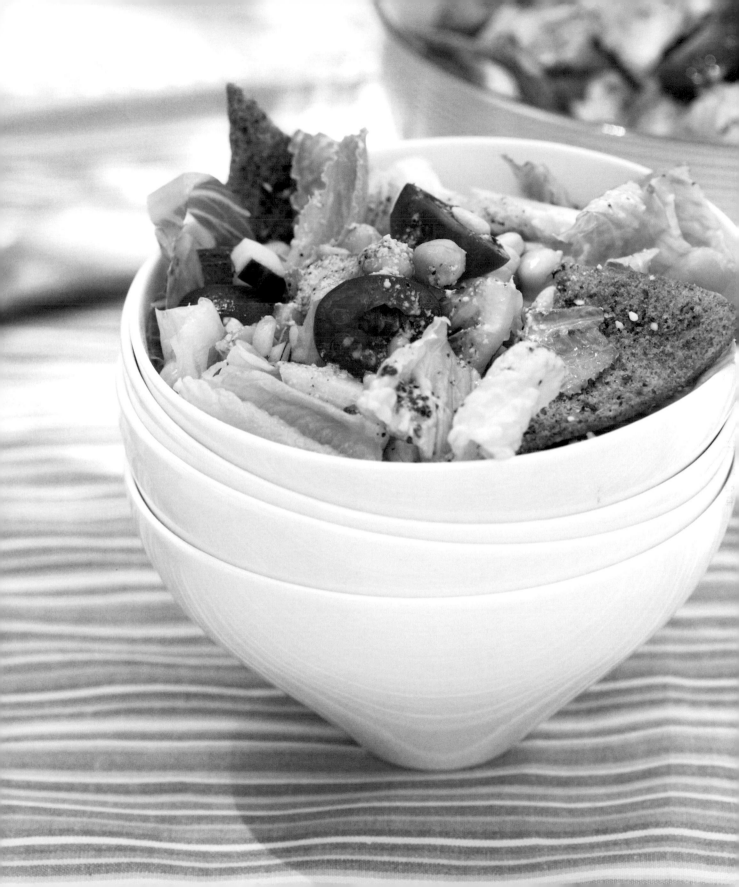

CHICKEN PANZANELLA

This classic Italian chopped salad is a traditional use for day-old bread.

MAKES 4 SERVINGS

FOR THE DRESSING

½ cup red wine vinegar

¼ cup water

½ teaspoon minced garlic

½ teaspoon sea salt

¼ teaspoon freshly ground black pepper

———

Four 4-ounce boneless, skinless chicken breast halves

1 cup grape tomatoes, cut in half

¾ cup peeled, diced cucumbers

⅓ cup minced red onions

2 tablespoons chopped kalamata olives

2 tablespoons capers, rinsed and drained

½ cup diced red bell peppers

2 tablespoons chiffonade of fresh basil

4 slices multigrain bread

1. Combine the vinegar, water, garlic, salt, and pepper in a small bowl. Set aside.

2. Preheat the grill or broiler.

3. Grill or broil the chicken breasts for 3 to 5 minutes on each side, or until the temperature at the center reaches 165°F. Cool completely and dice.

4. Combine tomatoes, cucumbers, onions, olives, capers, bell peppers, and basil in a large bowl. Add the diced chicken and the dressing and toss well.

5. Coat the bread slices on both sides with extra virgin olive oil spray. Grill until browned. Dice. Toss with the vegetables and chicken.

6. Divide the salad into four equal servings and place in salad bowls.

C COOK'S NOTE: *Three cups croutons (page 117) can be substituted for these home-made ones.*

EACH SERVING CONTAINS

385 calories

35 g carbohydrate

13 g fat

72 mg cholesterol

32 g protein

702 mg sodium

4 g fiber

CHOPPED SALAD WITH LOX

Look for lox (smoked salmon) made from wild-caught Pacific or organic-farmed salmon.

MAKES 4 SERVINGS

FOR THE CAPER DRESSING

1 tablespoon plus
1 teaspoon capers,
rinsed and drained

2 tablespoons diced
red onions

1½ teaspoons grated
lemon zest

3 tablespoons water

Pinch freshly ground
black pepper

½ pound lox

1 medium cucumber,
peeled and diced

½ cup chopped carrots

⅓ cup diced red
bell peppers

3 tablespoons minced
red onions

3 tablespoons minced
fresh flat-leaf parsley

½ cup chopped
baby arugula

1 cup crumbled bagel
crisps, preferably
whole wheat

1. Combine the capers, onions, lemon zest, water, and pepper in a blender and puree until smooth.

2. Chop the lox into ½-inch pieces.

3. Combine the lox, cucumbers, carrots, peppers, onions, parsley, arugula, and bagel chips in a large bowl. Add the dressing and toss lightly.

4. Divide the salad equally among four salad bowls.

n **NUTRITION NOTE:** *The omega-3 fat found in salmon combats inflammation more than any other dietary component.*

EACH SERVING CONTAINS

300 calories

38 g carbohydrate

8 g fat

31 mg cholesterol

20 g protein

625 mg sodium

6 g fiber

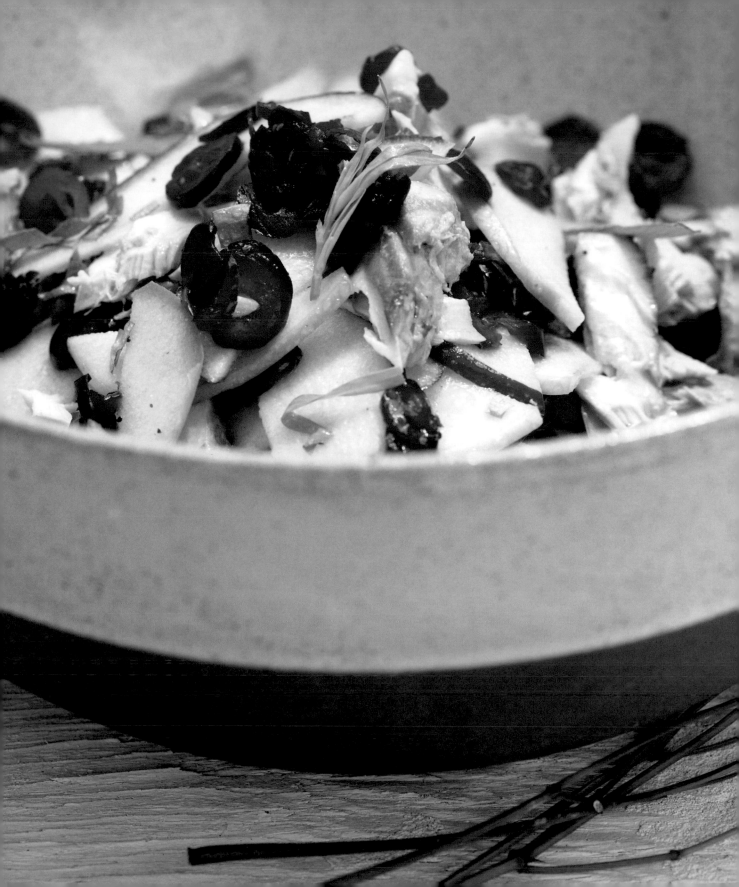

APPLE-CRANBERRY SALMON SALAD

*Apples are the main ingredient. Use the kinds suggested here
or any combination of tangy and sweet varieties.*

MAKES 4 SERVINGS

½ cup Mongolian BBQ
Sauce (page184)

Four 4-ounce
salmon fillets

FOR THE APPLE-
CRANBERRY SALAD

¼ cup fresh lemon juice

2 tablespoons honey

¼ teaspoon sea salt

Pinch freshly ground
black pepper

1 pound Gala apples

½ pound Granny
Smith apples

½ cup chopped fresh or
thawed frozen cranberries

2 tablespoons chopped
fresh tarragon

1. Combine the barbecue sauce and the salmon in a shallow glass baking dish. Cover with plastic wrap and place in the refrigerator for 30 minutes to 2 hours.

2. Combine the lemon juice, honey, salt, and pepper in a large bowl.

3. Core and thinly slice the Galas and Granny Smiths using a mandoline or a sharp knife. Add the sliced apples to the lemon-honey mixture and toss together to coat. Add the cranberries and tarragon and toss well.

4. Preheat the grill or broiler.

5. Grill or broil the salmon fillets for 3 to 5 minutes on each side, or until opaque at the center. Do not overcook.

6. Break apart the salmon into bite-size pieces. Add the salmon to the apple-cranberry salad and toss well.

7. Divide the salad evenly among four plates.

n NUTRITION NOTE: *Children need omega-3 fat for neurological development. They may love this salad with its combination of sweet flavor and crunchy texture.*

EACH SERVING CONTAINS

325 calories

38 g carbohydrate

11 g fat

54 mg cholesterol

20 g protein

223 mg sodium

6 g fiber

PAPRIKA-LEMON CHICKEN SALAD

*This delicious salad was created by one of our chefs
who hails from the former Czechoslovakia.*

MAKES 5 SERVINGS

FOR THE DRESSING

1 tablespoon Dijon mustard

2 tablespoons fresh lemon juice

2 tablespoons canola oil

¼ cup chopped fresh
flat-leaf parsley

Pinch evaporated cane juice

FOR THE GARLIC RUB

1 tablespoon paprika

2 teaspoons garlic granules

¾ teaspoon sea salt

2 teaspoons freshly
ground black pepper

¾ teaspoon fresh lemon juice

———

Five 4-ounce boneless, skinless
chicken breast halves

1½ cups thickly sliced mushrooms

1¼ cups baby spinach, washed

2 cups shredded romaine lettuce

Pinch sea salt

Pinch freshly ground black pepper

2 tablespoons chopped,
toasted walnuts

½ cup diced red onions

¼ teaspoon dried thyme
leaves, crushed

1 tablespoon plus 1
teaspoon lime zest

1. Preheat the oven to 400°F.

2. Mix the mustard, lemon juice, canola oil, parsley, and cane juice in a small bowl. Refrigerate until ready to use.

3. Combine the paprika, garlic granules, salt, pepper, and lemon juice in a small bowl.

4. Evenly rub 1½ teaspoons spice mixture over each chicken breast.

5. Heat a large sauté pan over medium-high heat. Spray a heavy-bottomed sauté pan with canola oil spray and sauté the chicken for 1 minute on each side.

6. Transfer to the oven and bake for 15 to 20 minutes, or until the internal temperature reaches 165°. Cool completely and cut into cubes.

7. Combine the mushrooms and the dressing in a large bowl and marinate 5 minutes. Add the spinach, romaine, salt, pepper, walnuts, onions, and thyme and mix well.

8. Divide the salad evenly among five plates and serve each diced chicken breast and sprinkle with 1 teaspoon lime zest to garnish.

n NUTRITION NOTE: *Walnuts are a good source of omega-3 fatty acids. They are wonderful in salads but also great eaten out of hand as a snack with a piece of fruit.*

EACH SERVING CONTAINS

290 calories

9 g carbohydrate

14 g fat

146 mg cholesterol

33 g protein

563 mg sodium

3 g fiber

TURKEY PINEAPPLE SALAD

MAKES 4 SERVINGS

2 cups peeled and sliced fresh pineapple

1 cup julienned sugar snap peas

1 cup julienned red bell peppers

¼ cup julienned jicama

½ cup shredded carrots

½ cup julienned red onions

½ cup chopped fresh cilantro

FOR THE DRESSING

½ cup frozen pineapple juice concentrate

¼ cup champagne vinegar

½ teaspoon sea salt

¼ teaspoon freshly ground black pepper

1 tablespoon chopped fresh mint

2 tablespoons extra virgin olive oil

12 ounces sliced roasted turkey breast

1 cup chopped leaf lettuce

1. Preheat the grill or broiler.

2. Grill or broil the pineapple slices to soften only slightly. Do not overcook. Dice into bite-size pieces and place in a medium bowl.

3. Add the snap peas, bell peppers, jicama, carrots, onions, and cilantro and toss well.

4. Combine the pineapple juice concentrate, vinegar, salt, pepper, and mint in a small bowl. Slowly whisk in the olive oil.

5. Chop the turkey into bite-size pieces and add to the pineapple salad. Add the dressing and toss well.

6. Divide the salad into four equal portions and serve each over chopped lettuce.

EACH SERVING CONTAINS

295 calories

28 g carbohydrate

8 g fat

71 mg cholesterol

28 g protein

292 mg sodium

3 g fiber

SHRIMP SALAD WITH MANGO VINAIGRETTE

The delicious dressing makes this dish spectacular.

MAKES 4 SERVINGS

FOR THE MANGO VINAIGRETTE

½ cup peeled fresh or thawed frozen mango pieces

2 tablespoons cane sugar

1 tablespoon minced shallots

½ teaspoon minced serrano chiles

¼ cup rice vinegar

1 tablespoon extra virgin olive oil

⅛ teaspoon sea salt

---

24 fresh asparagus spears, blanched (about 12 ounces)

1½ cups peeled orange sections, pith removed (about 2 medium oranges)

¾ pounds cooked shrimp

½ teaspoon sea salt

¼ teaspoon freshly ground black pepper

4 pieces Flatbreads (page 74) or crusty multigrain sourdough bread

1. Combine the mangoes and cane sugar in a blender and puree until smooth. Add the shallots, serranos, rice vinegar, olive oil, and salt and puree until smooth and well blended. (Wear gloves while handling hot chile peppers, or wash your hands thoroughly before touching your eyes, nose, or mouth.)

2. Mix together the asparagus, oranges, shrimp, salt, and pepper in a large bowl.

3. Pour the mango vinaigrette over the shrimp mixture and toss well.

4. Serve 1 cup shrimp salad with 1 crispy flatbread.

n **NUTRITION NOTE:** *The color of mango tells you it is rich in antioxidants from beta-carotene.*

EACH SERVING CONTAINS

230 calories

25 g carbohydrate

6 g fat

129 mg cholesterol

21 g protein

457 mg sodium

5 g fiber

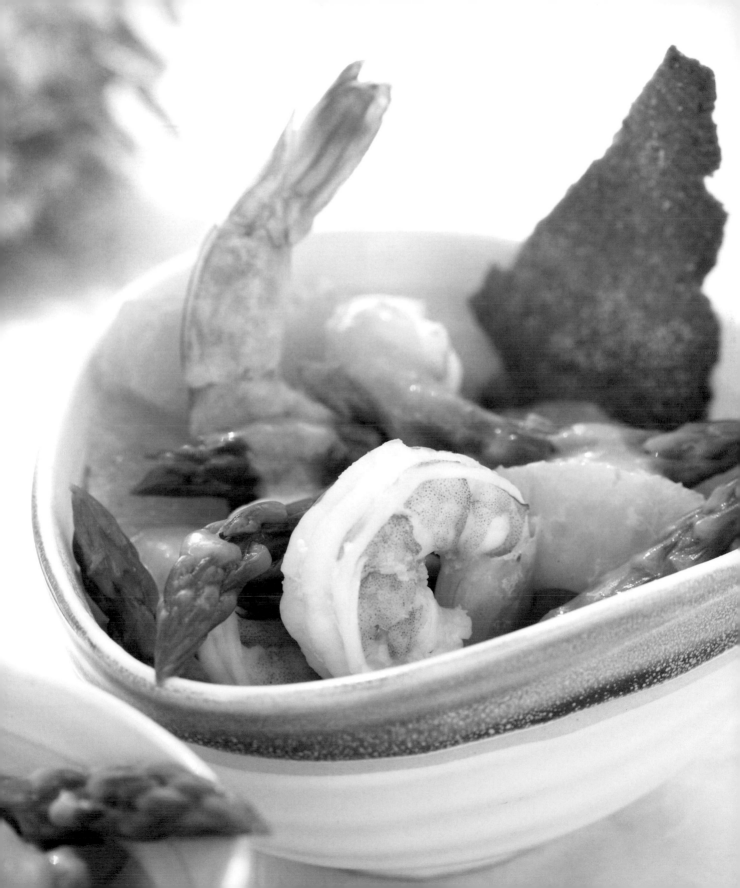

SMOKED SALMON, SPINACH, AND MUSHROOM SALAD

The ingredients list for this terrific dish is long, but the whole thing is easy to put together.

MAKES 4 SERVINGS

FOR THE SOY MARINADE

1 tablespoon light brown sugar

¼ cup low-sodium tamari sauce

⅜ cup water

¼ teaspoon sea salt

¼ teaspoon freshly ground black pepper

¾ teaspoon liquid smoke

———————

Four 4-ounce salmon fillets

FOR THE DRESSING

2 tablespoons extra virgin olive oil

2 tablespoons diced yellow onions

1 tablespoon champagne vinegar

1 tablespoon water

2 tablespoons light brown sugar

1 tablespoon Dijon mustard

½ teaspoon liquid smoke

½ teaspoon sea salt

½ teaspoon freshly ground black pepper

———————

5 cups baby spinach, washed

3 cups sliced button mushrooms

¾ cup diced tomatoes

¼ teaspoon sea salt

1. Combine the brown sugar, tamari, water, salt, pepper, and liquid smoke in a large bowl. Add the salmon, cover, and marinate overnight in the refrigerator.

2. Preheat the oven to 400°F.

3. Remove the salmon from the marinade and discard the marinade. Wrap the salmon in aluminum foil and bake for 15 to 20 minutes.

4. Heat the olive oil over medium-high heat in a small sauté pan. Sauté the onions until translucent. Cool.

5. Combine the onions with the vinegar, water, brown sugar, mustard, liquid smoke, salt, and pepper in a blender and puree until smooth.

6. Combine the spinach, mushrooms, tomatoes, and salt in a large bowl and toss well.

7. Place 2 cups spinach mixture on a plate. Top with 2 tablespoons dressing and 1 salmon fillet.

n NUTRITION NOTE: *The process of smoking salmon does result in some loss of the valuable omega-3 fatty acids, so we have come up with a marinade that imparts the flavor of smoking to a fresh salmon fillet. Use wild-caught Alaskan or Pacific salmon rather than Atlantic versions. The populations are healthier and the fishing methods are preferable to those in other waters.*

EACH SERVING CONTAINS

290 calories

13 g carbohydrate

14 g fat

51 mg cholesterol

28 g protein

605 mg sodium

3 g fiber

SALMON CITRUS SALAD

One mixture can often serve as both a marinade and a salad dressing. Here's a recipe that illustrates this principle.

MAKES 4 SERVINGS

FOR THE MARINADE

⅓ cup orange juice concentrate

⅓ cup fresh lemon juice

⅓ cup fresh lime juice

1 tablespoon honey

1 tablespoon extra virgin olive oil

½ cup diced yellow onions

2 tablespoons minced ginger

½ cup chopped fresh cilantro

Pinch sea salt

Pinch freshly ground black pepper

———

1 pound salmon fillets

4 cups spinach

¼ cup diced orange sections

¼ cup diced fresh pineapple

1. Combine the orange juice concentrate, lemon juice, lime juice, honey, olive oil, onions, ginger, cilantro, salt, and pepper in a small bowl. Divide in half.

2. Place the salmon in a shallow glass baking dish and pour one half of the marinade over the salmon. Cover and refrigerate for 1 hour. Set aside the other half of the marinade for later.

3. Wash, dry, and tear the spinach into bite-size pieces.

4. Preheat the grill or broiler.

5. Remove the salmon from the marinade and discard the marinade. Grill or broil the salmon for 3 to 5 minutes on each side.

6. Toss the spinach and the reserved marinade in a large bowl. Divide the spinach evenly among four large serving bowls. Garnish each serving with 1 tablespoon each diced oranges and pineapple and top with 3 ounces cooked, flaked salmon.

n NUTRITION NOTE: *Benefits in cardiovascular disease prevention have been seen with as few as one or two fish meals a week.*

EACH SERVING CONTAINS

265 calories

17 g carbohydrate

13 g fat

54 mg cholesterol

21 g protein

122 mg sodium

2 g fiber

STRAWBERRY, CHICKEN, AND ARUGULA SALAD

Strawberries are an excellent source of vitamin C and antioxidants. Choose organic strawberries to minimize your exposure to pesticides and herbicides.

MAKES 4 SERVINGS

FOR THE DRESSING

½ cup red wine vinegar

¼ cup water

½ teaspoon minced garlic

½ teaspoon sea salt

¼ teaspoon freshly ground black pepper

Four 4-ounce boneless, skinless chicken breast halves

4 slices multigrain bread

2 cups sliced strawberries

3 cups baby arugula, washed

415 calories
—
42 g carbohydrate
—
13 g fat
—
72 mg cholesterol
—
33 g protein
—
510 mg sodium
—
5 g fiber

EACH SERVING CONTAINS

1. Combine the vinegar, water, garlic, salt, and pepper in a small bowl. Set aside.

2. Preheat the grill or broiler.

3. Grill or broil the chicken breasts for 3 to 5 minutes on each side, or until the internal temperature reaches 165°F. Cool completely and dice.

4. Lightly spray the bread with canola oil spray on both sides. Grill until toasted. Dice the bread into bite-size pieces and set aside.

5. Combine the chicken, strawberries, and arugula in a large bowl. Whisk the dressing until well mixed. Toss the salad with the dressing and grilled bread.

6. Divide the salad evenly into four servings and place in salad bowls.

C COOK'S NOTE: *Three cups of croutons (page 117) can be substituted for the multigrain bread slices.*

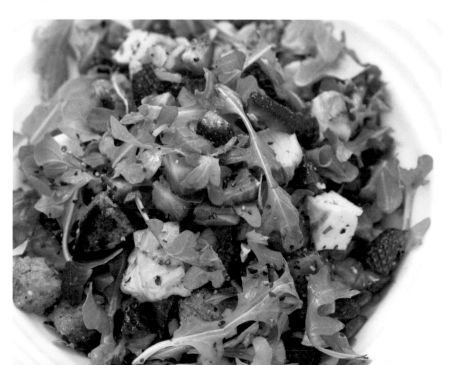

CLASSIC EGG SALAD SANDWICH

Juicy, dead-ripe summer tomatoes make this sandwich sublime.

MAKES 8 SERVINGS

7 hard-boiled large eggs

3 tablespoons diced celery

1 teaspoon Dijon mustard

⅓ cup canola oil mayonnaise

¼ cup diced red onions

¼ cup sweet pickle relish

3 tablespoons diced red bell peppers

2 teaspoons distilled white vinegar

¾ teaspoon sea salt

¼ teaspoon freshly ground black pepper

16 slices whole grain bread

8 large lettuce leaves

2 medium tomatoes, cut into 4 slices each

1. Coarsely chop the hard-boiled eggs and place in a large bowl. Add the celery, mustard, mayonnaise, onions, pickle relish, bell peppers, vinegar, salt, and pepper and mix well.

2. Place ⅓ cup egg salad between 2 slices bread. Top with a lettuce leaf and tomato slice.

n NUTRITION NOTE: *Eggs are a good source of protein, biotin, and lutein, a carotenoid that helps protect against macular degeneration. The best choice for the healthiest eggs is organic—it ensures good conditions and diet for the laying hens and no antibiotic use.*

EACH SERVING CONTAINS

325 calories

40 g carbohydrate

13 g fat

189 mg cholesterol

12 g protein

646 mg sodium

3 g fiber

CHAPTER SEVEN | *We love the zing and interest that salsas and sauces add to food and appreciate the way they can improve the nutritional profile of a dish. We recommend that you serve our pasta sauces with whole-grain pasta cooked in a generous amount of rapidly boiling water until just tender. Research has shown that the Italian insistence on al dente pasta is not only aesthetic but practical: Perfectly cooked pasta causes a much smaller rise in blood sugar than pasta that's overcooked and mushy.*

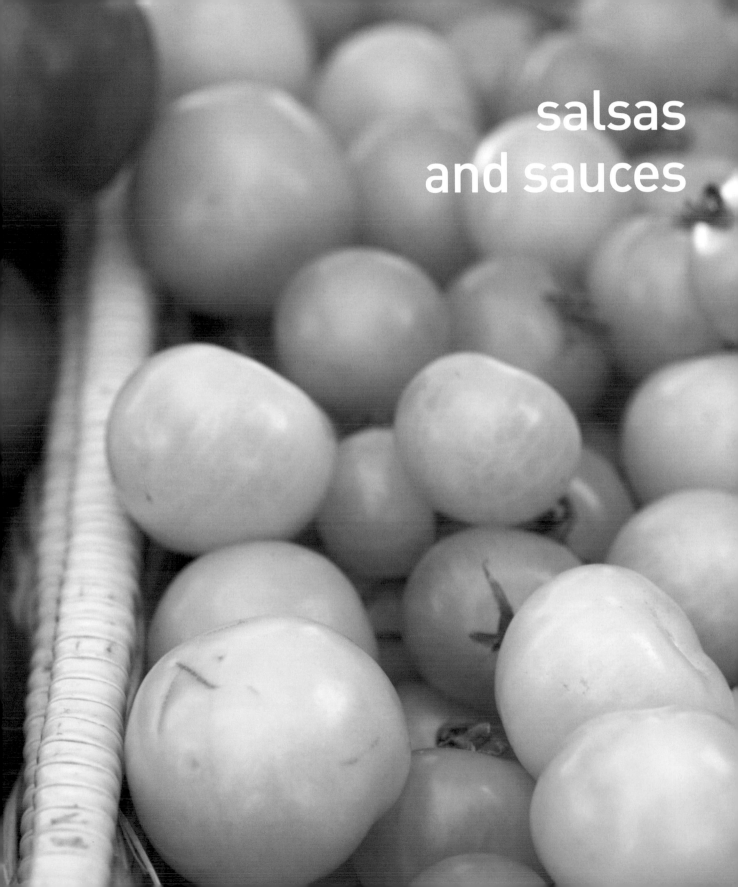

salsas
and sauces

FRESH MARINARA SAUCE

This flavorful sauce is a great way to use a bounty of fresh vine-ripened summer tomatoes. It freezes well and can be used in a dozen ways, so make plenty.

MAKES TWELVE ½-CUP SERVINGS

1 tablespoon extra virgin olive oil

2 cups diced onions

2 tablespoons minced garlic

1½ teaspoons dried basil

1 teaspoon dried oregano

¼ teaspoon dried thyme

¼ teaspoon freshly ground black pepper

5 pounds tomatoes, chopped

2 tablespoons honey

2 teaspoons sea salt

2 tablespoons minced fresh basil

1 tablespoon minced fresh oregano

1. Heat the olive oil in a large saucepan over medium heat. Sauté the onions until translucent. Add the garlic and brown slightly. Add the dried basil, dried oregano, thyme, and pepper and sauté briefly.

2. Add the tomatoes and reduce the heat to low. Simmer for 1 hour, or until thickened.

3. Stir in the honey and salt. (If you want a smooth sauce, puree with an immersion blender and strain the mixture through a large-mesh sieve.) Add the fresh basil and fresh oregano and simmer for 5 minutes.

n NUTRITION NOTE: *Although we often don't realize it, tomato-based sauces such as this marinara are all vegetables with all the associated benefits—vitamins, minerals, fiber, and antioxidants.*

EACH SERVING CONTAINS

75 calories

15 g carbohydrate

2 g fat

0 mg cholesterol

2 g protein

411 mg sodium

3 g fiber

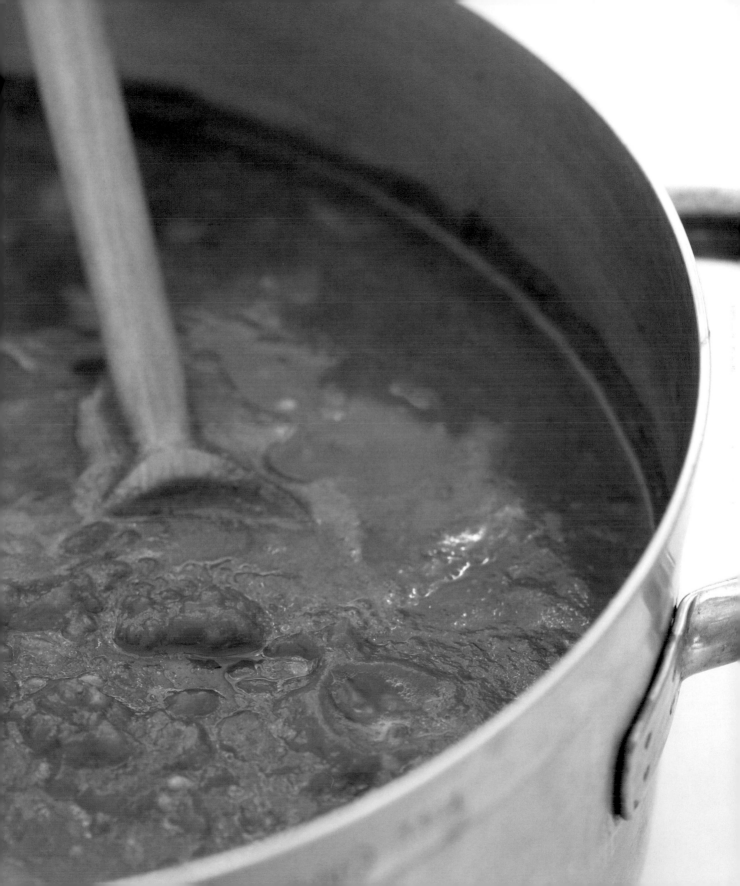

CHUNKY TOMATO SAUCE

Cooking tomatoes actually increases the availability of lycopene, a powerful antioxidant that helps fight heart disease and some forms of cancer, particularly prostate cancer. Canned organic tomatoes are a great choice here.

MAKES SIX ½-CUP SERVINGS

One 28-ounce can whole peeled tomatoes

1 teaspoon extra virgin olive oil

2 teaspoons minced garlic

½ cup chopped yellow onions

1 cup water

1 teaspoon dried basil

1 teaspoon dried oregano

Pinch dried thyme leaves, crushed

⅛ teaspoon sea salt

⅛ teaspoon freshly ground black pepper

1. Place the tomatoes in a medium bowl and lightly crush them with your hands.

2. Heat the olive oil over medium heat in a medium saucepan. Sauté the garlic and onions until the onions are translucent.

3. Add the crushed tomatoes, water, basil, oregano, thyme, salt, and pepper. Bring to a boil and reduce the heat to low. Simmer for 30 to 40 minutes, or until thickened.

EACH SERVING CONTAINS

40 calories

8 g carbohydrate

1 g fat

0 mg cholesterol

1 g protein

55 mg sodium

2 g fiber

BÉCHAMEL SAUCE

Our version of a kitchen basic. You'll find it used in Moussaka (page 206) and Macaroni and Cheese (page 110) and in more complex sauces as well.

MAKES 1 QUART SAUCE, EACH A ⅓-CUP SERVING

2 teaspoons canola oil

⅓ cup diced yellow onions

Pinch ground cloves

Pinch freshly ground
black pepper

2 bay leaves

3 tablespoons cornstarch

4 cups 2% milk

¾ teaspoon sea salt

1. Heat the canola oil over medium heat in a large saucepan. Sauté the onions in oil until translucent. Add the cloves, pepper, and bay leaves. Reduce the heat to low and sauté for 1 more minute.

2. Mix the cornstarch and milk in a large bowl with a wire whisk. Add to the onion mixture and bring to a simmer, whisking continuously. (This sauce will stick and burn on the bottom if you don't keep stirring.) Cook for 1 to 2 minutes, or until slightly thickened but still pourable.

3. Stir in the salt and strain the mixture through a large-mesh sieve.

n NUTRITION NOTE: *Our chefs have lightened the traditional recipe without compromising its rich flavor.*

EACH SERVING CONTAINS

55 calories

6 g carbohydrate

2 g fat

6 mg cholesterol

2 g protein

135 mg sodium

Trace fiber

CREAMY PARMESAN SAUCE

Traditionally served on pasta. Try it, though, with vegetables such as steamed broccoli or with chicken.

MAKES FIFTEEN ¼-CUP SERVINGS

½ cup diced shallots

½ cup white wine

6 tablespoons heavy cream

3 cups Béchamel Sauce (page175)

1 cup freshly grated Parmesan

¾ teaspoon sea salt

½ teaspoon freshly ground black pepper

3 tablespoons nonfat sour cream

1. Spray a large saucepan with canola oil spray. Sauté the shallots over medium heat until translucent. Add the white wine and reduce until almost dry.

2. Add the cream and béchamel and bring to a simmer. Remove from the heat and strain through a fine-mesh sieve into a large bowl.

3. Add the Parmesan, salt, pepper, and sour cream and mix well.

n   NUTRITION NOTE: *You may be surprised to find a Canyon Ranch recipe for a creamy Alfredo-type sauce that doesn't taste "light." Here's how we do it. First, we start with our own healthier béchamel sauce, adding a bit of heavy cream and a generous amount of freshly grated Parmesan for authentic flavor. The nonfat sour cream adds a silkiness to the sauce and stabilizes it. Also note that we suggest using only ¼ cup of the sauce with a portion of ½ cup of the cooked pasta rather than the ½ cup of sauce and 1 cup of pasta for vegetable-based sauces. Sometimes it takes several strategies like these to successfully transform a very high-fat, high-calorie recipe into one we are proud to put our name on.*

EACH SERVING CONTAINS

120 calories

6 g carbohydrate

6 g fat

18 mg cholesterol

6 g protein

320 mg sodium

Trace fiber

CREAMY PESTO SAUCE

The evocative flavor of basil makes this sauce special—and a great addition to your pasta sauce repertoire.

MAKES SIX ⅓-CUP SERVINGS

FOR THE PESTO

⅓ cup packed fresh basil leaves

3 tablespoons chopped fresh flat-leaf parsley

1½ teaspoons extra virgin olive oil

1½ teaspoons toasted pine nuts

2 garlic cloves, chopped

¼ cup freshly grated Parmesan

2 tablespoons water

FOR THE CREAM SAUCE

1½ teaspoons canola oil

¼ cup diced yellow onions

Pinch ground cloves

Pinch freshly ground black pepper

½ bay leaf

2 tablespoons cornstarch

2 cups 2% milk

1½ teaspoons sea salt

⅓ cup freshly grated Parmesan

1. Combine the basil, parsley, olive oil, pine nuts, garlic, Parmesan, and water in a blender and puree until smooth.

2. Heat the canola oil in a large saucepan. Sauté the onions over medium heat until translucent. Add the cloves, pepper, and bay leaf. Reduce the heat to low and sauté for 1 more minute.

3. Mix the cornstarch and milk in a large bowl with a wire whisk.

4. Add the cornstarch mixture to the onion mixture and bring to a simmer. Cook, stirring constantly, for 2 to 3 minutes, or until thickened. Add the salt, pesto, and Parmesan. Remove and discard the bay leaf.

n NUTRITION NOTE: *The pigments in plants that add color provide a wide range of health benefits with antioxidant, antiinflammatory, and anticancer properties. Many of the substances responsible for fragrance have similar effects. Basil has both.*

EACH SERVING CONTAINS

120 calories

7 g carbohydrate

8 g fat

11 mg cholesterol

6 g protein

239 mg sodium

Trace fiber

FENNEL AND GARLIC SALSA

Toss with pasta for a terrific starter or side dish.

MAKES FIVE 2-TABLESPOON SERVINGS

2 ounces fresh fennel
(about ¼ bulb)

12 garlic cloves

1 tablespoon chopped
toasted walnuts

1½ teaspoons extra
virgin olive oil

¼ teaspoon sea salt

⅛ teaspoon freshly
ground black pepper

1½ teaspoons fresh
lemon juice

1 tablespoon chopped
fresh chives

1½ teaspoons
chopped fresh basil

¼ teaspoon lemon
zest, minced

1. Preheat the oven to 350º. Lightly coat a small baking sheet with canola oil spray.

2. Place the fennel and garlic cloves on the baking sheet and roast for 10 minutes, or until golden brown. Cool completely.

3. Small dice the roasted fennel and garlic and transfer to a small bowl. Add the walnuts, olive oil, salt, pepper, lemon juice, chives, basil, and lemon zest and mix well.

n **NUTRITION NOTE:** *Garlic has long been studied for its ability to lower blood pressure. This is one of the more interesting ways to use it.*

EACH SERVING CONTAINS

35 calories

3 g carbohydrate

3 g fat

0 mg cholesterol

1 g protein

101 mg sodium

1 g fiber

BBQ SAUCE

This grilling favorite has much less sugar than most bottled sauces, and no gums, stabilizers, or preservatives.

MAKES SIXTEEN 2-TABLESPOON SERVINGS (SEE PHOTO PAGE 182.)

½ cup diced yellow onions

1 tablespoon minced garlic

1½ **teaspoons** chili powder

½ cup brewed coffee

¼ cup Worcestershire sauce

½ cup dark beer

2 tablespoons molasses

1½ cups low-sodium ketchup

3 tablespoons apple cider vinegar

⅓ cup firmly packed light brown sugar

½ teaspoon liquid smoke

1. Lightly coat a small sauté pan with canola oil spray. Sauté the onions and garlic over medium heat until soft and caramelized, 3 to 5 minutes.

2. Add the chili powder, coffee, Worcestershire, beer, molasses, ketchup, vinegar, brown sugar, and liquid smoke and simmer until the sauce begins to thicken, 5 to 10 minutes.

n **NUTRITION NOTE:** *This is a lower sodium BBQ sauce you can use on virtually anything. Remember, cooked tomato products, including ketchup, are rich in lycopene, which has been linked to protection against osteoporosis, prostate cancer, and breast cancer.*

EACH SERVING CONTAINS

40 calories

9 g carbohydrate

Trace fat

0 mg cholesterol

Trace protein

170 mg sodium

Trace fiber

GINGER PEACH HOT SAUCE

Make a double batch of this zippy sauce to enjoy on everything from chicken to tofu to vegetables. It keeps in an airtight glass jar in the refrigerator for up to a week.

MAKES EIGHT 2-TABLESPOON SERVINGS (SEE PHOTO PAGE 182.)

¾ cup sliced peaches

¼ cup chopped yellow onions

2 tablespoons minced red bell peppers

2 teaspoons minced garlic

1 tablespoon minced fresh ginger

1 tablespoon minced crystallized ginger

⅛ teaspoon crushed red pepper flakes

3 tablespoons apple cider vinegar

⅓ cup water

¼ teaspoon sea salt

⅛ teaspoon black peppercorns

¼ teaspoon cane sugar

1. Combine the peaches, onions, bell peppers, garlic, fresh ginger, crystallized ginger, red pepper flakes, vinegar, water, salt, peppercorns, and cane sugar in a small saucepan over medium heat. Simmer for 10 to 15 minutes until the peaches are tender and the volume of the liquid is approximately equal to that of the solids.

2. Remove from the heat and cool slightly.

3. Place the ginger-peach mixture in a blender and puree until smooth.

n NUTRITION NOTE: *Ginger, found here in two different forms, has many medicinal uses, from stomach soothing to fighting inflammation.*

c COOK'S NOTE: *Leave the peel on the peaches for more peach flavor and aroma. Frozen or canned peaches can be substituted if fresh are not available, but the sauce will not be quite as flavorful.*

EACH SERVING CONTAINS

25 calories

6 g carbohydrate

0 g fat

0 mg cholesterol

Trace protein

73 mg sodium

Trace fiber

ROASTED RED PEPPER RELISH

This makes an excellent dip or a wonderful topping for toasted bread.

MAKES FOUR 2-TABLESPOON SERVINGS

½ cup minced roasted
red peppers

½ cup chopped
kalamata olives

2 tablespoons
chiffonade of arugula

1 tablespoon red
wine vinegar

¼ teaspoon sea salt

¼ teaspoon freshly
ground black pepper

Combine the roasted peppers and olives in a small bowl. Fold in the arugula, vinegar, salt, and pepper.

n NUTRITION NOTE: *Red peppers are ripened green peppers but have more antioxidant carotenoids and are easier to digest.*

EACH SERVING CONTAINS

15 calories

2 g carbohydrate

1 g fat

0 mg cholesterol

Trace protein

149 mg sodium

1 g fiber

TOMATO FETA RELISH

Make this pretty, juicy relish two ways (see Cook's Note).

MAKES EIGHT 2-TABLESPOON SERVINGS

4 medium tomatoes, diced

3 tablespoons
champagne vinegar

3 tablespoons water

3 tablespoons
evaporated cane juice

2 tablespoons chopped
kalamata olives

Pinch dried basil

Pinch sea salt

Pinch freshly ground
black pepper

½ cup crumbled
feta cheese

1. Bring the tomatoes, vinegar, water, cane juice, olives, basil, salt, and pepper to a slow simmer in a small saucepan over medium heat. Cook until the mixture thickens. Cool completely.

2. Add the feta and mix thoroughly.

C COOK'S NOTE: *For a quicker fresh relish, combine the tomatoes, 1 tablespoon vinegar, the olives, basil, salt, pepper, and feta in a small bowl. Exclude the water and cane juice. Toss to combine.*

EACH SERVING CONTAINS

30 calories

4 g carbohydrate

1 g fat

3 mg cholesterol

1 g protein

77 mg sodium

Trace fiber

Top: Cucumber, Dill, and Goat Cheese Relish, page 191. Left: Thai Peanut Sauce, page 183. Right: BBQ Sauce, page 179. Bottom: Ginger Peach Hot Sauce, page 180.

THAI PEANUT SAUCE

This is the classic sauce you find in Thai restaurants. Toss it with noodles and peanuts for a quick, exotic side dish. Or serve it as a dipping sauce for chicken kebabs.

MAKES EIGHT 2-TABLESPOON SERVINGS (SEE PHOTO OPPOSITE.)

½ cup natural peanut butter

Pinch sea salt

1 tablespoon cane sugar

1 tablespoon light coconut milk

1 tablespoon fresh lime juice

1¼ teaspoons fresh ginger juice

½ teaspoon rice vinegar

½ teaspoon fish sauce

Dash Tabasco

½ cup water

1 tablespoon low-sodium tamari sauce

1. Place the peanut butter in a small bowl. Add the salt and cane sugar and mix until almost dissolved. Add the coconut milk, lime juice, ginger juice, rice vinegar, fish sauce, and Tabasco. Mix well to form a thick paste—an electric mixer works well.

2. Combine the water and tamari in a small saucepan and bring to a boil. Whisk in the peanut butter mixture. Cook until the mixture begins to thicken. Remove from the heat.

C COOK'S NOTE: *To make fresh ginger juice, grate fresh ginger using a cheese grater, collect the grated ginger in the palm of your hand, and squeeze out the juice.*

EACH SERVING CONTAINS

95 calories

5 g carbohydrate

7 g fat

0 mg cholesterol

4 g protein

178 mg sodium

1 g fiber

MONGOLIAN BBQ SAUCE

A terrific marinade as well as a great dipping sauce. Store in a tightly sealed container in the refrigerator for up to one week.

MAKES SIXTEEN 2-TABLESPOON SERVINGS

½ cup plus 2 tablespoons low-sodium tamari sauce

2 tablespoons cane sugar

¼ cup rice vinegar

1 tablespoon sesame oil

½ cup sake

⅓ cup plus 2 tablespoons water

⅓ cup low-sodium ketchup

Pinch ground coriander

Pinch ground ginger

¼ teaspoon crushed red pepper flakes

¼ cup minced leeks, white part only

2 teaspoons minced garlic

2 teaspoons minced fresh ginger

1. Combine the ½ cup tamari, the cane sugar, rice vinegar, sesame oil, sake, and the ⅓ cup water and bring to a boil over medium heat, then reduce to low. Add the ketchup, coriander, ground ginger, and red pepper flakes. Simmer for 10 minutes. Remove from the heat.

2. Combine the leeks, garlic, fresh ginger, the 2 tablespoons water, and the 2 tablespoons tamari.

3. Add the leek mixture to the sauce mixture and stir until combined.

n NUTRITION NOTE: *This sauce is lower in sodium than similar sauces. Garlic, ginger, and tomato ketchup are all rich sources of bioactive phytonutrients.*

EACH SERVING CONTAINS

35 calories

4 g carbohydrate

Trace fat

0 mg cholesterol

Trace protein

288 mg sodium

Trace fiber

PONZU SAUCE

A clean, tangy sauce that tastes especially good in hot weather.
Try it with grilled bok choy or stir-fry green vegetables.

MAKES EIGHT 1-TABLESPOON SERVINGS

2 tablespoons
fresh lime juice

2 tablespoons low-
sodium tamari sauce

2 tablespoons water

1 tablespoon plus 1
teaspoon rice vinegar

1 teaspoon minced
fresh ginger

2 teaspoons cane sugar

Combine the lime juice, tamari, water, rice vinegar, ginger, and cane sugar in a blender and puree until smooth. Strain through a fine-mesh sieve, if desired.

n NUTRITION NOTE: *Ginger, a predominant flavor in our Ponzu sauce, is an antiin-flammatory agent. Using it daily may help with minor aches and pains as well as help combat the systemic inflammation that seems to accompany heart disease, insulin resistance, and autoimmune diseases.*

EACH SERVING CONTAINS

15 calories

4 g carbohydrate

0 g fat

0 mg cholesterol

1 g protein

304 mg sodium

Trace fiber

GREEN CURRY PASTE

Try green curry on sandwiches instead of mayonnaise.
It keeps in a covered jar in the refrigerator for up to a week.

MAKES SIX 2-TABLESPOON SERVINGS

1 cup chopped
fresh cilantro

¼ cup chopped fresh mint

½ jalapeño pepper,
chopped

2 tablespoons fresh
lemon juice

2 tablespoons cane sugar

½ teaspoon sea salt

1 tablespoon water

Combine the cilantro, mint, jalapeño, lemon juice, cane sugar, salt, and pepper in a small food processor or blender and puree until a paste forms. (Wear gloves when handling hot chile peppers, or wash your hands thoroughly before touching your eyes, nose, or mouth.)

EACH SERVING CONTAINS

25 calories

6 g carbohydrate

Trace fat

0 mg cholesterol

1 g protein

241 mg sodium

1 g fiber

LATIN SPICE RUB

*Fantastic with chicken or fish. Store this spice rub in a cool,
dark place in a tightly covered glass jar up to 6 months.*

MAKES FORTY-TWO 1-TEASPOON SERVINGS

1 tablespoon black
peppercorns

2 tablespoons whole
coriander seed

2 tablespoons whole
cumin seed

1 tablespoon sea salt

¼ cup cane sugar

1. Preheat the toaster oven to 350°F. Place the peppercorns, coriander, and cumin on a baking tray. Toast for 5 to 7 minutes, or until the spices are slightly browned and aromatic. Cool completely.

2. Place in a spice or coffee grinder and grind until powdered.

3. Mix the ground spices with the salt and cane sugar.

EACH SERVING CONTAINS

5 calories

2 g carbohydrate

Trace fat

0 mg cholesterol

Trace protein

134 mg sodium

Trace fiber

GUACAMOLE

Avocados are full of heart-healthy monounsaturated fat, along with vitamins C and E, several B complex vitamins, and potassium. The added veggies help balance out the concentrated fat calories from the avocado.

MAKES EIGHTEEN 2-TABLESPOON SERVINGS

2 medium avocados, peeled, pitted, and diced

3 tablespoons fresh lime juice

¼ cup diced red onions

2 tablespoons chopped fresh cilantro

1 teaspoon minced, seeded jalapeño peppers

½ teaspoon sea salt

Pinch freshly ground black pepper

¾ cup diced tomatoes

½ teaspoon minced garlic

1. Lightly mash the avocados with the lime juice in a medium bowl.

2. Gently fold the onions, cilantro, jalapeños, salt, pepper, tomatoes, and garlic into the avocado mixture. (Wear gloves when handling hot chile peppers, or wash your hands thoroughly before touching your eyes, nose, or mouth.)

n NUTRITION NOTE: *Avocados are extremely wholesome, providing monounsaturated fat and fat-soluble vitamin E.*

EACH SERVING CONTAINS

25 calories

2 g carbohydrate

1 g fat

0 mg cholesterol

1 g protein

53 mg sodium

1 g fiber

PICO DE GALLO

Authentic Sonoran salsa, Canyon Ranch style. Store it immediately in a glass jar in the refrigerator up to a week.

MAKES 3 CUPS

4 medium fresh tomatoes, diced

1½ cups canned diced tomatoes

½ cup diced red onions

3 tablespoons chopped scallions

½ cup diced yellow bell peppers

1 tablespoon diced jalapeño peppers

¼ cup chopped fresh cilantro

1 tablespoon plus 1 teaspoon fresh lime juice

1 teaspoon sea salt

¼ teaspoon freshly ground black pepper

½ teaspoon dried oregano

¼ teaspoon garlic powder

Place the fresh tomatoes, canned tomatoes, onions, scallions, bell peppers, jalapeños, cilantro, lime juice, salt, pepper, oregano, and garlic powder in a food processor and pulse briefly to combine.

n NUTRITION NOTE: *There isn't a healthier condiment than salsa with its vitamin C, beta-carotene, and other antioxidants.*

EACH SERVING CONTAINS

10 calories

2 g carbohydrate

Trace fat

0 mg cholesterol

Trace protein

122 mg sodium

Trace fiber

OLIVE SALSA

Terrific with grilled lamb, grass-fed beef, or chicken.

MAKES FOUR ⅓-CUP SERVINGS

1 cup quartered grape tomatoes

½ cup diced Roasted Fennel (page 99)

½ cup chopped mixed olives—kalamatas, Niçoise, or other gourmet olives

1 tablespoon fresh lemon juice

1 teaspoon lemon zest, minced

¼ teaspoon sea salt

¼ teaspoon freshly ground black pepper

1 tablespoon minced fresh flat-leaf parsley

¼ teaspoon minced fresh oregano

Combine the tomatoes, fennel, olives, lemon juice, lemon zest, salt, pepper, parsley, and oregano in a medium bowl.

EACH SERVING CONTAINS

40 calories

6 g carbohydrate

2 g fat

0 mg cholesterol

1 g protein

342 mg sodium

2 g fiber

CUCUMBER, DILL, AND GOAT CHEESE RELISH

Spectacular with grilled salmon.

MAKES EIGHT ¼-CUP SERVINGS [SEE PHOTO PAGE 182]

⅓ cup low-fat sour cream

¼ cup crumbled goat cheese

2 tablespoons minced fresh dill

2 tablespoons minced fresh chives

1½ teaspoons fresh lemon juice

½ teaspoon sea salt

Pinch freshly ground black pepper

Dash Worcestershire sauce

1 medium cucumber, peeled and diced

Combine the sour cream, goat cheese, dill, chives, lemon juice, salt, pepper, and Worcestershire in a medium bowl, and mix well. Fold in the cucumbers.

EACH SERVING CONTAINS

30 calories

2 g carbohydrate

2 g fat

6 mg cholesterol

2 g protein

153 mg sodium

Trace fiber

BOLOGNESE SAUCE

MAKES SIX ½-CUP SERVINGS

2 teaspoons extra
virgin olive oil

8 ounces lean ground beef

1 small yellow onion, diced

2 minced garlic cloves

1 bay leaf

¾ teaspoon dried basil

½ teaspoon dried oregano

1 teaspoon sea salt

¼ teaspoon freshly
ground black pepper

1 teaspoon cane sugar

¼ cup red wine

¼ cup beef stock

1 cup Fresh Marinara
Sauce (page 172)

One 14½-ounce can (2
cups) whole tomatoes,
hand crushed

1. Heat ½ teaspoon of the olive oil in a large sauté pan. Sauté the ground beef over medium-high heat until cooked through. Drain well.

2. Heat the remaining olive oil in a large saucepan. Sauté the onions and garlic over medium-high heat until the onions are translucent. Add the beef, bay leaf, basil, oregano, salt, pepper, and cane sugar and sauté briefly. Add the red wine and reduce by half.

3. Add the beef stock, marinara sauce, and tomatoes. Bring to a boil, reduce the heat, and simmer for 15 minutes, or until the tomatoes are broken down and the sauce has thickened.

EACH SERVING CONTAINS

150 calories

10 g carbohydrate

5 g fat

23 g cholesterol

15 g protein

302 mg sodium

2 g fiber

BLACKENING SPICE

MAKES 30 TEASPOONS

1 tablespoon Old
Bay Seasoning

2 tablespoons
ground paprika

2 tablespoons chili powder

1 tablespoon
onion powder

1 tablespoon garlic
granules

1 teaspoon dried thyme

1 tablespoon Colman's
dry mustard

1 tablespoon dried basil

1 teaspoon dried oregano

½ teaspoon
cayenne pepper

¼ teaspoon freshly
ground black pepper

¼ teaspoon ground cumin

¼ teaspoon curry powder

Combine the Old Bay Seasoning, paprika, chili powder, onion powder, garlic, thyme, mustard, basil, oregano, cayenne pepper, black pepper, cumin and curry powder in a small bowl and mix well. Store any leftover spice mix in a tightly sealed container in a cool, dark place.

EACH SERVING CONTAINS

7 calories

1 g carbohydrate

Trace fat

0 mg cholesterol

Trace protein

56 mg sodium

1 g fiber

CHAPTER EIGHT | *We love organic, grass-fed beef, which is lower in fat and cholesterol and higher in disease-fighting nutrients than grain-fed beef. It is also a cleaner, tastier, and more humanely raised alternative to feedlot beef, which usually contains antibiotics and hormones. It's typically less tender, though, than conventional beef, and requires either quick or very long cooking—our recipes take that into account. Clean, locally sourced lamb is also available at many farmers' markets, although availability will vary throughout the year. Once again, your freezer can make life simpler and help you improve the quality of your diet.*

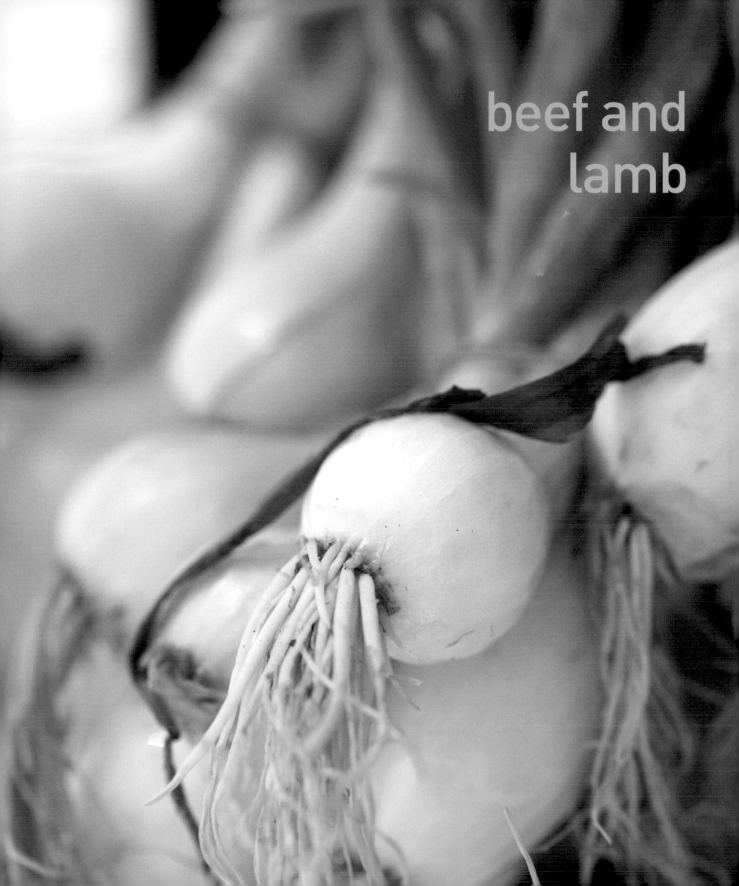

beef and
lamb

LONDON BROIL

*This is a quick-cooking dish that's perfect for a summer meal.
We like this with our Chilled Green Bean Salad (page 93).*

MAKES 4 SERVINGS

1 pound beef flank steak

**1 cup Mongolian BBQ
Sauce (page 184)**

1. Place the flank steak in a shallow glass baking dish. Pour the Mongolian BBQ sauce over the steak. Cover and refrigerate for at least 2 hours or overnight, turning the steak occasionally.

2. Preheat the grill or broiler.

3. Remove the steak from the marinade and discard the marinade. Grill or broil the steak for 4 to 6 minutes on each side, or to the desired doneness. Slice thinly across the grain to serve.

> **n** **NUTRITION NOTE:** *Red meat is a wonderful source of B vitamins, iron, and zinc. We recommend, however, small servings of 3 to 4 ounces and choosing grass-fed beef, which is higher in omega-3 fatty acids.*

EACH SERVING CONTAINS

175 calories

1 g carbohydrate

7 g fat

47 mg cholesterol

24 g protein

150 mg sodium

Trace fiber

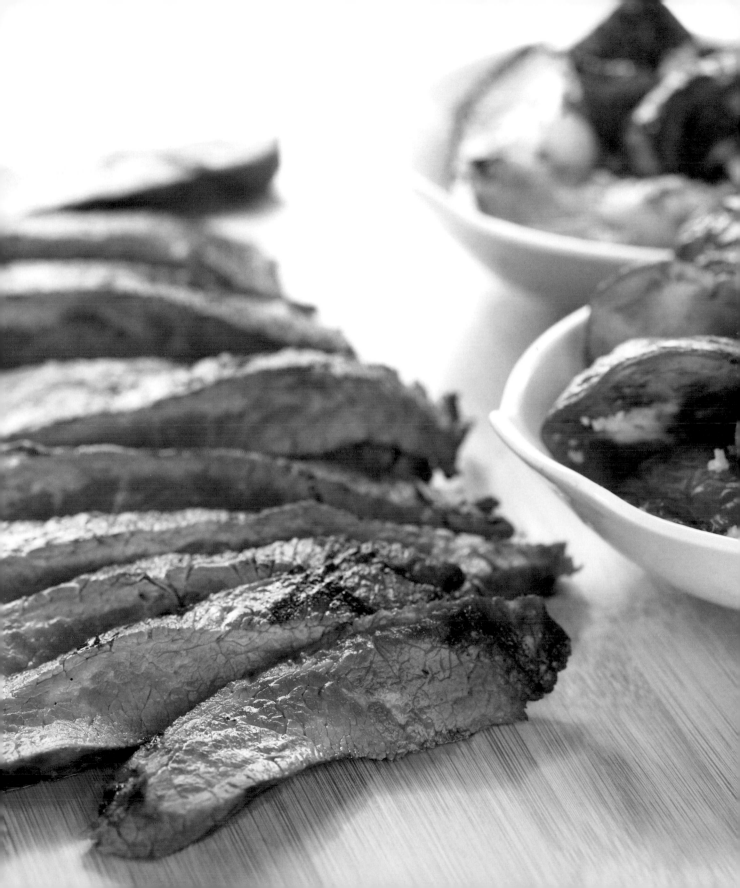

ASIAN BRAISED FLANK STEAK
WITH BOK CHOY AND BROWN RICE

Chef Scott's fabulous Mongolian BBQ Sauce is the key to this nourishing meal.

MAKES 4 SERVINGS

1 tablespoon plus
¼ teaspoon extra
virgin olive oil

2 cups diced yellow onions

1 pound beef flank steak

2 cups Mongolian BBQ
Sauce (page 184)

2 quarts water

¼ cup minced crimini
mushrooms

3 whole allspice berries

3 bay leaves

¼ teaspoon sea salt

Pinch plus ¼ teaspoon
freshly ground
black pepper

¾ pound cleaned
baby bok choy

2 cups cooked brown rice

1. Heat 1 tablespoon of the olive oil in a large saucepan over medium heat. Sauté the onions until lightly browned.

2. Pound out the steak with a meat mallet to ¼ inch thickness. Add to the onions and brown 1 to 2 minutes per side. Remove from the pan.

3. Deglaze the pan with the BBQ sauce and water over medium heat, scraping the bottom to remove the browned bits. Return the steak to the pan and stir in the mushrooms.

4. Wrap the allspice and bay leaves in cheesecloth and tie with thread or string to form a bouquet garni. Add the bouquet garni, salt, and pinch pepper to the pan. Bring to a boil over low heat, reduce the heat to a simmer, and cover with a lid. Cook for 2 to 2½ hours, or until the steak is tender. Remove and discard the bouquet garni.

5. Cut the bok choy lengthwise into quarters.

6. Heat the remaining ¼ teaspoon olive oil in a medium sauté pan over medium heat. Sauté the bok choy and ¼ teaspoon pepper until tender and crisp.

7. Divide the cooked bok choy evenly among four plates. Serve 4 ounces flank steak with ¼ cup sauce and ½ cup brown rice on each plate.

n NUTRITION NOTE: *Bok choy is rarely recognized as a good source of calcium, but it provides a generous amount for a vegetable.*

c COOK'S NOTE: *Allspice berries are the pea-size berry of the evergreen pimiento tree native to South America and the West Indies. The spice is so named because it tastes like a blend of cinnamon, nutmeg, and cloves. Store dried berries in a cool, dry place.*

EACH SERVING CONTAINS

385 calories
40 g carbohydrate
12 g fat
41 mg cholesterol
27 g protein
660 mg sodium
3 g fiber

STEAK PIZZAIOLA

Instead of steak and potatoes.

MAKES 4 SERVINGS

1 pound beef flank steak

2 cups Mongolian BBQ Sauce (page 184)

FOR THE BELL PEPPER MIXTURE

½ cup chopped red bell peppers

½ cup chopped yellow bell peppers

2 teaspoons minced garlic

2 cups thinly sliced red onions

1 cup canned fire-roasted tomatoes, chopped

5 fresh basil leaves

1 tablespoon low-sodium tamari sauce

¼ teaspoon sea salt

⅛ teaspoon freshly ground black pepper

2 teaspoons red wine vinegar

1 pound cooked spaghetti

1. Place the flank steak in a shallow glass baking dish. Pour the Mongolian BBQ sauce over the steak. Cover and refrigerate for at least 2 hours or overnight, turning the steak occasionally.

2. Preheat the grill or broiler.

3. Remove the steak from the marinade and discard the marinade. Grill or broil the steak for 4 to 6 minutes on each side, or to the desired doneness. Slice thinly across the grain to serve.

4. Spray a medium sauté pan with canola oil spray. Sauté the red bell peppers, yellow bell peppers, garlic, and onions over medium heat until the onions are translucent. Add the tomatoes and simmer for 2 to 3 minutes, stirring occasionally.

5. Chiffonade the basil leaves and add to the pan. Stir in the tamari, salt, pepper, and vinegar.

6. Arrange 3 ounces of cooked steak over 4 ounces of cooked spaghetti. Serve with ½ cup cooked bell pepper mixture.

NUTRITION NOTE: *You've heard, we're sure, the simple advice to "move more, eat less." The "eat less" part of the equation sounds simple, but how many of us know just how much to eat? This spicy pasta recipe provides a great opportunity to talk portions. Take pasta, for instance. A reasonable portion for an adult is a quarter pound, which translates into about one cup, cooked. A reasonable portion of red meat or chicken is a quarter pound raw. When it comes to vegetables, which are low in calories and rich in nutrients, we want you to splurge.*

EACH SERVING CONTAINS

420 calories

50 g carbohydrate

9 g fat

47 mg cholesterol

33 g protein

596 mg sodium

4 g fiber

BEEF TENDERLOINS
WITH BOURBON CHERRIES

A simple yet impressive dish for company.
It's great with Creamed Leeks (page 96).

MAKES 4 SERVINGS

½ cup dried cherries

¼ cup bourbon

Four 4-ounce beef
tenderloin fillets

Pinch sea salt

Pinch freshly ground
black pepper

1 teaspoon extra
virgin olive oil

2 cups low-sodium
beef stock

1. Soak the cherries in the bourbon in a small bowl for 5 to 10 minutes.

2. Lightly season the beef tenderloin fillets with the salt and pepper.

3. Heat the olive oil over medium-high heat in a large sauté pan. Sauté the fillets for 3 to 5 minutes on each side, or to desired doneness. Remove from the pan.

4. Deglaze the pan with the bourbon cherries. Cook until the pan is dry. Deglaze again with the beef stock and reduce by three-quarters.

5. Divide the bourbon cherries and sauce evenly over each beef tenderloin fillet.

n NUTRITION NOTE: *Cherries, especially tart ones, are a good source of beta-carotene, vitamins, and other nutrients. Their powerful antioxidants help fight inflammation, heart disease, and some cancers. Choose organic cherries whenever possible.*

EACH SERVING CONTAINS

375 calories

23 g carbohydrate

12 g fat

105 mg cholesterol

34 g protein

189 mg sodium

2 g fiber

GRILLED BEEF TENDERLOINS WITH TOMATO–BLUE CHEESE SALSA

A piquant salsa sets off the flavor of grilled tenderloin fillets.

MAKES 4 SERVINGS

FOR THE TOMATO BLUE CHEESE SALSA

1½ cups chopped tomatoes

¼ cup minced red onions

¼ cup blue cheese, crumbled

1 tablespoon chopped fresh flat-leaf parsley

1 teaspoon dried oregano

½ teaspoon sea salt

¼ teaspoon freshly ground black pepper

2 teaspoons fresh lemon juice

———————

Four 4-ounce beef tenderloin fillets

Pinch sea salt

Pinch freshly ground black pepper

1. Preheat the grill or broiler.

2. Combine the tomatoes, onions, blue cheese, parsley, oregano, salt, pepper, and lemon juice in a medium bowl and mix well. Set aside.

3. Season the fillets with the salt and pepper. Grill or broil the fillets for 3 to 5 minutes on each side, or until desired doneness.

4. Serve each fillet with ½ cup tomato–blue cheese salsa.

n NUTRITION NOTE: *One of the easiest foods to eat seasonally and locally is fresh tomatoes. In fact, you can grow your own even in containers.*

EACH SERVING CONTAINS

310 calories

6 g carbohydrate

15 g fat

115 mg cholesterol

37 g protein

673 mg sodium

1 g fiber

BEEF SHORT RIBS

Bison ribs are another good low-fat choice for this recipe.

MAKES 4 SERVINGS

2 pounds bone-in beef short ribs or 1 pound boneless short ribs

2 cups Mongolian BBQ Sauce (page 184)

2 cups water

¼ cup firmly packed brown sugar

Mashed Potatoes (page 105)

Braised Red Cabbage (page 92)

1. Preheat the oven to 350°F.

2. Sear the short ribs in a large heavy-bottomed pan over medium-high heat for 1 to 2 minutes on each side. Place in a shallow glass baking dish with a cover.

3. Combine the BBQ sauce, water, and brown sugar in a medium bowl and mix well. Pour over ribs. Cover tightly and roast for 2 to 3 hours, or until tender.

4. Serve 2 ribs with 2 tablespoons sauce, ½ cup mashed potatoes and ½ cup braised red cabbage.

n **NUTRITION NOTE:** *The tenderness of short ribs comes more from the breakdown of connective tissue than from the fat.*

EACH SERVING CONTAINS

370 calories

35 g carbohydrate

15 g fat

58 mg cholesterol

22 g protein

740 mg sodium

4 g fiber

POT ROAST

The thick, rich sauce here consists mostly of vegetables, so the one-quarter-cup portion of sauce is actually a vegetable serving. This is a terrific example of how Canyon Ranch cuisine delivers both great nutrition and fantastic flavor.

MAKES 4 SERVINGS

¼ teaspoon dried thyme

¼ teaspoon black peppercorns

1 bay leaf

1 teaspoon extra virgin olive oil

1 pound beef eye round

½ teaspoon sea salt

⅛ teaspoon freshly ground black pepper

¼ cup chopped red onions

¾ cup chopped carrots

¼ cup chopped celery

2 teaspoons minced garlic

1 cup chicken stock

One 14½-ounce can diced tomatoes (about 2 cups)

2 teaspoons red wine

2 medium Red Bliss potatoes, quartered

1 medium parsnip, chopped

1 medium yellow onion, chopped

1. Preheat the oven to 350°F.

2. Wrap the thyme, peppercorns, and bay leaf in cheesecloth and tie with thread or string to form a bouquet garni.

3. Heat the olive oil in a large saucepan over medium heat. Evenly sprinkle the roast with ¼ teaspoon of the salt and the pepper. Brown on all sides.

4. Place the roast in an ovenproof casserole and add the red onions, carrots, celery, garlic, chicken stock, tomatoes, red wine, and bouquet garni. Tightly cover and cook for 2 hours, or until the roast is fork-tender.

5. Place the potatoes, parsnips, yellow onions, and remaining carrots in a steamer and steam until tender. Set aside.

6. Remove the roast and the bouquet garni from the casserole. Discard the bouquet garni. Transfer the remaining contents of the casserole to a blender and puree until smooth. Add the remaining ¼ teaspoon salt.

7. Return the pureed vegetables to the saucepan and cook briefly. Add the steamed vegetables and cook until well coated.

8. Divide the beef and vegetable sauce mixture evenly among four plates.

n **NUTRITION NOTE:** *It is worth looking for a source of grass-fed beef for this recipe, but even if that isn't available, minimize the fat by using lean eye of round rather than chuck roast.*

EACH SERVING CONTAINS

275 calories

29 g carbohydrate

5 g fat

63 mg cholesterol

27 g protein

424 mg sodium

6 g fiber

BAKED ZITI

This is great served up family style, too. Toss the pasta and sauce and place in a 9 x 13-inch baking dish. Top with the cheeses, and bake until the cheeses brown. Serve Sautéed Spinach and Garlic (page 101) alongside.

MAKES 6 SERVINGS

1 pound ziti

1 cup shredded mozzarella (about 4 ounces)

⅓ cup freshly grated Parmesan

Bolognese Sauce (page 192)

1. Preheat the oven to 350°F.

2. Cook the pasta according to the package instructions.

3. Mix the mozzarella and Parmesan together in a small bowl.

4. Place 1 cup of the cooked pasta in a 1-cup ovenproof bowl. Top with ½ cup of the Bolognese Sauce and 3 tablespoons of the cheese mixture. Bake until the cheeses melt and are bubbling.

n   NUTRITION NOTE: *We make this delicious comfort food healthier by using a reasonable portion of pasta with just enough cheese and meat for flavor, and portion the recipe into six servings. Serving size matters.*

EACH SERVING CONTAINS

495 calories

67 g carbohydrate

10 g fat

39 mg cholesterol

31 g protein

650 mg sodium

4 g fiber

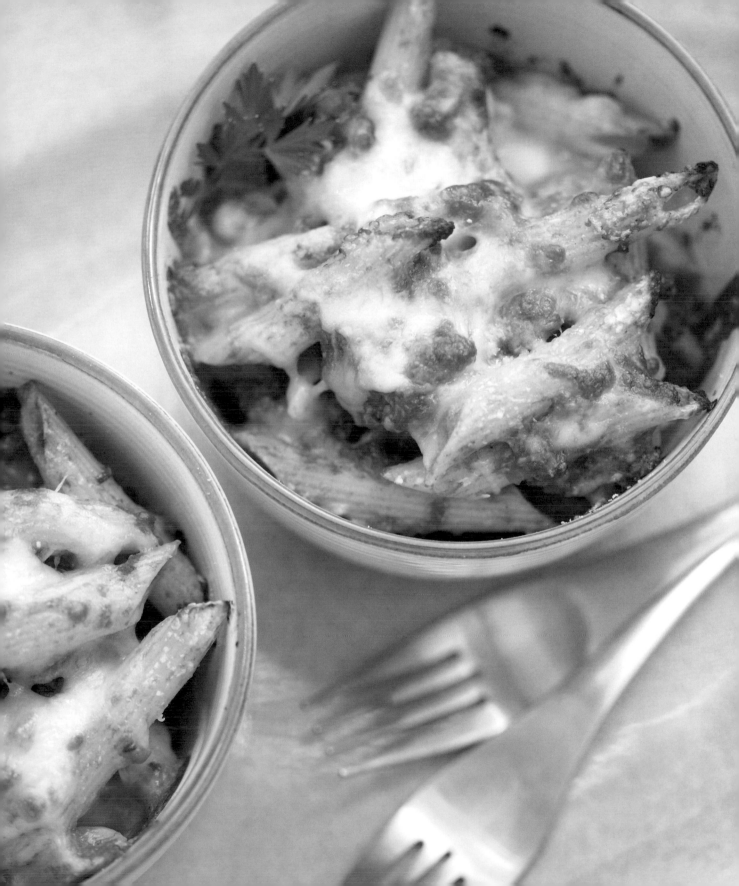

MOUSSAKA

This is wonderful served family style.

MAKES 9 SERVINGS   (SEE PHOTO ON PAGE 208.)

2 cups Béchamel
Sauce (page 175)

¼ cup egg yolks (4)

———————

2 tablespoons extra
virgin olive oil

1½ pounds lean
ground lamb

1 large yellow onion, diced

1½ teaspoons
minced garlic

1 teaspoon freshly
ground black pepper

Four 14½-ounce cans
(6 cups) diced tomatoes,
with their liquid

4 bay leaves

½ teaspoon whole cloves

2 cinnamon sticks

1 cup beef stock

1 teaspoon sea salt

1½ teaspoons cane sugar

3 medium eggplants
(about 4 pounds)

½ cup dried bread crumbs

½ teaspoon sea salt

½ pound feta, crumbled

1. Preheat the oven to 375ºF. Lightly coat a 9 x 13-inch baking pan with canola oil spray.

2. Remove the slightly warm Béchamel sauce from the heat and whisk in the egg yolks, mixing well. Set aside.

3. Heat 1 tablespoon of the olive oil in a large saucepan over medium heat. Brown the lamb, drain the fat, and remove from the pan. Add the remaining olive oil and sauté the onions and garlic until the onions are translucent. Return the meat to the pan and add the pepper. Sauté briefly. Add the tomatoes and simmer for 5 minutes.

4. Wrap the bay leaves, cloves, and cinnamon in cheesecloth and tie with thread or string to form a bouquet garni. Add to the lamb mixture along with the beef stock, salt, and cane sugar. Simmer until all the liquid has evaporated.

5. Pierce the eggplant skin with a fork and place on a baking sheet and roast for 30 minutes. Remove from the oven and cover with aluminum foil and let sit for 15 minutes. Uncover, cool, and peel. Slice the eggplant into ½-inch slices.

6. Spread the bread crumbs in the bottom of the baking pan. Layer half the eggplant slices over the bread crumbs and season with ¼ teaspoon of the salt. Top with the lamb sauce.

7. Layer the remaining eggplant over the sauce in the opposite direction and season with the remaining salt. Pour the cream sauce over the eggplant and top with feta.

9. Bake for 35 to 45 minutes, or until bubbly. Cut into 9 equal portions.

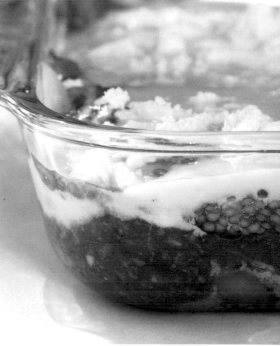 NUTRITION NOTE: *Lamb is a healthy red meat because it comes from animals fed on grass rather than grain and is higher in healthy omega-3 fats.*

EACH SERVING CONTAINS

325 calories

27 g carbohydrate

15 g fat

150 mg cholesterol

22 g protein

638 mg sodium

7 g fiber

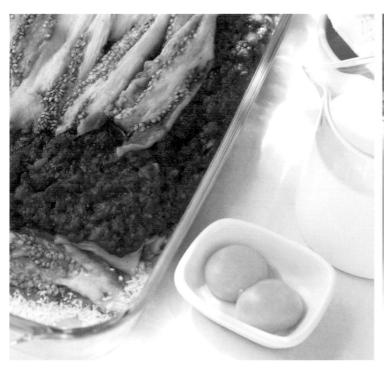

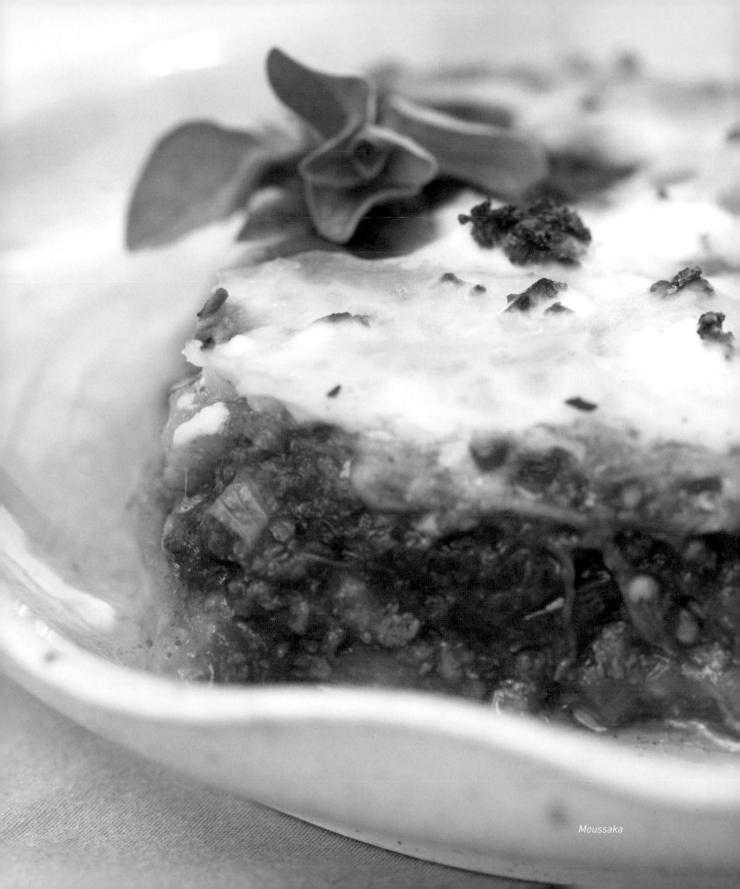

Moussaka

BEEF CANNELLONI

A light, fresh version of an Italian classic. This is great with a Rainbow Vegetable Salad (page 98).

MAKES SIX 2-CANNELLONI SERVINGS

Three 8 x 10-inch pasta sheets

1 cup Bolognese Sauce (page 192)

3 cups Fresh Marinara Sauce (page 172)

¾ cup shredded mozzarella (about 3 ounces)

1. Preheat the oven to 350°F. Lightly coat a 9 x 13-inch baking pan with canola oil spray.

2. Slice the pasta sheets into quarters. Spread ¼ cup Bolognese Sauce onto each pasta sheet quarter. Roll up each quarter and place seam side down in the baking pan. Spread the marinara sauce over the tops of the cannelloni rolls and sprinkle with mozzarella. Cover with aluminum foil.

3. Bake for 20 to 25 minutes, or until the cheese melts.

n NUTRITION NOTE: *One trick to making this dish more wholesome is using only half a pound of meat for the whole recipe of bolognese sauce. Another is careful portioning.*

c COOK'S NOTE: *Pasta sheets can be found frozen in Italian grocery stores or in the frozen foods section of your favorite supermarket.*

EACH SERVING CONTAINS

380 calories

46 g carbohydrate

12 g fat

63 mg cholesterol

22 g protein

739 mg sodium

5 g fiber

BAKED LASAGNE WITH MEAT SAUCE

Perfect for a party.

MAKES 8 SERVINGS

FOR THE MEAT SAUCE

1½ teaspoons extra virgin olive oil

¾ pound lean ground beef, drained

¾ cup chopped yellow onions

1 tablespoon minced garlic

2 teaspoons dried basil

1 teaspoon dried oregano

1 teaspoon ground fennel seed

2 tablespoons chopped fresh flat-leaf parsley

2 cups Fresh Marinara Sauce (page 172)

_____

2 cups fat-free ricotta

2 egg yolks

1 teaspoon garlic granules

1 teaspoon dried basil

½ teaspoon dried oregano

½ teaspoon sea salt

⅛ teaspoon freshly ground black pepper

3 cups Fresh Marinara Sauce (page 172)

1 8-ounce package oven-ready lasagna noodles

¾ cup freshly grated Parmesan

¾ cup shredded mozzarella

1. Preheat the oven to 350°F. Lightly coat a 9 x 13-inch baking pan with canola oil spray.

2. Heat ½ teaspoon of the olive oil in a large sauté pan over medium high heat and brown the beef until cooked through. Drain well.

3. Heat the remaining olive oil over medium heat in a large saucepan. Sauté the onions and garlic until the onions are translucent. Add the beef, basil, oregano, fennel seed, and parsley and sauté briefly. Add the marinara sauce and bring to a boil. Reduce the heat to low and simmer until the sauce thickens, about 15 minutes.

4. In a medium bowl, combine the ricotta, egg yolks, garlic, basil, oregano, salt, and pepper.

5. To assemble the lasagne, spread ½ cup marinara sauce on the bottom of the baking pan. Place 1½ lasagna noodles over the marinara. Add half the ricotta mixture, spreading the ricotta evenly over the noodles. Top with 1 cup meat sauce and sprinkle over ¼ cup Parmesan.

6. Repeat using 1½ noodles, ½ cup marinara sauce, 1 cup meat sauce. Sprinkle over ¼ cup mozzarella.

7. Top with another 1½ noodles, the remaining ricotta mixture, 1 cup meat sauce, and ¼ cup Parmesan.

8. Repeat using 1½ noodles, ½ cup marinara sauce, 1 cup meat sauce, and ¼ cup mozzarella.

9. Finally, top with the remaining lasagna noodle, ½ cup marinara sauce, ¼ cup mozzarella, and ¼ cup Parmesan. Cover with aluminum foil and bake for 45 to 50 minutes, until the cheeses brown. Cool slightly. Cut into 8 servings.

EACH SERVING CONTAINS

435 calories

46 g carbohydrate

13 g fat

144 mg cholesterol

37 g protein

749 mg sodium

4 g fiber

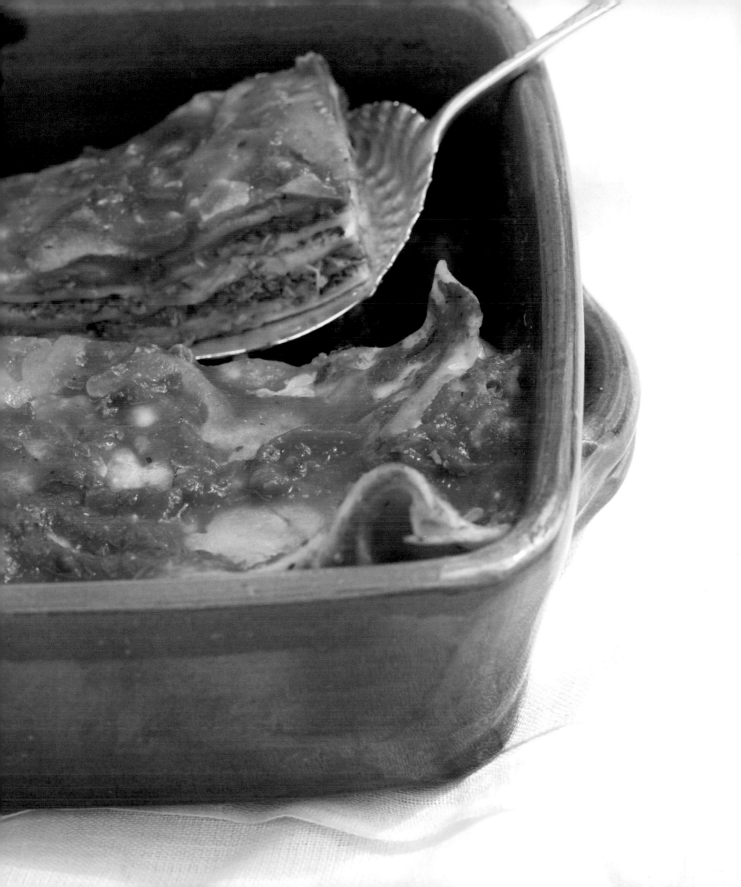

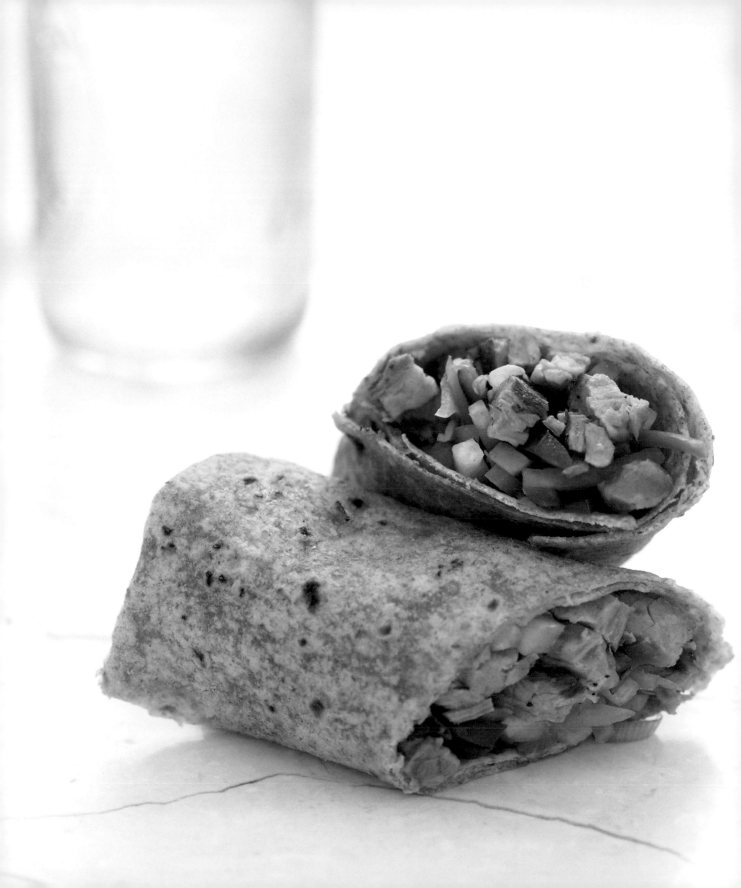

SPICY THAI BEEF WRAP

This is also terrific served over rice noodles.

MAKES 6 SERVINGS

1 pound beef flank steak

1 cup Mongolian BBQ Sauce (page 184)

FOR THE DRESSING

¼ cup fresh lime juice

1 tablespoon water

½ teaspoon low-sodium tamari sauce

2 teaspoons minced jalapeño peppers

3 tablespoons minced fresh cilantro

2 tablespoons minced fresh ginger

1 tablespoon fish sauce

½ teaspoon minced garlic

1 teaspoon sesame oil

⅛ teaspoon crushed red pepper flakes

1 teaspoon rice vinegar

2½ cups julienned vegetables of choice—bell peppers, red onions, snap peas

Six 10-inch whole wheat tortillas

1. Place the flank steak in a shallow glass baking dish. Pour the Mongolian BBQ sauce over the steak. Cover and refrigerate for at least 2 hours or overnight, turning the steak occasionally.

2. Combine the lime juice, water, tamari, jalapeños, cilantro, ginger, fish sauce, garlic, sesame oil, red pepper flakes, and vinegar in a small bowl. Whisk together and set aside. (Wear gloves when handling hot chile peppers, or wash your hands thoroughly before touching your eyes, nose, or mouth.)

3. Preheat the grill or broiler.

4. Remove the steak from the marinade and discard the marinade. Grill or broil the steak for 4 to 6 minutes on each side, or to the desired doneness. Slice thinly across the grain.

5. Toss the vegetables with the dressing.

6. Place the tortillas on a flat surface. Place about 2 ounces steak and evenly divided vegetables on each tortilla. Roll up burrito-style.

n NUTRITION NOTE: *Besides soothing the tummy, ginger contains potent antioxidants and antiinflammatory compounds. Add minced ginger to your tea after a meal for a nourishing and warming natural digestive.*

EACH SERVING CONTAINS

315 calories

34 g carbohydrate

12 g fat

26 mg cholesterol

19 g protein

710 mg sodium

4 g fiber

ZA'ATAR-CRUSTED LAMB CHOPS WITH POMEGRANATE MOLASSES

Serve with Soft Corn Polenta (page 115) and Roasted Fennel (page 99).

MAKES 4 SERVINGS

FOR THE ZA'ATAR
SPICE MIXTURE

¼ cup sesame seeds

3 tablespoons
sumac powder

2 tablespoons
dried oregano

1 tablespoon dried
marjoram

1½ teaspoons sea salt

1½ teaspoons ground
fennel seed

½ teaspoon cayenne

¼ teaspoon dried thyme

Four 4-ounce lamb chops

3 tablespoons
pomegranate molasses
or pomegranate syrup

1. Preheat the oven to 350°F.

2. Spread the sesame seeds evenly on a baking sheet and toast for about 5 minutes, or until golden. Cool completely.

3. Combine the sesame seeds, sumac powder, oregano, marjoram, salt, fennel, cayenne, and thyme in a clean coffee grinder or a mortar and pestle. Grind briefly. Do not overmix; mixture should be coarse.

4. Dust each chop with 2 teaspoons spice mixture.

5. Preheat the grill or broiler.

6. Grill or broil the lamb until cooked through, about 5 minutes per side.

7. Drizzle 2 teaspoons pomegranate molasses over each grilled lamb chop.

n NUTRITION NOTE: *We generally think of vegetables, fruit, tea, and chocolate as the main sources of antioxidants in our diets. But spices are rich in these healthful phytonutrients as well. Although very little is used in any given recipe, using these aromatic spices regularly can contribute to your intake of phytonutrients with their varied health benefits. As an example, fennel contains limonene, which has been studied for its anticancer benefits. Even the flavorful pomegranate molasses, made from pomegranate seeds, is rich in antioxidants.*

c COOK'S NOTE: *You can find sumac powder and pomegranate molasses at Middle Eastern specialty shops and online. Store any leftover za'atar spice mixture in an airtight container in a cool, dry place.*

EACH SERVING CONTAINS

280 calories

7 g carbohydrate

13 g fat

99 mg cholesterol

31 g protein

546 mg sodium

1 g fiber

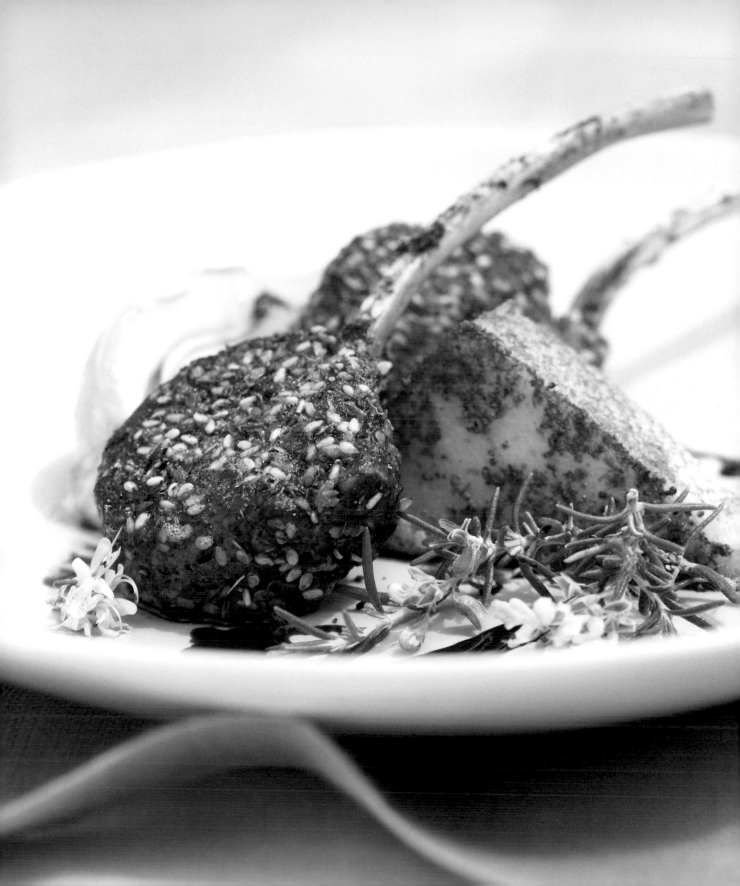

CHAPTER NINE | *Fish is fantastic, but even more than with most foods, awareness is key. It pays to know your fishmonger—and to know when he gets his shipments. Seafood must be fresh, sourced from reputable fishermen, and sustainably caught. Once you've done your homework, enjoy a variety of fish and shellfish two to three times a week.*

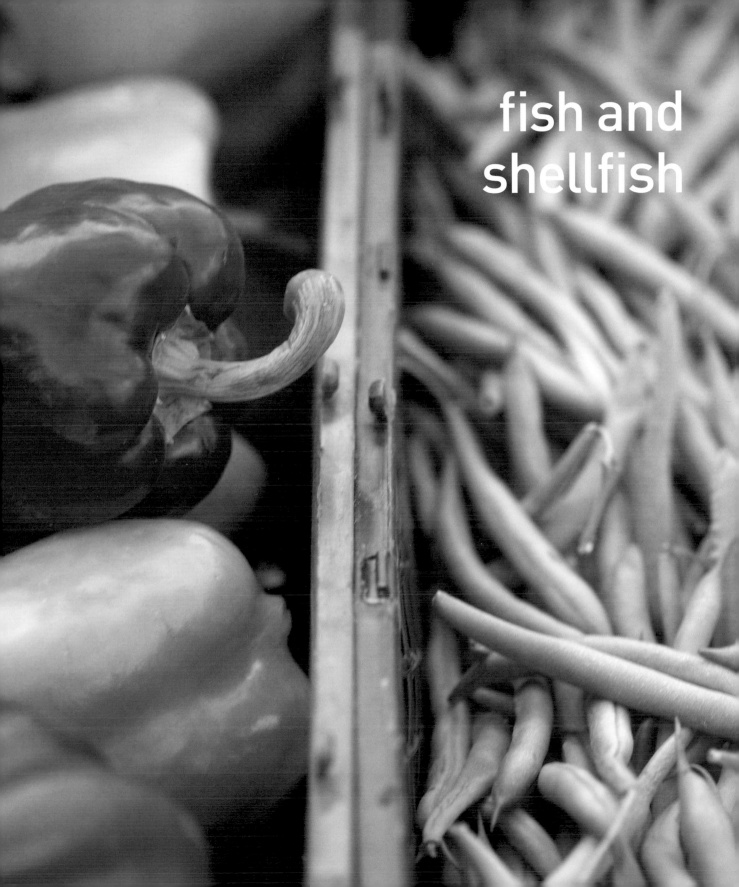

fish and
shellfish

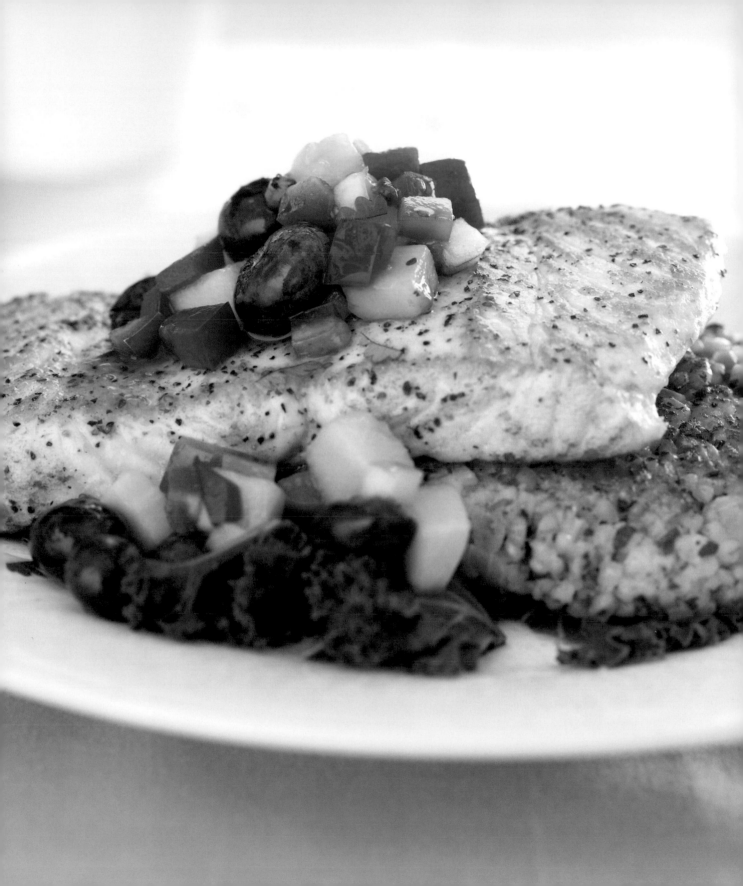

SALMON
WITH BLUEBERRY MANGO SALSA

Blueberries are rich in anthocyanins, which show potential for preventing glaucoma, heart disease, and cancer. Mangoes are rich in vitamins A and C and carotenoids. Salmon is a great source of disease-fighting omega-3 fatty acids. (We prefer wild-caught Pacific or organic farm-raised salmon.) In short, this dish delivers amazing nutritional value along with wonderful flavor. We serve it at our Superfoods Dinner alongside Sautéed Kale (page 100) and Oat Cakes (page 111).

MAKES 4 SERVINGS

FOR THE BLUEBERRY
MANGO SALSA

⅓ cup blueberries

⅓ cup peeled, diced mangoes

2 tablespoons minced
red onions

2 tablespoons minced
red bell peppers

1 tablespoon minced
fresh cilantro

1 tablespoon fresh lime juice

½ teaspoon minced
jalapeño peppers

2 teaspoons evaporated
cane juice

¼ teaspoon sea salt

_____

½ teaspoon extra
virgin olive oil

Four 4-ounce salmon fillets

Pinch sea salt

Pinch freshly ground
black pepper

1. Combine the blueberries, mangoes, onions, bell peppers, cilantro, lime juice, jalapeños, cane juice, and salt in a medium bowl. Lightly crush with a fork to release the juices. Set aside. (Wear gloves when handling hot chile peppers, or wash your hands thoroughly before touching your eyes, nose, or mouth.)

2. Heat the olive oil in a large sauté pan over medium-high heat. Season the salmon with salt and pepper and sear for 3 to 5 minutes on each side, or until just cooked through.

3. Serve each salmon fillet with ¼ cup blueberry mango salsa.

EACH SERVING CONTAINS

205 calories

6 g carbohydrate

11 g fat

54 mg cholesterol

19 g protein

216 mg sodium

1 g fiber

BROILED SALMON
WITH CUCUMBER LEMONGRASS SALSA

One of the recipes most frequently requested by Canyon Ranch guests.

MAKES 4 SERVINGS

Four 4-ounce salmon fillets

1 cup Mongolian BBQ
Sauce (page 184)

FOR THE CUCUMBER
LEMONGRASS SALSA

1 cup peeled, diced cucumbers

½ tablespoon finely minced
fresh lemongrass

½ tablespoon minced
fresh ginger

1 tablespoon chopped
fresh cilantro

½ tablespoon chopped
fresh mint

2 tablespoons fresh lime juice

⅛ teaspoon crushed
red pepper flakes

½ tablespoon low-
sodium tamari sauce

¼ teaspoon sea salt

½ teaspoon extra virgin olive oil

½ cup julienned carrots

¼ cup julienned red
bell peppers

¼ cup julienned yellow
bell peppers

⅛ teaspoon sea salt

Pinch freshly ground
black pepper

Coconut Black Rice (page107)

1. Place the salmon in a shallow glass baking dish. Pour the Mongolian BBQ sauce over the salmon and marinate for 30 minutes to 2 hours. Cover and refrigerate.

2. Combine the cucumbers, lemongrass, ginger, cilantro, mint, lime juice, red pepper flakes, tamari, and salt in a medium bowl and mix well. Set aside.

3. Preheat the broiler.

4. Remove the salmon from the marinade and discard the marinade. Broil the salmon fillets for 3 to 5 minutes on each side, or until cooked through. Cover and keep warm.

5. Heat the olive oil in a hot wok or sauté pan and stir-fry the carrots and peppers until tender-crisp. Season with the salt and pepper.

6. Serve each salmon fillet with ⅓ cup coconut black rice and ¼ cup vegetables. Top with ¼ cup cucumber lemongrass salsa.

n NUTRITION NOTE: *Only 5 percent of the population gets enough omega-3 fatty acid to have a beneficial effect on health. Regular consumption of salmon will ensure you're in that 5 percent.*

EACH SERVING CONTAINS

325 calories

27 g carbohydrate

13 g fat

56 mg cholesterol

22 g protein

596 mg sodium

3 g fiber

ORANGE-GLAZED SALMON
WITH SCREAMIN' GINGER SALSA

Vegetable Nori Rolls (page 86) are a nice starter with this.

MAKES 4 SERVINGS

FOR THE SCREAMIN' GINGER SALSA

¼ cup chopped crystallized ginger

1 tablespoon minced fresh ginger

2 tablespoons minced red bell peppers

1 tablespoon minced scallions

1 tablespoon minced fresh basil

¼ teaspoon low-sodium tamari sauce

⅓ cup frozen orange juice concentrate

¼ cup honey

¼ cup low-sodium tamari sauce

1 teaspoon five-spice powder

½ teaspoon minced garlic

Four 4-ounce salmon fillets

1. Preheat the grill or broiler.

2. Combine the crystallized ginger, fresh ginger, bell peppers, scallions, basil, and tamari in a medium bowl and mix well.

3. Combine the orange juice concentrate, honey, tamari, five-spice powder, and garlic in a medium bowl. Brush thoroughly over the salmon.

4. Grill or broil the salmon fillets for 3 to 5 minutes on each side.

5. Serve each salmon fillet with 2 tablespoons ginger salsa.

n NUTRITION NOTE: *This is truly food as medicine—omega-3 fat and ginger both fight inflammation.*

c COOK'S NOTE: *Five-spice powder, which is often used in Asian cuisines, consists of equal amounts of ground cinnamon, anise, cloves, fennel, and black pepper.*

EACH SERVING CONTAINS

350 calories

43 g carbohydrate

11 g fat

54 mg cholesterol

21 g protein

613 mg sodium

1 g fiber

SALMON EN CROUTE

This spectacular dish is actually very easy to make, and it's great for entertaining—once it's in the oven, you're done.

MAKES 4 SERVINGS

FOR THE CRUST

1 cup unbleached all-purpose flour

½ teaspoon sea salt

½ teaspoon cane sugar

2 tablespoons cold unsalted butter, cubed

4 to 6 tablespoons ice water

FOR THE CAPER SAUCE

2 teaspoons capers, rinsed and drained

1 tablespoon minced fresh chives

1¼ teaspoons chopped fresh dill

3 tablespoons plus 1 teaspoon nonfat sour cream

¼ teaspoon grated lemon zest

⅛ teaspoon sea salt

⅛ teaspoon freshly ground black pepper

¼ teaspoon Worcestershire sauce

(continued)

1. Preheat the oven to 375°F. Lightly spray a baking sheet with canola oil.

2. For the crust, combine the flour, salt, and cane sugar in a medium bowl and mix well. Cut the butter into the flour, using a pastry cutter, until the butter is the size of small peas. Add the water, 1 tablespoon at a time, mixing gently with a fork after each addition. The dough will begin to form a ball when enough water has been added. Gather the dough with dry hands and form into a ball. Let rest for 5 minutes.

3. Combine the capers, chives, dill, sour cream, lemon zest, salt, pepper, and Worcestershire in a medium bowl. Set aside.

4. Season the salmon with the salt and pepper. Spread with mustard.

5. On a lightly floured surface, roll out the dough into an 8 x 12-inch rectangle. Spread the shallots and spinach over the center of the pastry. Place the salmon mustard side down on top of the spinach, so that the mustard is in contact with the vegetables. Wrap the dough around the salmon, sealing the edges, then flip the pastry upside down so that the salmon is on the bottom and the vegetables are on top. Place on the baking sheet.

6. Beat the egg in a small bowl and brush over the top of the pastry. With a sharp knife, score the pastry evenly.

7. Bake for 20 minutes, or until golden brown.

8. Cut into four equal portions and serve each portion with 2 tablespoons caper sauce.

One 1-pound salmon
fillet, skin and
pinbones removed

⅛ teaspoon sea salt

⅛ teaspoon freshly
ground black pepper

2 tablespoons
Dijon mustard

2 tablespoons
minced shallots

⅔ cup spinach, washed

1 large egg

EACH SERVING CONTAINS

370 calories

26 g carbohydrate

17 g fat

78 mg cholesterol

26 g protein

691 mg sodium

4 g fiber

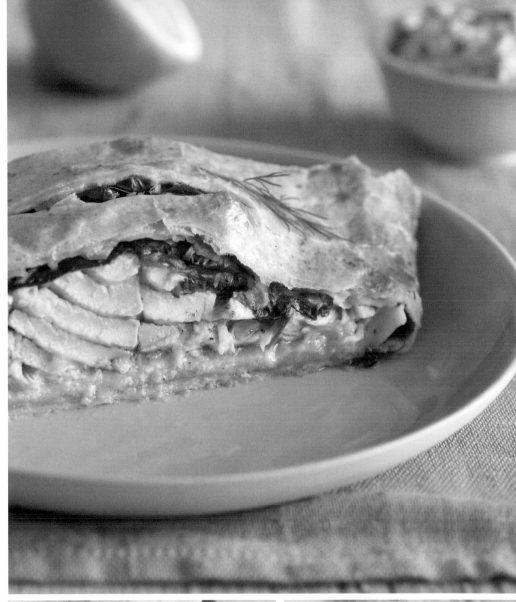

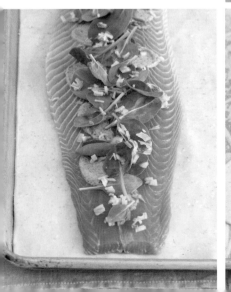

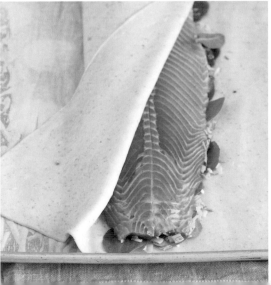

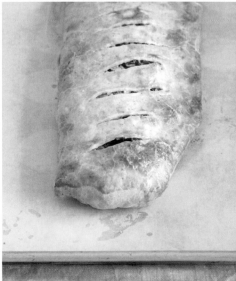

POACHED SALMON WRAP
WITH YOGURT DILL SAUCE

This works in a wrap or as a salad. Make extra.

MAKES 4 SERVINGS

Two 4-ounce salmon fillets

1 lemon, sliced

Pinch sea salt

Pinch freshly ground
black pepper

1 tablespoon capers,
rinsed and drained

2 tablespoons julienned daikons

½ cup peeled, diced cucumbers

½ cup diced jicama

FOR THE YOGURT DILL SAUCE

2 teaspoons chopped fresh dill

2 teaspoons canola
oil mayonnaise

2 tablespoons low-fat sour cream

2 tablespoons nonfat plain yogurt

2 teaspoons chopped scallions

1½ teaspoons whole
grain mustard

1 tablespoon distilled
white vinegar

1 teaspoon prepared horseradish

Pinch ground turmeric

Four 10-inch whole wheat tortillas

1. Bring water to a boil in a large saucepan that will accommodate a steamer basket.

2. Lightly spray a steamer basket with canola oil. Lay the salmon fillets in the basket, top with the lemon slices, and season with the salt and pepper.

3. Place the steamer basket in the saucepan and cook covered until opaque, about 8 minutes. Remove and discard the lemons. Allow the salmon to cool, then shred by hand.

4. Toss together the salmon, capers, daikons, cucumbers, and jicama in a medium bowl.

5. For the yogurt dill sauce, combine the dill, mayonnaise, sour cream, yogurt, scallions, mustard, vinegar, horseradish, and turmeric in a small bowl.

6. Place the tortillas on a flat surface. Place one-quarter salmon mixture on each tortilla and top each with 2 tablespoons yogurt dill sauce. Roll up burrito style.

C COOK'S NOTE: *Quite often, woks come as a set that includes a small steamer basket and wok cover.*

EACH SERVING CONTAINS

320 calories

34 g carbohydrate

14 g fat

30 mg cholesterol

15 g protein

411 mg sodium

5 g fiber

BAKED HADDOCK
WITH ZUCCHINI TOMATO SALAD

This is an ideal combination of flavors and textures. Fresh, juicy vegetables enhanced by herbs, simply prepared haddock, and the mild, comforting goodness of Macaroni and Cheese come together for a deeply satisfying meal.

MAKES 4 SERVINGS

FOR THE ZUCCHINI
TOMATO SALAD

1¼ cups diced zucchini

¾ cup diced tomatoes

1 teaspoon dried basil

¼ teaspoon dried oregano

¼ teaspoon sea salt

Pinch freshly ground
black pepper

1 teaspoon extra
virgin olive oil

2 tablespoons
unsalted butter

2 teaspoons fresh
lemon juice

1 tablespoon minced
fresh flat-leaf parsley

Pinch sea salt

Pinch freshly ground pepper

¾ cup toasted panko
bread crumbs

Four 4-ounce haddock fillets

Macaroni and Cheese
(page 110)

1. Preheat the oven to 375°F. Lightly spray a baking sheet with canola oil spray.

2. Combine the zucchini, tomatoes, basil, oregano, salt, and pepper in a medium bowl and toss together. Heat the olive oil in a sauté pan over medium-high heat. Add the zucchini mixture and sauté for 1 minute. Set aside.

3. Melt the butter in a small saucepan over low heat.

4. Combine the melted butter, lemon juice, parsley, salt, and pepper in a medium bowl and mix well. Add the bread crumbs and mix well.

5. Coat each haddock fillet with 3 tablespoons bread crumb mixture. Place the breaded fillets on the baking sheet and bake for 8 to 10 minutes, or until opaque at the center.

6. Serve each fillet with ⅓ cup zucchini tomato salad and one 4-ounce square macaroni and cheese.

n NUTRITION NOTE: *This is a good dish for summer, when young, tender zucchini and ripe tomatoes are available.*

c COOK'S NOTE: *Panko bread crumbs, which can be found in the Asian section of most supermarkets, stay crisp and crunchy during baking. Look for whole wheat panko crumbs.*

EACH SERVING CONTAINS

415 calories

36 g carbohydrate

15 g fat

101 mg cholesterol

33 g protein

643 mg sodium

3 g fiber

COD WITH OLIVE SALSA
AND ARTICHOKE FRITTERS

Serve with Roasted Fennel (page 99) alongside.

MAKES 4 SERVINGS

1 teaspoon extra
virgin olive oil

Four 4-ounce cod fillets

¼ teaspoon sea salt

¼ teaspoon freshly
ground black pepper

1⅓ cups Olive Salsa
(page 190)

4 Artichoke Fritters
(page 91)

1. Heat the olive oil a large sauté pan over medium-high heat. Season the cod fillets with the salt and pepper. Sauté the cod for 3 to 5 minutes on each side, or until opaque throughout.

2. Serve each cod fillet topped with ⅓ cup olive salsa and 1 artichoke fritter.

EACH SERVING CONTAINS

245 calories

15 g carbohydrate

6 g fat

67 mg cholesterol

32 g protein

684 mg sodium

4 g fiber

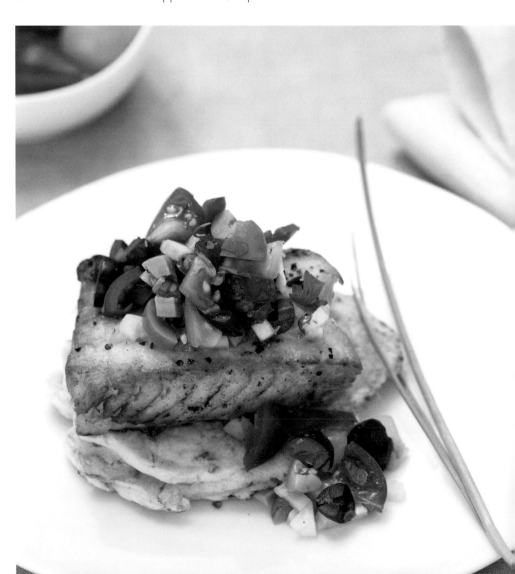

COD WITH CAULIFLOWER TOMATO BROTH

*The broth does double-duty as both sauce and
vegetable in this easily put together one-dish meal.*

MAKES 4 SERVINGS

FOR THE CAULIFLOWER
TOMATO BROTH

1 teaspoon extra virgin olive oil

⅓ cup diced yellow onions

1 teaspoon minced garlic

¾ cup diced cauliflower

One 14½-ounce can
whole tomatoes with
their liquid (1½ cups)

2 bay leaves

1 teaspoon chopped
fresh flat-leaf parsley

⅔ cup water

⅛ teaspoon lemon
zest, minced

¼ teaspoon sea salt

⅛ teaspoon freshly
ground black pepper

½ teaspoon cane sugar

½ teaspoon
Worcestershire sauce

—

Four 4-ounce cod fillets

½ teaspoon sea salt

½ teaspoon freshly
ground black pepper

2 teaspoons canola oil

FOR THE GARLIC BREAD

2 teaspoons extra
virgin olive oil

2 teaspoons minced garlic

Four 1-ounce slices
multigrain bread

2 tablespoons freshly
grated Parmesan

1. Heat the olive oil over medium heat in a large sauté pan. Sauté the onions, garlic, and cauliflower until the onions are translucent.

2. Crush tomatoes by hand in a medium bowl.

3. Add the tomatoes with their liquid to the sauté pan. Add the bay leaves and parsley, then the water, lemon zest, salt, pepper, cane sugar, and Worcestershire. Simmer for 20 to 25 minutes. Remove and discard the bay leaves.

4. Season the cod fillets with the salt and pepper. Heat the canola oil in a large sauté pan over medium heat. Sauté the cod for 3 to 5 minutes on each side, or until opaque throughout.

5. Preheat the broiler.

6. Combine the olive oil and garlic and brush on the bread. Sprinkle each slice with ½ tablespoon Parmesan. Broil until golden brown.

7. Divide the cauliflower tomato broth evenly among four bowls. Place a cod fillet in each bowl and serve with a slice of garlic bread.

EACH SERVING CONTAINS

260 calories

22 g carbohydrate

8 g fat

50 mg cholesterol

25 g protein

556 mg sodium

4 g fiber

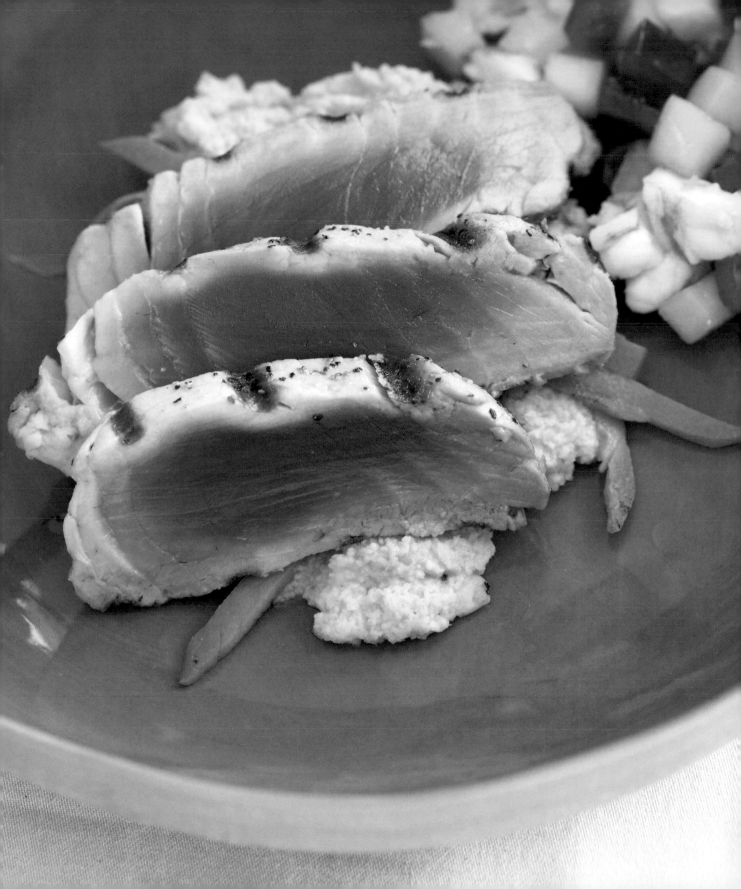

AHI TUNA WITH SHRIMP JICAMA SALSA

If you don't have shrimp on hand, just increase the mango and jicama in this wonderful fresh salsa.

MAKES 4 SERVINGS

FOR THE SHRIMP
JICAMA SALSA

½ cup cooked,
diced shrimp

¼ cup diced mangoes

¼ cup diced jicama

2 tablespoons minced
red bell peppers

1 tablespoon
minced scallions

2 tablespoons
fresh lime juice

1 tablespoon plus 1
teaspoon low-sodium
tamari sauce

Pinch crushed red pepper
flakes, or more to taste

¼ teaspoon sea salt

———

Four 4-ounce ahi
tuna fillets

1 teaspoon canola oil

1 cup julienned carrots

1. Preheat the oven to 350°F.

2. Combine the shrimp, mangoes, jicama, bell peppers, scallions, lime juice, tamari sauce, red pepper flakes, and salt in a large bowl and mix well. Set aside.

3. Preheat the grill or broiler.

4. Grill or broil the tuna fillets for 3 to 4 minutes on each side, or to desired doneness. Cover with aluminum foil and keep warm.

5. Heat the canola oil in a wok or sauté pan over high heat. Stir-fry the carrots until tender.

6. Serve each tuna fillet with ¼ cup stir-fried carrots and ¼ cup shrimp jicama salsa.

Serving suggestion: Mashed Sesame Soybeans (page 106)

n **NUTRITION NOTE:** *The tropical sunset colors in this recipe are signs of health benefits. The naturally occurring pigments of pink, red, orange, and yellow act as antioxidants. (We recommend eating fresh tuna no more often than once a week because of concerns about mercury. Pregnant women should avoid it.)*

EACH SERVING CONTAINS

205 calories

11 g carbohydrate

3 g fat

106 mg cholesterol

34 g protein

461 mg sodium

3 g fiber

RED CURRY-CRUSTED GROUPER WITH RAINBOW VEGETABLE SALAD

You can find red curry paste in the Asian foods section of most supermarkets: Choose a brand that's free of additives, colorings, and monosodium glutamate (MSG). Look for grouper caught off the Hawaiian Islands. It's sometimes sold as sea bass. Complement this delicious combination with a lavash cracker.

MAKES 4 SERVINGS

Four 4-ounce grouper fillets

2 teaspoons red curry paste

Rainbow Vegetable Salad (page 98)

1. Preheat the oven to 400°F.

2. Rub each fish fillet with ½ teaspoon red curry paste. Lightly coat a large sauté pan with canola oil spray. Sear the fish for 1 minute on each side over medium-high heat.

3. Transfer to a baking sheet and bake for 5 to 10 minutes, or until the fish is opaque at the center.

4. Serve each fish fillet with ⅓ cup rainbow vegetable salad.

EACH SERVING CONTAINS

160 calories

6 g carbohydrate

2 g fat

53 mg cholesterol

29 g protein

316 mg sodium

1 g fiber

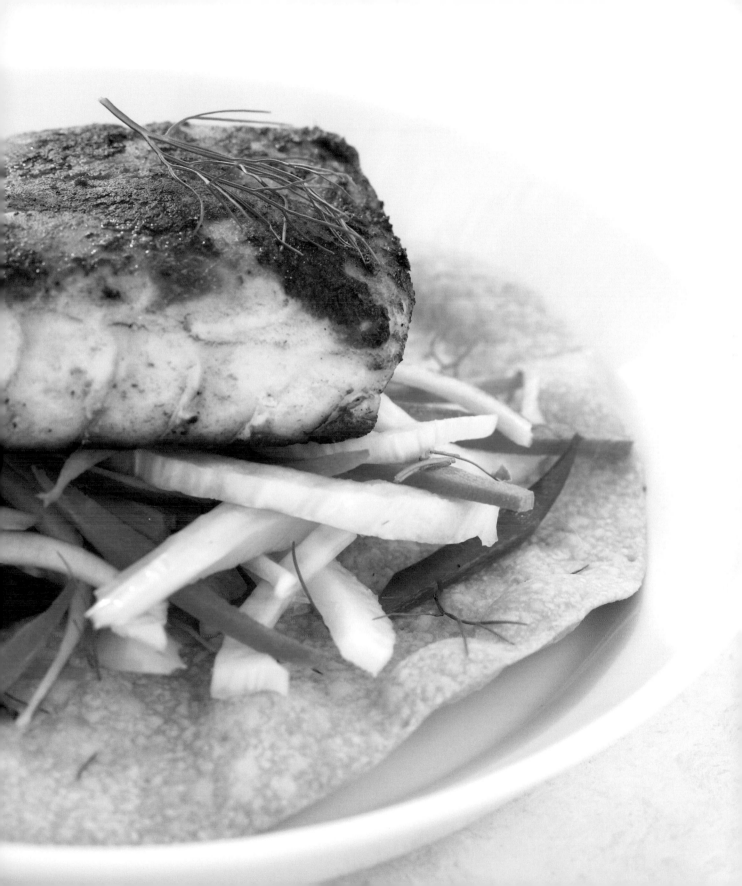

GROUPER WITH TOMATILLO SALSA

Tomatillos are small cousins of tomatoes, as their name suggests. Look for them in the produce sections of well-stocked markets, usually near the chiles.

MAKES 4 SERVINGS

FOR THE TOMATILLO SALSA

4 medium tomatillos, husks and stems removed

1 Roma tomato, diced

1½ teaspoons chopped fresh oregano

½ teaspoon minced jalapeño peppers

1½ teaspoons fresh lime juice

1½ teaspoons rice vinegar

¼ teaspoon sea salt

———

4 corn tortillas

1 tablespoon canola oil

Four 4-ounce grouper fillets

4 teaspoons Latin Spice Rub (page 187)

4 cups Southwest Green Cabbage Salad (page 102)

1. Preheat the oven to 375°F. Lightly coat a baking sheet with canola oil spray.

2. Place the tomatillos on the baking sheet and roast for 15 to 20 minutes, or until brown and soft. Cool completely. Coarsely chop.

3. Combine the tomatillos, tomatoes, oregano, jalapeños, lime juice, vinegar, and salt in a medium bowl. Set aside.

4. Preheat the grill.

5. Brush the tortillas with canola oil. Julienne. Spread the strips evenly on a baking sheet and bake until crispy, 5 to 10 minutes.

6. Rub each grouper fillet with 1 teaspoon spice rub. Grill for 3 to 5 minutes on each side, or until opaque throughout.

7. For each serving, place 1 cup Southwest green cabbage salad on a plate. Top with ¼ cup tomatillo salsa and a fish fillet. Sprinkle tortilla strips over the grouper.

n NUTRITION NOTE: *Grouper has at times been the subject of a heavy-metal advisory. A good substitute is mahi mahi, but you could choose any mild, firm-textured fish.*

EACH SERVING CONTAINS

275 calories

31 g carbohydrate

6 g fat

42 mg cholesterol

27 g protein

603 mg sodium

5 g fiber

SNAPPER WITH KUMQUAT VINAIGRETTE

Look for yellow snapper out of United States waters. Some snapper from other fisheries is not sustainable. Pair this dish with a side of seasonal baby vegetables.

MAKES 4 SERVINGS

2 corn tortillas, cut into thin strips

FOR THE KUMQUAT VINAIGRETTE

½ cup minced kumquat peel

2 tablespoons minced shallots

¼ cup rice vinegar

¼ cup water

2 teaspoons cane sugar

¼ teaspoon sea salt

¼ teaspoon freshly ground black pepper

¼ cup extra virgin olive oil

_____

Four 4-ounce yellow snapper fillets

½ teaspoon sea salt

½ teaspoon freshly ground black pepper

1 tablespoon plus 1 teaspoon whole fennel seed

2 teaspoons extra virgin olive oil

1. Preheat the oven to 400°F.

2. Brush the tortillas with canola oil. Julienne. Spread the strips evenly on a baking sheet and bake until crisp, 5 to 10 minutes.

3. Combine the kumquat peel, shallots, rice vinegar, water, cane sugar, salt, and pepper in a blender and puree for 10 seconds to combine. While the blender is running, slowly drizzle in the olive oil. (Refrigerate any left over vinaigrette in a tightly sealed glass container for about 1 week.)

4. Sprinkle the snapper with the salt and pepper. On each side of the fish, press in ½ teaspoon fennel seed. Heat a sauté pan to medium-high heat and add the olive oil. Sear the fish for 3 to 5 minutes on each side, or until opaque at the center.

5. Drizzle 1 tablespoon kumquat vinaigrette over each portion of snapper and top with tortilla strips.

n NUTRITION NOTE: *Some foods have a surprising natural sweetness and this recipe uses three of them. Corn tortillas, the peel of little kumquats, and fennel seed all have a sweetness you can appreciate if you haven't overloaded your taste buds with a regular diet of sugary foods.*

EACH SERVING CONTAINS

235 calories

9 g carbohydrate

8 g fat

53 mg cholesterol

31 g protein

330 mg sodium

2 g fiber

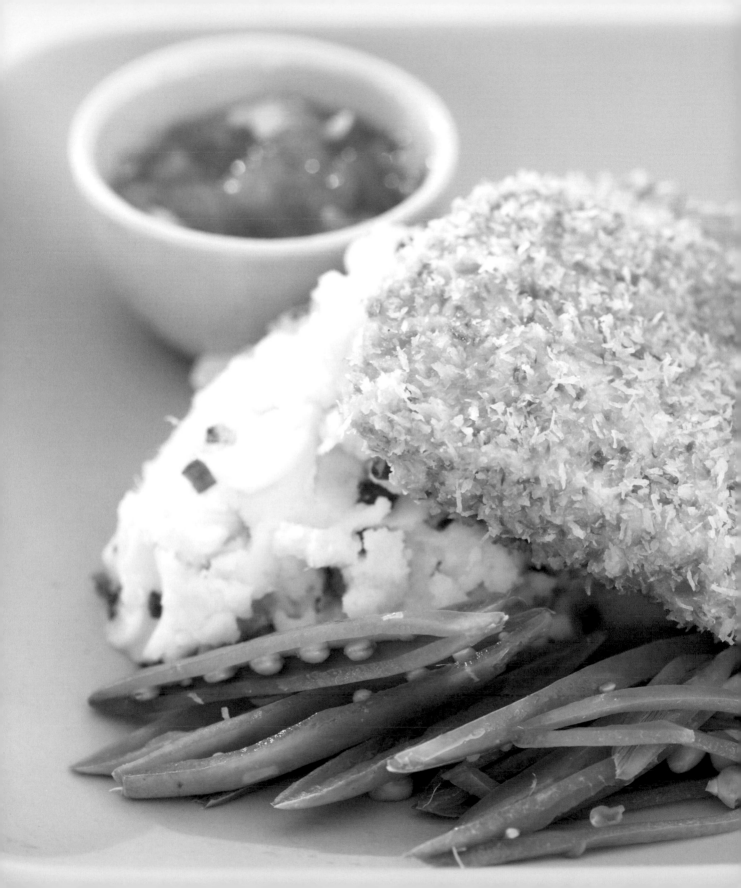

COCONUT-CRUSTED MAHI-MAHI WITH HORSERADISH ORANGE MARMALADE

This unusual flavor combination really works. It's delicious served with sautéed bok choy and Coconut Black Rice (page 107).

MAKES 4 SERVINGS

FOR THE HORSERADISH ORANGE MARMALADE

2 tablespoons cane sugar

2 tablespoons water

2 tablespoons distilled white vinegar

¼ cup diced orange slices, peel and membranes intact

2 teaspoons prepared horseradish

2 tablespoons unbleached all-purpose flour

½ teaspoon sea salt

½ teaspoon ground ginger

½ teaspoon freshly ground black pepper

1 large egg, beaten

½ cup toasted unsweetened coconut flakes

Four 4-ounce mahi-mahi fillets

1. Preheat the oven to 375°F. Lightly coat a baking dish with canola oil spray.

2. Bring the cane sugar, water, and vinegar to a boil in a small pan over medium-high heat. Add the orange and simmer until very thick and most of the liquid has been absorbed. Allow to cool. Fold in the horseradish. Set aside.

3. Mix together the flour, salt, ginger, and pepper in a small bowl. Put the egg and coconut in a bowl and dredge the mahi-mahi fillets in the flour mixture, then the egg, then the coconut. Place in the baking dish and bake for 8 to 10 minutes, or until cooked through.

4. Serve each fillet with 1 tablespoon horseradish orange marmalade.

n NUTRITION NOTE: *Choose organic oranges for this sauce because you are using the peel. Pesticide residues are harbored in citrus peels.*

EACH SERVING CONTAINS

210 calories

14 g carbohydrate

7 g fat

86 mg cholesterol

22 g protein

151 mg sodium

1 g fiber

WASABI-CRUSTED MAHI-MAHI WITH PONZU SAUCE

Dried wasabi-coated peas—a favorite Asian snack—can be purchased in the Asian foods section of well-stocked supermarkets and in specialty stores.

MAKES 4 SERVINGS

½ cup wasabi peas

Four 4-ounce mahi-mahi fillets

2 large eggs, beaten

1 teaspoon canola oil

1 cup julienned yellow bell peppers

1 cup julienned carrots

½ cup Ponzu Sauce (page 185)

2 cups cooked brown rice

1. Preheat the oven to 350°F.

2. Grind ¼ cup of the wasabi peas into a fine flour using a coffee grinder or spice grinder. Crush the remaining ¼ cup of the wasabi peas to make coarse crumbs. Dredge the mahi fillets in the wasabi flour, then the eggs, and then the wasabi crumbs.

3. Lightly coat a large sauté pan with canola oil spray. Heat over medium heat. Gently place the fish in the hot pan and cook until golden brown, about 2 minutes on each side.

4. Transfer to a baking pan and bake for 5 to 8 minutes, or until the fish is cooked through.

5. Heat the canola oil in a large sauté pan over medium heat. Sauté the bell peppers and carrots until tender.

6. Top each fillet with scant 2 tablespoons ponzu sauce. Serve with ½ cup stir-fried bell peppers and carrots and ½ cup brown rice.

n NUTRITION NOTE: *Use care when buying tilapia. Look for fish that has been farmed in the United States or Central America rather than Asia, where farming techniques are not as environmentally responsible.*

EACH SERVING CONTAINS

380 calories
42 g carbohydrate
7 g fat
213 mg cholesterol
36 g protein
577 mg sodium
2 g fiber

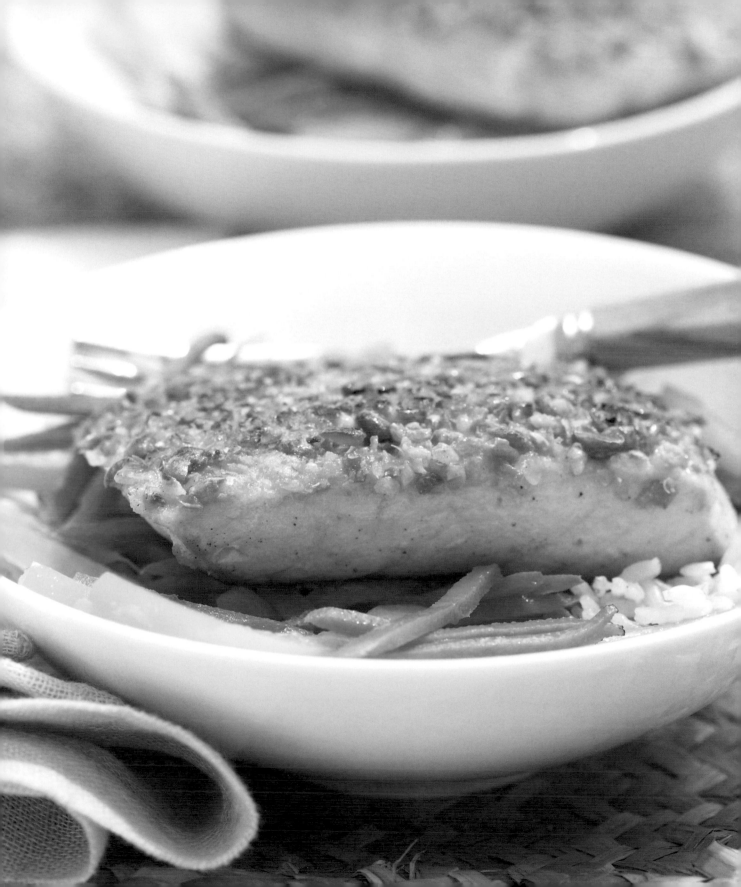

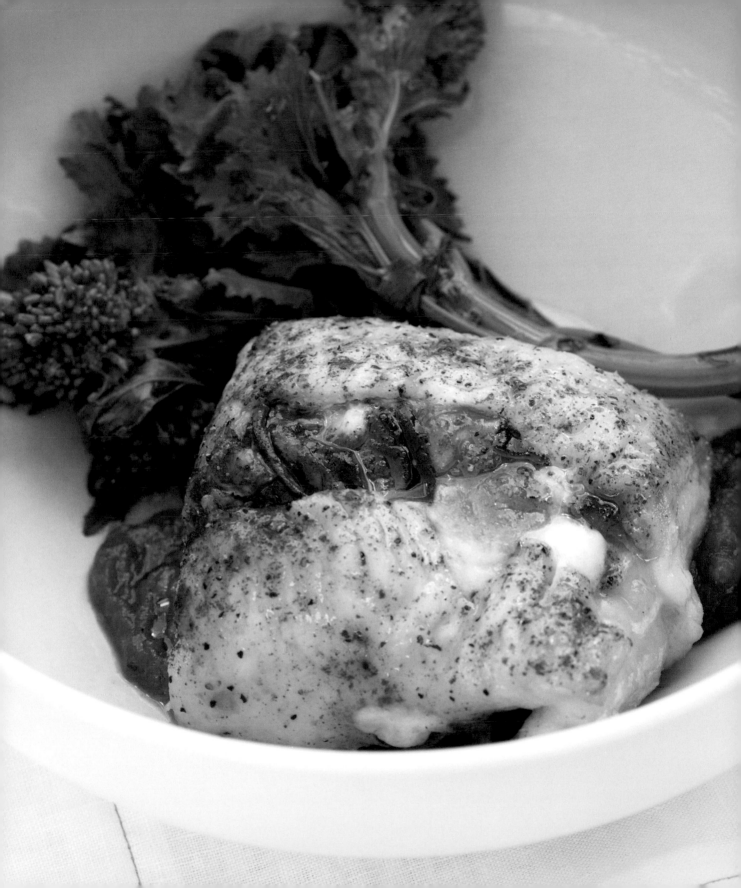

SOLE FLORENTINE

MAKES 6 SERVINGS

Six 4-ounce sole fillets

1 tablespoon extra virgin olive oil

1 medium yellow onion, diced

1 medium tomato, diced

5 cups spinach, washed

1 cup shredded mozzarella (about 4 ounces)

1 cup nonfat ricotta

½ teaspoon sea salt

3 cups cooked spaghetti

1½ cups Fresh Marinara Sauce (page 172)

3 cups Broccolini with Garlic and Olive Oil (page 94)

1.   Preheat the oven to 350°F. Lightly spray a baking sheet with canola oil.

2.   Place the sole fillets between two pieces of plastic wrap and tap lightly with a mallet until flat, about ¼ inch thick, being careful not to tear the fillets. Remove the plastic wrap and lay the fillets on the baking sheet.

3.   Heat the olive oil over medium-high heat in a medium sauté pan. Sauté the onions until translucent. Add the tomatoes and spinach. Cook until the spinach is wilted. Drain, if necessary. Cool completely. Fold in the mozzarella, ricotta, and salt.

4.   Place ¼ cup spinach mixture on each fillet. Roll up the fillets lengthwise and place on the baking sheet.

5.   Bake for 10 minutes, or until the fillet is opaque at the center and the cheese is melted.

6.   Serve each roll with ½ cup spaghetti, ¼ cup marinara sauce, and ½ cup Broccolini.

EACH SERVING CONTAINS

430 calories

42 g carbohydrate

15 g fat

67 mg cholesterol

34 g protein

705 mg sodium

7 g fiber

SOLE FRANÇAISE

An easy and delicious treatment for one of our favorite fish. Pasta, marinara sauce, and sautéed spinach round out the nutritional profile.

MAKES 4 SERVINGS

FOR THE BATTER

2 large eggs

2 tablespoons freshly grated Parmesan

3 tablespoons unbleached all-purpose flour

¼ teaspoon sea salt

⅛ teaspoon freshly ground black pepper

2 teaspoons minced fresh flat-leaf parsley

---

2 tablespoons unbleached all-purpose flour

Four 4-ounce sole fillets

1 tablespoon extra virgin olive oil

1⅓ cups cooked spaghetti

1 cup Fresh Marinara Sauce (page 172)

2 cups Sautéed Spinach and Garlic (page 101)

1. Combine the eggs and Parmesan in a medium bowl and mix well. Stir in the flour, 1 tablespoon at a time, until well combined. Whisk in the salt, pepper, and parsley.

2. Put flour in a shallow bowl, dredge the sole fillets in the flour, then dip in the batter. Let excess batter drip off.

3. Heat the olive oil in a large sauté pan over medium-high heat. Sauté the sole for 2 minutes on each side, or until golden brown.

4. Serve each sole fillet with ⅓ cup cooked spaghetti, ¼ cup marinara sauce, and ½ cup sautéed spinach. Garnish with fresh lemon wedges, if desired.

n NUTRITION NOTE: *Seafood Watch reports that Atlantic sole populations are dwindling and the floor trawling methods used to catch them are damaging the sea floor environment. They suggest you use sole exclusively wild caught in Pacific waters off Canada or the western United States.*

EACH SERVING CONTAINS

430 calories

40 g carbohydrate

13 g fat

193 mg cholesterol

37 g protein

714 mg sodium

5 g fiber

GRILLED MARINATED TROUT

Trout is one of the cold-water fish that's rich in omega-3 fatty acids.
Farmed trout is environmentally sustainable.

MAKES 4 SERVINGS

FOR THE MARINADE

1 tablespoon extra virgin olive oil

¼ cup diced shallots

2 tablespoons fresh lemon juice

¼ teaspoon sea salt

2 tablespoons minced fresh flat-leaf parsley

Four 4-ounce trout fillets

Horseradish Mashed Potatoes (page 105)

Chilled Green Bean Salad (page 93)

335 calories
28 g carbohydrate
14 g fat
61 mg cholesterol
25 g protein
504 mg sodium
6 g fiber

EACH SERVING CONTAINS

1. Combine the olive oil, shallots, lemon juice, salt, and parsley in a medium bowl.

2. Place the trout fillets in a shallow glass baking dish. Pour the marinade over the trout. Cover and refrigerate for 30 minutes to 2 hours, or overnight.

3. Preheat the grill.

4. Remove the trout from the marinade and discard the marinade. Grill the trout for 2 to 3 minutes on each side, or until cooked through.

5. Serve each fillet with about ½ cup of horseradish mashed potatoes and ¾ cup green bean salad.

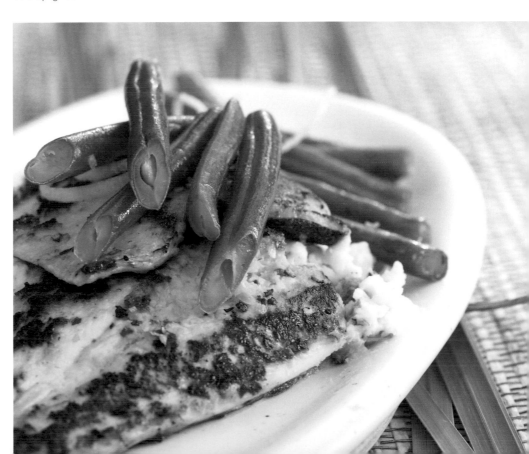

SCALLOPS WITH MASHED ARTICHOKES AND TOMATO CONFIT

One of our most-requested recipes. Frozen artichoke hearts make it a snap.

MAKES 6 SERVINGS

FOR THE TOMATO CONFIT

1 tablespoon extra virgin olive oil

1 medium yellow onion, diced

1 tablespoon minced garlic

4 medium tomatoes, peeled and diced

⅓ cup red wine

3 tablespoons chopped fresh flat-leaf parsley

½ teaspoon sea salt

¼ teaspoon freshly ground black pepper

FOR THE MASHED ARTICHOKES

1 pound frozen artichoke hearts or bottoms

¼ cup diced red onions

¼ cup freshly grated Parmesan

2 tablespoons fresh lemon juice

2 teaspoons extra virgin olive oil

¼ teaspoon sea salt

¼ teaspoon freshly ground black pepper

---

2 teaspoons extra virgin olive oil

1½ pounds scallops

1. Heat the olive oil over medium heat in a medium saucepan. Sauté the onions until translucent. Add the garlic and cook until soft. Add the tomatoes and cook briefly. Add the red wine and cook until almost dry. Add the parsley, salt, and pepper. Set aside.

2. Boil the artichokes in a large stockpot filled with water for 15 to 20 minutes, or until tender. Drain and place in a large mixing bowl.

3. Add the onions, Parmesan, lemon juice, olive oil, salt, and pepper. With an electric mixer on medium speed beat until well mashed and smooth.

4. Heat the olive oil in a large sauté pan over medium-high heat. Sear the scallops for 2 or 3 minutes on each side, or until golden brown. Do not overcook.

5. Serve 3 scallops with ½ cup mashed artichokes for each portion. Top each with 3 tablespoons tomato confit.

n   **NUTRITION NOTE:** *Artichokes are loaded with potassium, folic acid, and fiber. They have less carbohydrate than most vegetables you mash.*

EACH SERVING CONTAINS

235 calories

17 g carbohydrate

8 g fat

40 mg cholesterol

24 g protein

525 mg sodium

5 g fiber

SEARED SCALLOPS
WITH CRANBERRY GINGER VINAIGRETTE

We love cranberries for their tangy flavor, huge helping of vitamin C, and spectacular color.

MAKES 8 SERVINGS

FOR THE CRANBERRY GINGER VINAIGRETTE

½ cup fresh or frozen cranberries, thawed

½ teaspoon minced fresh ginger

2 tablespoons diced shallots

⅓ cup apple cider

1 tablespoon plus 1 teaspoon cane sugar

2 teaspoons canola oil

2 teaspoons extra virgin olive oil

———

2 tablespoons extra virgin olive oil

2 pounds scallops

Pinch sea salt

Pinch freshly ground black pepper

4 cups Sautéed Spinach and Garlic (page 101)

4 cups Parsnip Carrot Puree (page 97)

1. Combine the cranberries, ginger, shallots, apple cider, cane sugar, canola oil, and olive oil in a blender and puree until smooth.

2. Heat the olive oil over medium-high heat in a large sauté pan. Season the scallops with salt and pepper, then sear the scallops for 2 to 3 minutes on each side, until golden. Do not overcook.

3. Divide the scallops evenly among eight plates. Serve each portion with 2 tablespoons cranberry ginger vinaigrette, ½ cup sautéed spinach and ½ cup parsnip carrot puree.

EACH SERVING CONTAINS

295 calories

23 g carbohydrate

13 g fat

47 mg cholesterol

23 g protein

641 mg sodium

6 g fiber

CRAB SOUFFLÉS
WITH CARAMELIZED CARROT SAUCE

Cooked carrots are actually more nutritious than raw ones—heat helps release beta-carotene, the antioxidant compound that gives them their brilliant color.

MAKES 8 SERVINGS

½ cup egg yolks
(about 6 large yolks)

2 tablespoons fresh lemon juice

1 teaspoon Old Bay Seasoning

2 teaspoons Dijon mustard

1 teaspoon Worcestershire sauce

¼ cup unbleached
all-purpose flour

14 ounces fresh or canned
lump crabmeat, well drained

1 tablespoon chopped fresh chives

½ cup egg whites
(about 4 large whites)

1 teaspoon cream of tartar

FOR THE CARAMELIZED
CARROT SAUCE

½ teaspoon extra virgin olive oil

2 cups chopped carrots

1 cup diced yellow onions

1 tablespoon cane sugar

1 tablespoon apple cider vinegar

½ teaspoon sea salt

⅛ teaspoon freshly
ground black pepper

1¾ cups chicken stock

1. Preheat the oven to 350°F. Lightly spray eight 4-ounce individual ramekins or soufflé dishes with canola oil spray and dust with flour.

2. With an electric mixer with a whisk attachment, whip the yolks, lemon juice, Old Bay Seasoning, mustard, and Worcestershire at high speed until slightly thickened and lemon yellow in color. Reduce the mixer speed and beat in the flour until well combined.

3. Squeeze all the liquid out of the crabmeat. Fold the crabmeat and chives into the egg yolk mixture.

4. Whisk the egg whites and cream of tartar in a small bowl until soft peaks form. Fold the egg whites into the crabmeat mixture.

5. Place ½ cup crabmeat mixture in each ramekin. Bake for 15 to 20 minutes, or until firm to the touch.

6. Heat a medium saucepan over low heat. Add the olive oil, carrots, onions, cane sugar, vinegar, salt, and pepper. Caramelize the onion mixture for 20 to 30 minutes. Add the chicken stock and bring to a boil. Reduce to a simmer and cook for 5 to 10 minutes, or until slightly reduced.

7. Serve ⅓ cup carrot sauce with each soufflé.

C COOK'S NOTE: *Add more chicken stock to the carrot sauce if it is too thick.*

EACH SERVING CONTAINS

205 calories

15 g carbohydrate

7 g fat

303 mg cholesterol

19 g protein

512 mg sodium

2 g fiber

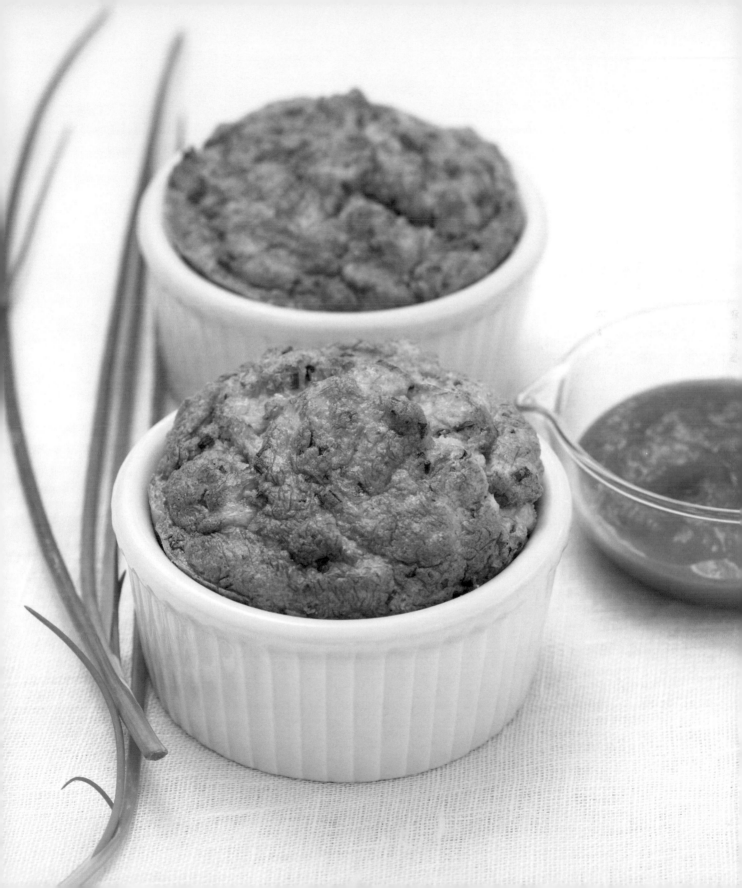

CRAB AND POBLANO QUESADILLA

The mild, dark green poblano chile—which you may know as the foundation of chiles rellenos—is to Mexican cuisine what the bell pepper is to European cooking, but poblanos have much more flavor and bite. The darkest poblanos are the tastiest. This quesadilla goes great with our Southwest Green Cabbage Salad (page 102).

MAKES 4 SERVINGS

8 ounces lump crabmeat, well drained

½ cup roasted, peeled, seeded, and diced poblano pepper

¼ cup minced fresh cilantro

2 tablespoons fresh lime juice

¼ teaspoon sea salt

4 ounces goat cheese, divided into 4 equal portions

Four 10-inch whole wheat tortillas

1. Combine the crabmeat, poblanos, cilantro, lime juice, and salt in a medium bowl.

2. Spread one portion goat cheese down half of each tortilla. Evenly divide the crab mixture into four portions and spread over the cheese.

3. Fold the tortilla in half and place it on a griddle pan. Cook, turning once, until the tortillas are slightly crisp. Cut each quesadilla into quarters.

320 calories

31 g carbohydrate

13 g fat

57 mg cholesterol

21 g protein

627 mg sodium

3 g fiber

EACH SERVING CONTAINS

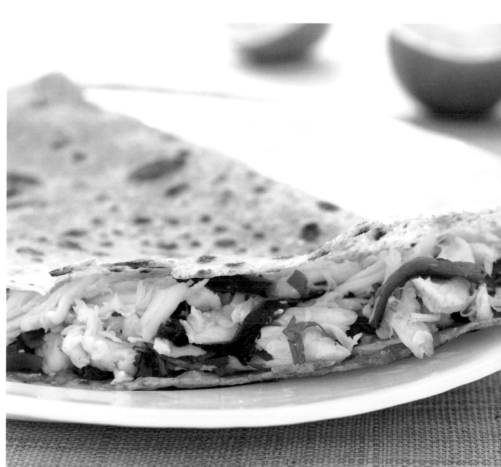

CHILI-RUBBED TEQUILA SHRIMP

Ten minutes from start to finish. We like these tangy,
fiery shrimp alongside Pomegranate Couscous (page 112)
and Southwest Green Cabbage Salad (page 102).

MAKES 4 SERVINGS

¼ teaspoon sea salt

¼ teaspoon crushed
red pepper flakes

½ teaspoon chili powder

¼ teaspoon ground cumin

¼ teaspoon freshly
ground black pepper

1 teaspoon water

1 pound large shrimp
(about 16 shrimp),
peeled and deveined

1 teaspoon canola oil

2 teaspoons minced garlic

¼ cup tequila

2 tablespoons minced
fresh cilantro

1 tablespoon fresh
lime juice

1. Combine the salt, red pepper flakes, chili powder, cumin, pepper, and water in a small bowl and form a paste. Rub the shrimp with the paste until well coated.

2. Heat a large sauté pan over medium-high heat. Add the oil and sear the shrimp for 1 minute per side. Add the garlic and sauté for 1 minute.

3. Remove from the heat and add the tequila, cilantro, and lime juice. Return to the heat. (Be careful: Tequila may flame.) Sauté for 1 minute, or until opaque at the center. Do not overcook.

EACH SERVING CONTAINS

170 calories

1 g carbohydrate

3 g fat

221 mg cholesterol

24 g protein

375 mg sodium

Trace fiber

GREEN CURRY SHRIMP WRAP

MAKES 6 SERVINGS

6 tablespoons Green Curry Paste (page 186)

1½ pounds medium shrimp (about 24 shrimp), peeled and deveined

¾ cup diced fresh tomatoes

¼ cup julienned jicama

¼ cup julienned carrots

FOR THE YOGURT CURRY SAUCE

½ cup nonfat plain yogurt

2 tablespoons Green Curry Paste (page 186)

¼ cup chopped tomatoes

¼ cup peeled, diced cucumbers

1 tablespoon minced red onions

⅛ teaspoon sea salt

———————

Six 10-inch whole wheat tortillas

1½ cups shredded romaine lettuce

1. Heat a large sauté pan over medium heat. Add the curry paste and sauté the shrimp until just pink. Keep warm.

2. Toss together the tomatoes, jicama, and carrots in a small bowl.

3. Combine the yogurt, curry paste, tomatoes, cucumbers, onions, and salt in a small bowl.

4. Lay the tortillas on a flat surface. Place 4 shrimp, 2 tablespoons tomato mixture, and ¼ cup shredded lettuce on each. Top with 3 tablespoons yogurt curry sauce. Roll up burrito style.

EACH SERVING CONTAINS

300 calories

34 g carbohydrate

5 g fat

173 mg cholesterol

29 g protein

632 mg sodium

3 g fiber

SHRIMP COCKTAIL WRAP

A favorite appetizer becomes a meal to go. Look for shrimp farmed in the United States or caught wild in the Gulf of Mexico.

MAKES 5 SERVINGS

½ pound cooked medium shrimp (about 10 shrimp), peeled and deveined, tails removed

½ cup peeled, diced cucumbers

2 tablespoons diced red onions

½ cup diced tomatoes

½ cup chopped romaine lettuce

FOR THE COCKTAIL SAUCE

½ cup ketchup

1 tablespoon prepared horseradish

1 teaspoon Worcestershire sauce

1 teaspoon Tabasco

1 teaspoon fresh lime juice

Five 10-inch whole wheat tortillas

1. Combine the shrimp, cucumbers, onions, tomatoes, and lettuce in a large bowl.

2. Combine the ketchup, horseradish, Worcestershire, Tabasco, and lime juice in a small bowl and mix well.

3. Place the tortillas on a flat surface. Spread 2 tablespoons cocktail sauce on each tortilla. Place ½ cup shrimp mixture on each. Roll up burrito style.

EACH SERVING CONTAINS

270 calories

37 g carbohydrate

7 g fat

69 mg cholesterol

14 g protein

701 mg sodium

3 g fiber

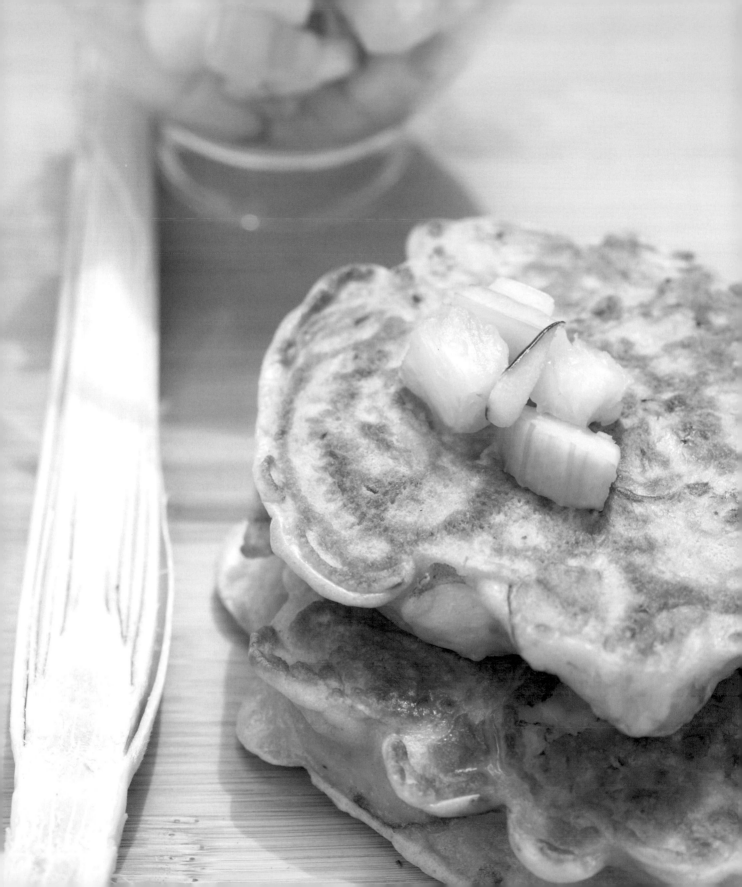

SHRIMP FRITTERS
WITH CUCUMBER PINEAPPLE SALAD

Fritters are appealing little fried cakes. We cook them in a tiny amount of healthy oil to reduce fat and calories. They're fun to make and taste terrific.

MAKES 4 SERVINGS

FOR THE CUCUMBER PINEAPPLE SALAD

2 tablespoons rice vinegar

Pinch sea salt

1 tablespoon cane sugar

1 tablespoon grated fresh ginger

1 teaspoon finely minced fresh lemongrass

1 cup diced pineapple

1 cup peeled, diced cucumber

¼ cup diced red onions

_____

½ cup lightly packed chopped scallions

2 teaspoons water

1 tablespoon plus 1 teaspoon low-sodium tamari sauce

¼ teaspoon crushed red pepper flakes

2 large eggs, beaten

1 pound well-drained raw shrimp (about 16 shrimp), peeled and deveined, tails removed

¾ cup whole wheat flour

½ teaspoon aluminum-free baking powder

1. Whisk the rice vinegar, salt, cane sugar, ginger, and lemongrass together in a medium bowl. Add the pineapple, cucumber, and onions and toss until well combined. Set aside.

2. Whisk the scallions, water, tamari, red pepper flakes, and eggs in a large bowl.

3. Cut the shrimp into thirds and stir into the egg mixture.

4. Combine the flour and baking powder in a small bowl. Slowly stir the flour mixture into the shrimp mixture, stirring constantly until the mixture reaches the consistency of thick pancake batter.

5. Heat a large sauté pan over medium heat and lightly spray with canola oil spray. Using a ⅓-cup measure for each fritter, pour the batter into the pan. Sauté the fritters for 3 to 5 minutes on each side, or until golden brown and crispy and the shrimp is cooked through.

6. Serve 2 fritters with ½ cup cucumber pineapple salad for each serving.

> **n** NUTRITION NOTE: *Most fritters are deep-fried, but these are cooked perfectly using only a spray of canola oil.*

EACH SERVING CONTAINS

245 calories

20 g carbohydrate

5 g fat

278 mg cholesterol

29 g protein

698 mg sodium

3 g fiber

SHRIMP SALAD SANDWICH

MAKES 4 SERVINGS

FOR THE DRESSING

2 tablespoons prepared horseradish, drained

2 tablespoons canola oil mayonnaise

2 tablespoons ketchup

¼ teaspoon Worcestershire sauce

⅛ teaspoon sea salt

⅛ teaspoon freshly ground black pepper

1 tablespoon chopped fresh chives

1 tablespoon fresh lemon juice

¾ pound cooked medium shrimp (about 12 shrimp), peeled and deveined

2 tablespoons minced red onions

½ cup diced celery

½ cup grape or cherry tomatoes, quartered

8 slices whole grain bread

1. Combine the horseradish, mayonnaise, ketchup, Worcestershire, salt, pepper, chives, and lemon juice in a small bowl. Set aside.

2. Dice the shrimp into 1-inch pieces.

3. Combine the shrimp, onions, celery, tomatoes, and dressing in a medium bowl and toss together.

4. Serve ¾ cup shrimp salad between 2 slices of bread.

n **NUTRITION NOTE:** *Dressing this shrimp salad with a remoulade-type sauce rather than mayonnaise alone and adding the fresh vegetables makes it more wholesome. Horseradish, an essential part of the dressing, is well known in botanical medicine for its potency against a variety of health problems.*

EACH SERVING CONTAINS

345 calories

39 g carbohydrate

10 g fat

132 mg cholesterol

25 g protein

446 mg sodium

6 g fiber

TUNA MELT WITH MUSTARD SAUCE

*When buying canned tuna, look for light tuna instead of white—
it's lower in mercury. Serve this classic sandwich alongside
Italian Vegetable Soup with Cannellini Beans (page 129).*

MAKES 4 SERVINGS

One 6-ounce can water-
packed light tuna, drained

2 tablespoons minced
red bell peppers

2 tablespoons minced
yellow bell peppers

2 tablespoons sweet
pickle relish

2 tablespoons minced celery

2 tablespoons canola
oil mayonnaise

½ teaspoon Dijon mustard

Pinch sea salt

Pinch freshly ground
black pepper

FOR THE MUSTARD SAUCE

1 tablespoon whole
grain mustard

1 tablespoon Dijon mustard

1 teaspoon honey

½ teaspoon Colman's
dry mustard

2 tablespoons plain
lowfat yogurt

4 slices rye bread

Four 1-ounce slices Swiss

1. Preheat the broiler.

2. Combine the tuna, red bell peppers, yellow bell peppers, pickle relish, celery, mayonnaise, mustard, salt, and pepper in a medium bowl and mix well.

3. Combine the whole grain mustard, Dijon mustard, honey, dry mustard, and yogurt in a small bowl or cup.

4. Spread ⅓ cup tuna salad on each slice of bread. Top with a slice of Swiss. Repeat with the remaining ingredients.

5. Place the sandwiches under the broiler for 1 to 2 minutes, or until the cheese melts.

6. Serve each sandwich with 1 tablespoon mustard sauce.

C COOK'S NOTE: *Tuna salad makes a great wrap filling.*

EACH SERVING CONTAINS

325 calories

28 g carbohydrate

12 g fat

17 mg cholesterol

24 g protein

663 mg sodium

2 g fiber

CHAPTER TEN | *Chicken and turkey are lean and wonderfully versatile meats—as the wide range of treatments here illustrates— but not all chickens are created equal. While we exclusively use organic chicken, there are other options like cage-free, vegetarian- fed chicken, and turkey from your local farmers' market, which, besides being better for you, are closer in taste and texture to the healthy, flavorful farmyard birds that our grandparents enjoyed. When selecting cooked chicken and turkey breast and sausages, look for reduced sodium, and nitrite- and nitrate-free products. More varieties are available all the time.*

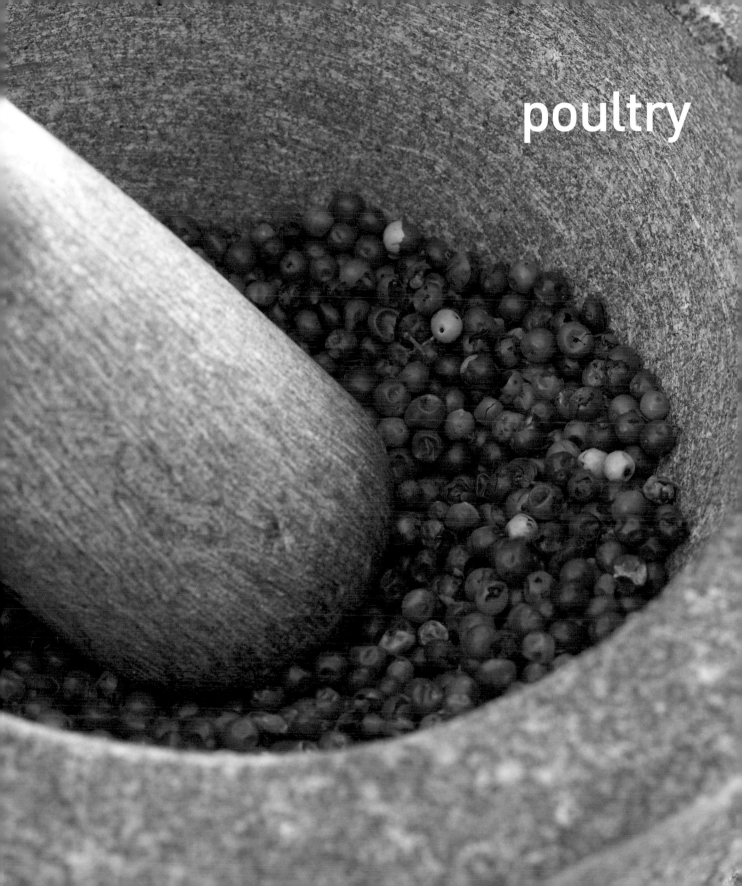

poultry

PEPPERED CHICKEN MEDALLIONS WITH MUSHROOMS

A company-pleasing variation on a calorie-laden classic. It's terrific with our Potato Medley (page 113) and grilled or roasted zucchini.

MAKES 4 SERVINGS

FOR THE PEPPER SAUCE

1 teaspoon dried
green peppercorns

1 tablespoon white wine

1 teaspoon extra
virgin olive oil

2 tablespoons
minced shallots

¼ cup dry sherry

⅔ cup beef stock

2 teaspoons Dijon mustard

1 tablespoon plus 1
teaspoon heavy cream

———

Four 4-ounce boneless,
skinless chicken
breast halves

½ teaspoon sea salt

1 teaspoon freshly
ground black pepper

1 tablespoon extra
virgin olive oil

1 cup fresh crimini
mushrooms or seasonal
wild mushrooms

1⅓ cups chicken stock

1. Combine the peppercorns and white wine in a small sauté pan. Cook over low heat until the wine has evaporated. Cool the peppercorns and coarsely chop in a coffee or spice grinder. (If using jarred green peppercorns, skip the cooking step and simply chop.)

2. Heat the olive oil over low heat in a large sauté pan. Cook the shallots until slightly browned. Add the peppercorns and the sherry. Simmer for 1 minute.

3. Add the beef stock and bring to a boil. Reduce the heat and whisk in the mustard. Remove from the heat and whisk in the cream. Set aside.

4. Cut the chicken breasts in half to form medallions. Pound with a meat mallet until ¼ inch thick. Season with the salt and pepper.

5. Heat the olive oil in a large sauté pan over medium heat. Sauté the chicken medallions until golden brown on one side. Turn the chicken and add the mushrooms. Sauté briefly. Add the chicken stock and cook until the internal temperature of the chicken reaches 165°F. Stir in the pepper sauce and cook until slightly thickened.

6. Serve 2 chicken medallions with ¼ cup pepper sauce.

n   NUTRITION NOTE: *Did you know chicken is a major source of vitamin K thanks to the vitamins added to chickens' diets? K is linked to protection against cardiovascular disease, osteoporosis, and prostate cancer.*

EACH SERVING CONTAINS

265 calories

6 g carbohydrate

12 g fat

79 mg cholesterol

30 g protein

340 mg sodium

Trace fiber

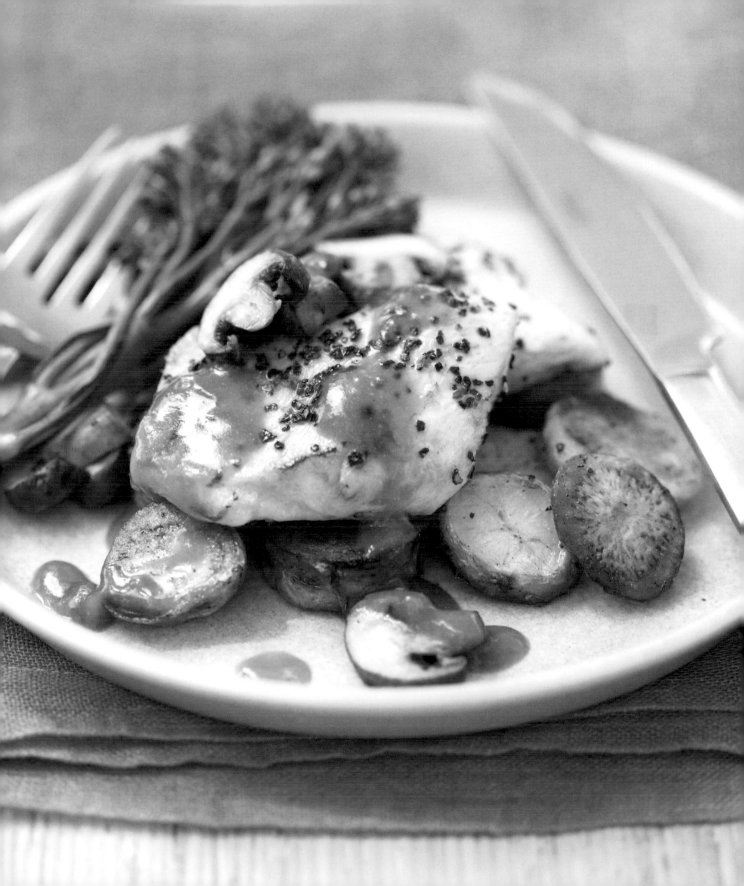

HONEY BALSAMIC–GLAZED CHICKEN

This tangy sweet-and-sour glaze showcases the culinary magic of balsamic vinegar. The dish pairs up beautifully with Broccolini with Garlic and Olive Oil (page 94) and Soft Corn Polenta (page 115).

MAKES 4 SERVINGS

FOR THE HONEY BALSAMIC GLAZE

3 tablespoons white balsamic vinegar

2 tablespoons honey

¼ cup chicken stock

Four 4-ounce boneless, skinless chicken breast halves

½ teaspoon sea salt

½ teaspoon freshly ground black pepper

1½ tablespoons unbleached all-purpose flour

1. Mix together the vinegar, honey, and chicken stock in a small bowl. Set aside.

2. Pound each chicken breast with a meat mallet until ¼ inch thick. Season with the salt and pepper.

3. Spread the flour on a small plate. Dredge the chicken in the flour.

4. Lightly coat a large sauté pan with canola oil spray. Sear the chicken breasts on each side over medium-high heat.

5. Deglaze the pan with the glaze. Reduce the heat to medium-low. Continue to cook the chicken until the internal temperature reaches 165°F, about 3 to 5 minutes total.

EACH SERVING CONTAINS

185 calories

11 g carbohydrate

3 g fat

73 mg cholesterol

27 g protein

185 mg sodium

Trace fiber

CHICKEN WITH ORANGE MARMALADE

A favorite of our guests, delicious with Sautéed Spinach and Garlic (page 101).

MAKES 4 SERVINGS

¼ cup orange marmalade

2 teaspoons fresh lemon juice

Four 4-ounce boneless, skinless chicken breast halves

¼ teaspoon sea salt

¼ teaspoon freshly ground black pepper

2 teaspoons extra virgin olive oil

1⅓ cups Cranberry Orzo (page 116)

1. Preheat the oven to 400°F.

2. Stir together orange marmalade and lemon juice in a small bowl. Set aside.

3. Season the chicken breasts with the salt and pepper.

4. Heat the olive oil in a large sauté pan over medium-high heat. Sear the chicken for 1 minute on each side.

5. Transfer the chicken breasts to a baking dish and bake for 15 to 20 minutes, or until the internal temperature reaches 165°F.

6. Serve each chicken breast topped with 1 tablespoon orange marmalade mixture and ⅓ cup cranberry orzo.

n NUTRITION NOTE: *Orange peel, found in marmalade, is a rich source of limonene, which has potent anticancer effects.*

EACH SERVING CONTAINS

320 calories

34 g carbohydrate

6 g fat

74 mg cholesterol

31 g protein

294 mg sodium

1 g fiber

CHICKEN MEDALLIONS
WITH MUSHROOM TARRAGON SAUCE

You can substitute crimini mushrooms for
the oyster mushrooms in this dish if you like.

MAKES 4 SERVINGS

1 pound boneless, skinless chicken breast halves

1 tablespoon diced shallots

1 cup oyster mushrooms

⅓ cup white wine

2 teaspoons dried tarragon

½ cup chicken stock

½ teaspoon sea salt

¼ teaspoon freshly ground black pepper

¼ cup heavy cream

¼ teaspoon Worcestershire sauce

2 cups Mashed Potatoes (page 105)

2 cups steamed fresh green beans

1. Cut the chicken breasts into 2-ounce medallions (8 pieces). Pound with a meat mallet until ¼ inch thick.

2. In a large sauté pan lightly sprayed with canola oil spray, over medium heat, sauté the chicken for 1 minute on each side. Remove and set aside. Add the shallots and sauté briefly. Add the mushrooms and sauté.

3. Deglaze the pan with the white wine. Add the tarragon and cook until almost dry. Stir in the chicken stock and chicken back into the pan and cook until the sauce is slightly thickened and the internal temperature of the chicken reaches 165°F, 3 to 5 minutes.

4. Stir in the salt and pepper, the cream, and Worcestershire sauce. Immediately remove from the heat.

5. Serve 2 chicken medallions and a quarter of the sauce on each plate, along with ½ cup mashed potatoes and ½ cup green beans.

EACH SERVING CONTAINS

395 calories

29 g carbohydrate

11 g fat

121 mg cholesterol

41 g protein

588 mg sodium

6 g fiber

SPINACH-STUFFED CHICKEN WITH ARTICHOKE CAPER SAUCE

Terrific with steamed asparagus and orzo.

MAKES 4 SERVINGS

Four 4-ounce boneless, skinless chicken breast halves

2 cups baby spinach, washed

¼ cup crumbled feta

FOR THE ARTICHOKE CAPER SAUCE

1 tablespoon extra virgin olive oil

2 tablespoons minced garlic

½ cup water-packed canned artichoke hearts, chopped

¼ cup capers, rinsed and drained

½ cup chicken stock

¼ cup fresh lemon juice

1. Preheat the oven to 400°F.

2. Pound the chicken breasts with a meat mallet to ¼ inch thick. Set aside.

3. Sauté the spinach over medium heat in a medium sauté pan until wilted. Remove from the pan and refrigerate until cool.

4. Place one quarter spinach and 1 tablespoon feta on each chicken breast and roll burrito style.

5. Sear the chicken in a large sauté pan over medium-high heat for 1 minute on each side.

6. Transfer the chicken to a baking dish and cook for 18 to 22 minutes, until the internal temperature is 165°F.

7. Heat the olive oil in a medium sauté pan. Sauté the garlic, artichokes, and capers. Add the chicken stock and lemon juice and simmer for 3 to 5 minutes, until slightly thickened.

8. Serve each stuffed chicken breast topped with ¼ cup artichoke caper sauce.

n NUTRITION NOTE: *Feta cheeses vary in sodium content. Compare labels to find a lower-sodium brand.*

220 calories
6 g carbohydrate
9 g fat
81 mg cholesterol
30 g protein
579 mg sodium
2 g fiber

EACH SERVING CONTAINS

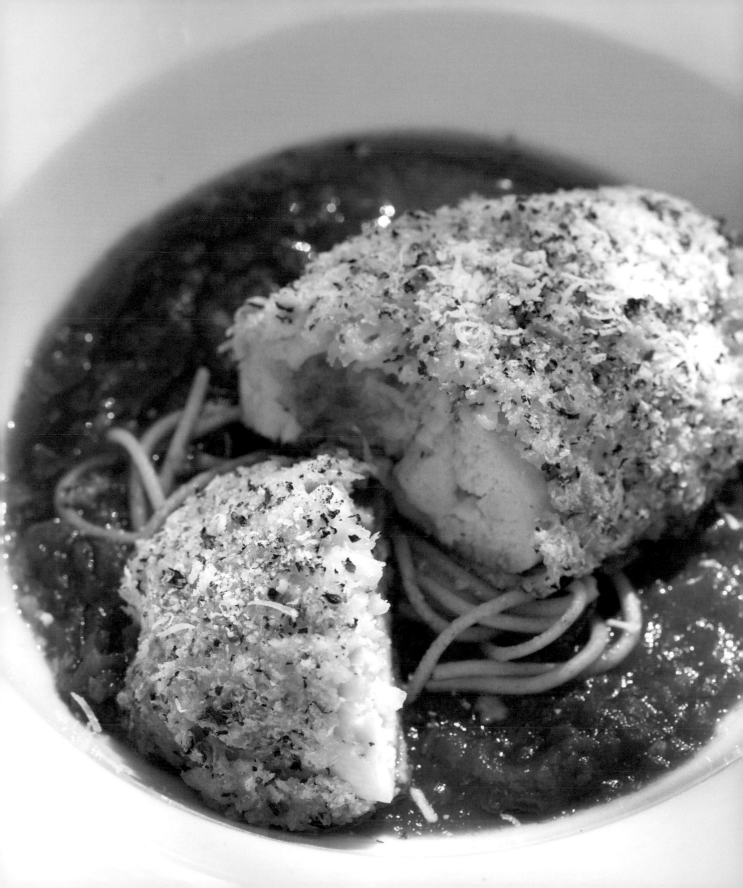

CHICKEN STUFFED WITH CARAMELIZED GARLIC

Chunky Tomato Sauce doubles as a vegetable in this recipe.

MAKES 4 SERVINGS

FOR THE
CARAMELIZED GARLIC

1 cup garlic cloves

½ teaspoon extra
virgin olive oil

⅛ teaspoon sea salt

⅛ teaspoon freshly
ground black pepper

1 teaspoon honey

½ teaspoon white
balsamic vinegar

————

Four 4-ounce boneless,
skinless chicken
breast halves

2 tablespoons freshly
grated Parmesan

½ cup whole wheat
bread crumbs

¼ teaspoon sea salt

⅛ teaspoon freshly
ground black pepper

¼ cup unbleached
all-purpose flour

1 egg, beaten

2 cups cooked
angel hair pasta

2 cups Chunky Tomato
Sauce (page 174)

1. Preheat the oven to 250°F.

2. Toss the garlic with the olive oil, salt, and pepper in a small bowl. Spread evenly on a baking pan that has been lightly sprayed with canola oil spray. Cover with aluminum foil and roast for 2 hours, stirring occasionally. Remove the pan from the oven, uncover, and allow to cool completely.

3. Combine the caramelized garlic with the honey and vinegar and puree in a blender until smooth.

4. Increase the oven temperature to 400°F.

5. Pound the chicken breasts with a meat mallet until ¼ inch thick. Place 1 tablespoon of the garlic mixture on each chicken breast and roll burrito style.

6. In a small bowl, combine the Parmesan, bread crumbs, salt, and pepper. Dredge each chicken breast in flour, then the egg, followed by the bread crumb mixture.

7. Spray each roll with canola oil. Bake for 10 to 15 minutes until the chicken reaches an internal temperature of 165°F.

8. Serve each stuffed chicken breast with ½ cup pasta and ½ cup tomato sauce.

EACH SERVING CONTAINS

435 calories

50 g carbohydrate

9 g fat

119 mg cholesterol

39 g protein

485 mg sodium

4 g fiber

CHICKEN WITH ARTICHOKE–SUN-DRIED TOMATO PESTO

An intriguing variation on traditional pesto. A great starter for this is Napoleon of Heirloom Tomatoes and Mozzarella (page 155).

MAKES 4 SERVINGS

FOR THE ARTICHOKE–
SUN-DRIED TOMATO PESTO

⅓ cup water-packed
canned artichoke
hearts, chopped

5 garlic cloves

¼ cup reconstituted sun-
dried tomatoes, chopped

¼ cup chopped red onions

⅓ cup freshly grated
Parmesan

1 teaspoon minced
fresh oregano

1 tablespoon fresh
lime juice

———————

Four 4-ounce boneless,
skinless chicken
breast halves

¼ teaspoon sea salt

¼ teaspoon freshly
ground black pepper

2 teaspoons extra
virgin olive oil

1. Preheat the oven to 400°F.

2. Spread the artichoke hearts and garlic evenly over a baking sheet and lightly spray with canola oil spray. Roast for 15 to 25 minutes, or until golden brown.

3. Place the roasted artichokes and garlic in a food processor. Add the sun-dried tomatoes, onions, Parmesan, oregano, and lime juice and pulse until well combined. Add water, 1 tablespoon at a time, until the pesto is smooth and reaches a spreadable consistency.

4. Season the chicken with the salt and pepper.

5. Heat the olive oil in a large sauté pan over medium heat. Sauté the chicken for 3 to 5 minutes on each side, or until the internal temperature reaches 165°F.

6. Serve each chicken breast with ¼ cup pesto.

EACH SERVING CONTAINS

225 calories

7 g carbohydrate

8 g fat

80 mg cholesterol

31 g protein

425 mg sodium

2 g fiber

CASHEW CHICKEN STIR-FRY

A flavorful, nutritionally balanced stir-fry.

MAKES 4 SERVINGS

¼ cup low-sodium
tamari sauce

1 teaspoon minced garlic

2 tablespoons
diced shallots

2 tablespoons firmly
packed light brown sugar

2 tablespoons rice vinegar

⅓ cup water

¼ teaspoon crushed
red pepper flakes

1 teaspoon minced
fresh ginger

½ pound boneless, skinless
chicken breast halves

¾ cup button mushrooms,
stems removed and
discarded, diced small

¾ cup carrots, diced small

¾ cup jicama, diced small

¾ cup thawed frozen peas

¾ cup unsalted
toasted cashews

3 tablespoons cornstarch

2 cups cooked brown rice

1. Combine the tamari, garlic, shallots, brown sugar, rice vinegar, water, red pepper flakes, and ginger in a blender and puree until smooth. Set aside.

2. Dice the chicken breasts. Dice should be the size of peas.

3. Lightly spray a wok or large sauté pan with canola oil spray. Do not preheat. Turn heat to medium-high, add the chicken and stir-fry until cooked through, 3 to 5 minutes. Add the mushrooms, carrots, jicama, peas, and cashews and stir-fry briefly.

4. Stir the cornstarch into the stir-fry sauce. Add the sauce to the pan and cook until thickened, only a few seconds.

5. Serve 1 cup stir-fried chicken with ½ cup brown rice.

n NUTRITION NOTE: *Sometimes healthy cooking is about changing proportions. In this recipe we use 3 full cups of vegetables to ½ pound of chicken, and portion the rice carefully.*

EACH SERVING CONTAINS

420 calories

55 g carbohydrate

13 g fat

36 mg cholesterol

23 g protein

700 mg sodium

5 g fiber

CHICKEN WITH
BLACK BEAN–CHIPOTLE SAUCE

One of our many entrées in which the sauce doubles as a side dish. (Freeze any remaining sauce for another use.) Serve with roasted summer squash (see page 17).

MAKES 4 SERVINGS

FOR THE BLACK BEAN–CHIPOTLE SAUCE

3 tablespoons diced yellow onions

1½ teaspoons minced garlic

One 14-ounce can black beans, rinsed and drained

2 teaspoons ground chipotle chile pepper

1 cup chicken stock

¼ cup diced tomatoes

½ teaspoon minced fresh cilantro

1 teaspoon sea salt

---

1 tablespoon extra virgin olive oil

2 tablespoons chili powder

Four 4-ounce skinless, boneless chicken breast halves

1. Lightly spray a large saucepan with canola oil spray. Sauté the onions and garlic over medium heat until the onions are translucent.

2. Add the black beans, chipotle, chicken stock, tomatoes, cilantro, and salt and slowly simmer for 10 to 20 minutes or until the beans are slightly thickened. Remove from the heat and cool slightly.

3. Place the black bean mixture in a blender and puree until smooth.

4. Preheat the grill or broiler.

5. Combine the olive oil and chili powder in a small bowl and mix to form a paste. Rub the paste over the chicken breasts.

6. Grill or broil the chicken for 3 to 5 minutes on each side, or until the internal temperature reaches 165°F.

7. Serve each chicken breast with 4 tablespoons black bean sauce.

n **NUTRITION NOTE:** *Canned beans are a good alternative to cooking beans from scratch. Look for a high quality, organic brand.*

c **COOK'S NOTE:** *You can leave the beans whole rather than pureed.*

EACH SERVING CONTAINS

330 calories

29 g carbohydrate

8 g fat

73 mg cholesterol

37 g protein

586 mg sodium

11 g fiber

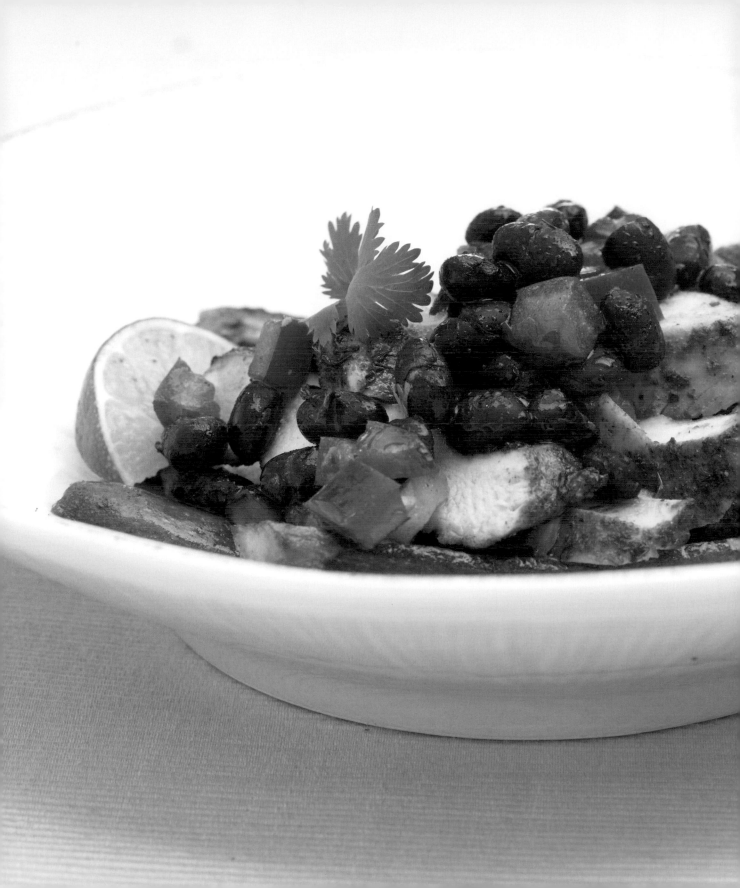

ROAST CHICKEN WITH GRAVY

For a real comfort-food meal, serve with green beans. Use leftover chicken to make Chicken Salad Sandwiches (page 274).

MAKES 4 SERVINGS

½ cup chopped celery

½ cup chopped carrots

½ cup chopped yellow onions

One 3- to 4-pound roasting chicken

½ teaspoon sea salt

½ teaspoon freshly ground black pepper

FOR THE GRAVY

1 teaspoon canola oil

2 tablespoons unsalted butter

⅓ cup diced yellow onions

2 tablespoons unbleached all-purpose flour

1 cup chicken stock

¼ teaspoon sea salt

⅛ teaspoon freshly ground black pepper

½ teaspoon minced fresh sage

Garlic Mashed Potatoes (page 105)

1. Preheat the oven to 350°F.

2. Mix together the celery, carrots, and onions.

3. Stuff the chicken with the celery mixture and season with the salt and pepper. Place the chicken in a roasting pan, cover with aluminum foil, and roast for 1 to 1½ hours, or until the temperature deep in the thigh reaches 165°F. Let rest for 10 minutes.

4. Cut the roasted chicken in half. Remove the back, ribs, wings, and drumsticks. Separate the thighs, legs, and breasts and remove the skin. Cut the breast halves in half.

5. Heat the oil and butter over a medium heat in a medium sauté pan. Sauté the onions until translucent. Add the flour and cook for 3 to 5 minutes. Add the chicken stock and whisk until the mixture begins to boil and becomes thick. Add the salt, pepper, and sage.

6. Serve 4 ounces of chicken (includes ¼ chicken breast and 1 thigh or drumstick per plate), evenly divided vegetables, ⅓ cup garlic mashed potatoes, and ¼ cup gravy.

n NUTRITION NOTE: *Look for an organic hen for this dish. You'll be guaranteed that the bird hasn't been fed antibiotics and has been raised in more acceptable conditions.*

EACH SERVING CONTAINS

280 calories

21 g carbohydrate

10 g fat

77 mg cholesterol

25 g protein

599 mg sodium

3 g fiber

RUSTIC CHICKEN

A deeply good, peasant-style chicken dish. You can also serve with asparagus: Simply chop steamed asparagus into 1-inch pieces and toss them in with the pasta and chicken.

MAKES 4 SERVINGS

1½ cups whole fresh pearl onions

3 tablespoons extra virgin olive oil

Four 4-ounce boneless, skinless chicken breast halves

¼ teaspoon sea salt

¼ teaspoon freshly ground black pepper

¼ cup minced shallots

1 cup chopped seasonal wild mushrooms

2 cups chicken stock

¼ teaspoon minced fresh rosemary

¼ teaspoon minced fresh sage

1 teaspoon sea salt

¼ teaspoon freshly ground black pepper

4 cups cooked pasta

1 tablespoon plus 1 teaspoon grated pecorino Romano

1. Preheat the oven to 350°F. Light coat a baking sheet with canola oil spray.

2. Spread the pearl onions evenly on the baking sheet and roast for 10 minutes, or until slightly browned. After roasting, cool and peel the onions.

3. Heat the olive oil over medium heat in a large sauté pan. Season the chicken breasts with salt and pepper and sauté them until the internal temperature reaches 165°F. Set aside.

4. Sauté the shallots and mushrooms in the same pan until the shallots are translucent. Deglaze with the chicken stock and reduce by half.

5. Add the rosemary, sage, onions, salt, and pepper. Add the chicken and cook until heated through. Remove from the heat. Add the pasta and toss together until well combined.

6. Divide the pasta mixture evenly among four bowls. Sprinkle each with 1 teaspoon pecorino Romano.

n NUTRITION NOTE: *We often recommend eating colorful foods, but not all those colors are bright. The golds, whites, and browns of onions and mushrooms are also associated with health benefits.*

c COOK'S NOTE: *You can substitute frozen peeled pearl onions for fresh. Simply thaw and add to the pan with the herbs.*

EACH SERVING CONTAINS

445 calories

41 g carbohydrate

14 g fat

115 mg cholesterol

37 g protein

694 mg sodium

2 g fiber

CHICKEN POT PIES

These pot pies are a great way to use up leftover chicken: Cut up cooked chicken and sauté it in the saucepan with the vegetables.

MAKES 6 SERVINGS

FOR THE CRUST

1⅓ cups unbleached all-purpose flour

½ teaspoon sea salt

½ teaspoon cane sugar

4 tablespoons (½ stick) chilled unsalted butter, diced

4 to 6 tablespoons ice water

---

3 tablespoons unsalted butter

Four 4-ounce boneless, skinless chicken breast halves, diced

2 cups diced yellow onions

1 cup diced carrots

1 cup diced celery

1 tablespoon minced garlic

⅓ cup unbleached all-purpose flour

4¼ cups chicken stock

¼ teaspoon dried crushed thyme

(continued)

1. Preheat the oven to 375°F.

2. For the crust, place the flour in a medium bowl. Add the salt and cane sugar and mix well. Cut the butter into the flour, using a pastry cutter, until the butter is the size of small peas. Add the water, 1 tablespoon at a time, mixing gently after each addition. The dough will begin to form a ball when enough water has been added. Gather the dough with dry hands and form into a ball. Let rest for 5 minutes.

3. Divide the dough into 6 pieces. On a lightly floured surface, roll out each piece into a circle large enough to fit the top of an 8-ounce ramekin.

4. Melt the butter in a large saucepan over medium heat. Brown the chicken on all sides. Add onions, carrots, celery, and garlic. Sauté until the onions are translucent. Sprinkle the flour over the chicken and vegetables and cook for 5 to 7 minutes, or until slightly golden in color.

5. Whisk 4 cups of the chicken stock, the thyme, and sage into the chicken mixture. Bring to a boil and simmer for 10 minutes.

6. Combine the cornstarch and the remaining ¼ cup of the chicken stock in a small bowl. Mix well. Slowly whisk the paste into the chicken and vegetable mixture and cook over medium heat until thickened. Stir continuously to avoid burning.

7. Add the salt, pepper, Worcestershire, parsley, and lemon juice and remove from the heat.

8. Place 1 cup chicken mixture in each of six individual 8-ounce ramekins and top each with a dough circle. Place the ramekins on a baking sheet. Bake for 15 to 20 minutes, or until the crusts are golden brown.

n **NUTRITION NOTE:** *We use a little bit of chicken to a lot of vegetables. That's real balance.*

2 teaspoons chopped
fresh sage

3 tablespoons cornstarch

1½ teaspoons sea salt

¼ teaspoon freshly
ground black pepper

2 teaspoons
Worcestershire sauce

2 tablespoons chopped
fresh flat-leaf parsley

1 tablespoon fresh
lemon juice

400 calories

40 g carbohydrate

15 g fat

86 mg cholesterol

24 g protein

734 mg sodium

3 g fiber

EACH SERVING CONTAINS

MOJITO-MARINATED CHICKEN FAJITAS

The sweetness of the rum gives chicken fajitas a whole new character.
Great with our Southwest Green Cabbage Salad (page 102).

MAKES 4 SERVINGS

FOR THE MOJITO
MARINADE

¾ cup fresh lime juice

½ cup rum

½ cup chiffonade of
fresh mint leaves

1 tablespoon extra
virgin olive oil

1 tablespoon sea salt

2 teaspoons cane sugar

———————

Four 4-ounce boneless,
skinless chicken
breast halves

½ cup sliced red
bell peppers

½ cup sliced yellow
bell peppers

1 cup sliced yellow onions

Four 10-inch whole
wheat flour tortillas

½ cup Guacamole
(page 188)

½ cup Pico de Gallo
(page 189)

½ cup fat-free sour cream

1. Combine the lime juice, rum, mint, olive oil, salt, and cane sugar in a shallow glass baking dish and mix well.

2. Place the chicken in the marinade and turn to coat evenly. Cover and refrigerate for at least 15 minutes or up to 1 hour.

3. Preheat the grill or broiler.

4. Remove the chicken from the marinade and discard the marinade. Grill or broil the chicken for 3 to 5 minutes per side, or until the internal temperature reaches 165°F.

5. While the chicken is cooking, lightly spray a medium sauté pan with canola oil. Sauté the red bell peppers, yellow bell peppers, and onions over medium heat until just tender. Set aside and keep warm.

6. Cut the cooked chicken into strips and divide the strips into four portions. Serve each portion with one whole wheat tortilla, a quarter of the sautéed vegetables, and 2 tablespoons each guacamole, pico de gallo, and sour cream.

n NUTRITION NOTE: *Our fajitas are a colorful lesson in proportions—4 ounces chicken, a tortilla providing a serving of whole grain, and a full ¾ cup vegetables.*

EACH SERVING CONTAINS

425 calories

43 g carbohydrate

12 g fat

76 mg cholesterol

34 g protein

584 mg sodium

5 g fiber

MEDITERRANEAN CHICKEN WRAP

This juicy, fresh-tasting wrap is very popular at our resorts in summer.

MAKES 6 SERVINGS

1 tablespoon minced
red onions

1 tablespoon canola
oil mayonnaise

1½ teaspoons Dijon mustard

1 tablespoon freshly
grated Parmesan

2 tablespoons red
wine vinegar

½ teaspoon garlic granules

1 teaspoon minced fresh basil

¼ teaspoon dried oregano

1 teaspoon minced fresh
flat-leaf parsley

⅛ teaspoon sea salt

⅛ teaspoon freshly
ground black pepper

―――――――――――

1 pound boneless, skinless
chicken breast halves

2 medium Roma
tomatoes, diced

½ cup chopped water-packed
canned artichoke hearts

¼ cup chopped
kalamata olives

Six 10-inch whole
wheat tortillas

1. Preheat the oven to 350°F. Lightly spray a baking sheet with canola oil.

2. Combine the onions, mayonnaise, mustard, Parmesan, vinegar, garlic, basil, oregano, parsley, salt, and pepper in a small bowl. Set aside.

3. Place the chicken breasts on the baking sheet and bake for 15 to 20 minutes, or until the internal temperature reaches 165°F. Let cool. Cut into bite-size pieces.

4. Combine the chicken, tomatoes, artichokes, and olives in a large bowl. Pour the dressing over the mixture and toss gently until fully coated.

5. Place ½ cup chicken mixture on each tortilla. Roll up burrito style.

EACH SERVING CONTAINS

350 calories

25 g carbohydrate

13 g fat

77 mg cholesterol

33 g protein

607 mg sodium

6 g fiber

CHICKEN SALAD SANDWICHES

The next time you cook chicken, make some extra and use it to make these.

MAKES 6 SERVINGS

1 pound boneless, skinless chicken breast halves

FOR THE DRESSING

½ cup low-fat Greek-style yogurt

3 tablespoons canola oil mayonnaise

1 tablespoon Dijon mustard

1 teaspoon cane sugar

¼ teaspoon garlic powder

½ teaspoon sea salt

¼ teaspoon freshly ground black pepper

⅓ cup minced yellow onions

½ cup minced celery

12 slices whole grain bread

6 large lettuce leaves

2 medium tomatoes, cut into 12 slices

1. Place the chicken breasts in a medium saucepan and cover with water. Bring to a boil on high heat, reduce the heat to low, and simmer for 7 to 10 minutes, or until the internal temperature reaches 165°F. Cool completely and cut into small cubes.

2. Combine the yogurt, mayonnaise, mustard, cane sugar, garlic powder, salt, and pepper in a large bowl. Add the onions and celery and mix well. Fold in the chicken.

3. Place ½ cup chicken salad on each of 6 slices of bread. Garnish each with a lettuce leaf and 2 tomato slices. Top each with a remaining bread slice.

n **NUTRITION NOTE:** *The combination of thick Greek yogurt with a little real mayonnaise makes this classic chicken salad lower in fat and calories. The whole grain bread, lettuce, and tomato make it a full meal.*

EACH SERVING CONTAINS

410 calories

44 g carbohydrate

12 g fat

73 mg cholesterol

34 g protein

601 mg sodium

5 g fiber

TURKEY APPLE WRAP

A scrumptious way to use holiday leftovers.

MAKES 6 SERVINGS

½ pound cooked turkey breast, chopped

2 tablespoons minced red onions

¼ cup chopped celery

¼ cup chopped apples of your choice

2 tablespoons minced dried cranberries

½ teaspoon garlic granules

3 tablespoons canola oil mayonnaise

1 tablespoon nonfat sour cream

½ teaspoon Dijon mustard

1 tablespoon distilled white vinegar

Pinch dried thyme

Pinch sea salt

Pinch freshly ground black pepper

Six 10-inch whole wheat tortillas

1½ cups spinach, washed

1. Combine the turkey, onions, celery, apples, cranberries, garlic granules, mayonnaise, sour cream, mustard, vinegar, thyme, salt, and pepper in a large bowl and mix well.

2. Place the turkey mixture in a food processor and pulse for 2 to 3 seconds at a time until the mixture is finely diced.

3. Lay the tortillas on a flat surface. Spread ¼ cup spinach on each. Place ¼ cup turkey mixture on top of the spinach. Roll up burrito style.

n NUTRITION NOTE: *Everything in this whole meal wrap is available in the cold weather months, making it easy to eat by the seasons.*

EACH SERVING CONTAINS

305 calories

32 g carbohydrate

12 g fat

32 mg cholesterol

16 g protein

363 mg sodium

4 g fiber

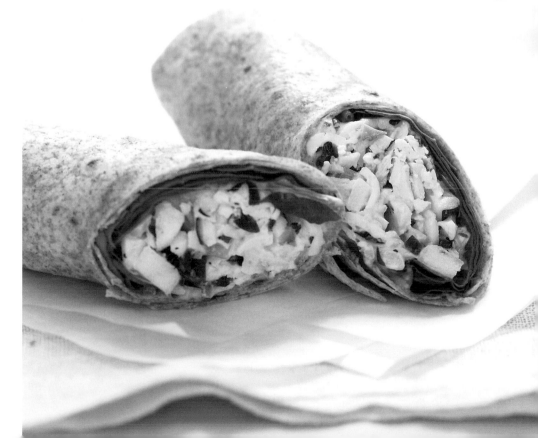

TURKEY MUFFALETTA

This zesty sandwich is a particular favorite of both guests and staff.

MAKES 4 SERVINGS

FOR THE OLIVE SPREAD

2 tablespoons minced green olives

1 tablespoon capers, rinsed and drained

1 tablespoon minced celery

⅛ teaspoon minced garlic

1 tablespoon minced red onions

¼ teaspoon dried oregano

1 teaspoon minced fresh flat-leaf parsley

2 tablespoons minced roasted red peppers

1½ teaspoons red wine vinegar

⅛ teaspoon freshly ground black pepper

1 teaspoon extra virgin olive oil

———

4 whole grain rolls

Eight 1-ounce slices roasted turkey breast

Four 1-ounce slices pepper Jack

1. Preheat the broiler.

2. Toss together the olives, capers, celery, garlic, and onions in a small bowl. Add the oregano, parsley, roasted peppers, vinegar, pepper, and olive oil and mix well.

3. Slice the rolls in half and toast each side. Evenly spread 2 tablespoons olive spread on one half of each toasted roll. Place 2 slices turkey breast and 1 slice pepper Jack on top of the olive spread. Repeat for the remaining sandwiches.

4. Lay the open-face sandwiches on a baking sheet. Broil for 1 to 2 minutes, or until the cheese is melted. Top each sandwich with the other half of the roll.

n   NUTRITION NOTE: *We have reduced the sodium in the olive salad by using fewer olives and more celery and red pepper. You can reduce the sodium in the sliced turkey by carefully choosing what you buy.*

c   COOK'S NOTE: *Organic whole wheat rolls can be purchased online or at natural foods stores in your area.*

EACH SERVING CONTAINS

400 calories

41 g carbohydrate

8 g fat

89 mg cholesterol

40 g protein

611 mg sodium

4 g fiber

WARM TURKEY
AND ASPARAGUS SANDWICH

Look for low-sodium deli turkey that's free of nitrites or nitrates.

MAKES 4 SERVINGS

FOR THE MUSTARD SAUCE

⅓ cup low-fat sour cream

1 teaspooon fresh
lemon juice

1 tablespoon
Dijon mustard

4 slices rye bread

¾ pound deli-sliced
turkey breast

12 asparagus
spears, blanched

1 tomato, sliced,
about ½ inch thick

Four 1-ounce slices Swiss

1. Preheat the broiler.

2. Combine the sour cream, lemon juice, and mustard and mix well.

3. Toast the bread.

4. Place 3 ounces sliced turkey on each slice of toasted bread. Top the turkey with 3 asparagus spears, 1 tomato slice, 2 teaspoons mustard sauce, and 1 slice of Swiss.

5. Place the sandwiches under the broiler or in a toaster oven until the cheese melts.

n NUTRITION NOTE: *An open-face sandwich using only one slice of bread saves you about 100 calories.*

EACH SERVING CONTAINS

365 calories

29 g carbohydrate

9 g fat

99 mg cholesterol

39 g protein

371 mg sodium

3 g fiber

TURKEY MEDALLIONS
WITH HONEY CHIPOTLE SAUCE

Easy to prepare and a favorite of children.

MAKES 4 SERVINGS

FOR THE HONEY
CHIPOTLE SAUCE

1¼ tablespoons honey

2 tablespoons cold
unsalted butter

¼ teaspoon sea salt

¼ teaspoon ground
chipotle chile pepper

---

1 pound boneless, skinless
turkey breast halves

¼ teaspoon sea salt

¼ teaspoon freshly
ground black pepper

½ teaspoon extra
virgin olive oil

Potato Medley (page 113)

Sautéed Kale (page 100)

1. Preheat the oven to 400°F.

2. Warm the honey in a small saucepan over medium heat. Whisk in the butter, being careful not to let the mixture boil. Remove from the heat and add the salt and ground chipotle. Mix well.

3. Cut the turkey breasts into 2-ounce medallions (8 pieces). Pound with a meat mallet until ¼ inch thick. Season with the salt and pepper.

4. Heat the olive oil over medium heat in a large sauté pan. Sauté the turkey for 2 to 3 minutes on each side, or until golden brown. Remove the turkey medallions from the pan.

5. Add the honey chipotle sauce to the pan and cook until the sauce is slightly thickened.

6. Place 2 turkey medallions on each plate and top with 1 tablespoon honey chipotle sauce. Serve with ¾ cup potato medley and 1 cup sautéed kale.

EACH SERVING CONTAINS

390 calories

45 g carbohydrate

11 g. fat

81 mg cholesterol

29 g protein

448 mg sodium

7 g fiber

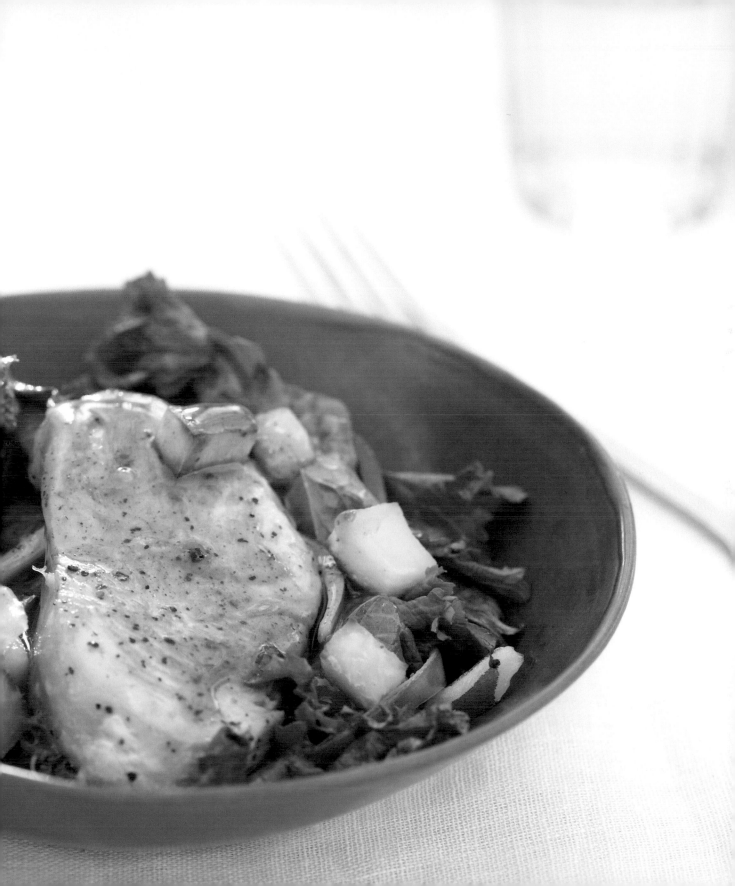

CHAPTER ELEVEN | *All the world's great cuisines offer terrific vegetable-, grain-, dairy-, and bean-based dishes, and we've tapped them in creating vegetarian main dishes that will tempt and satisfy even committed omnivores. Of course, many of our soups, starters, and side dishes are also vegetarian—don't overlook them when you're planning meatless meals.*

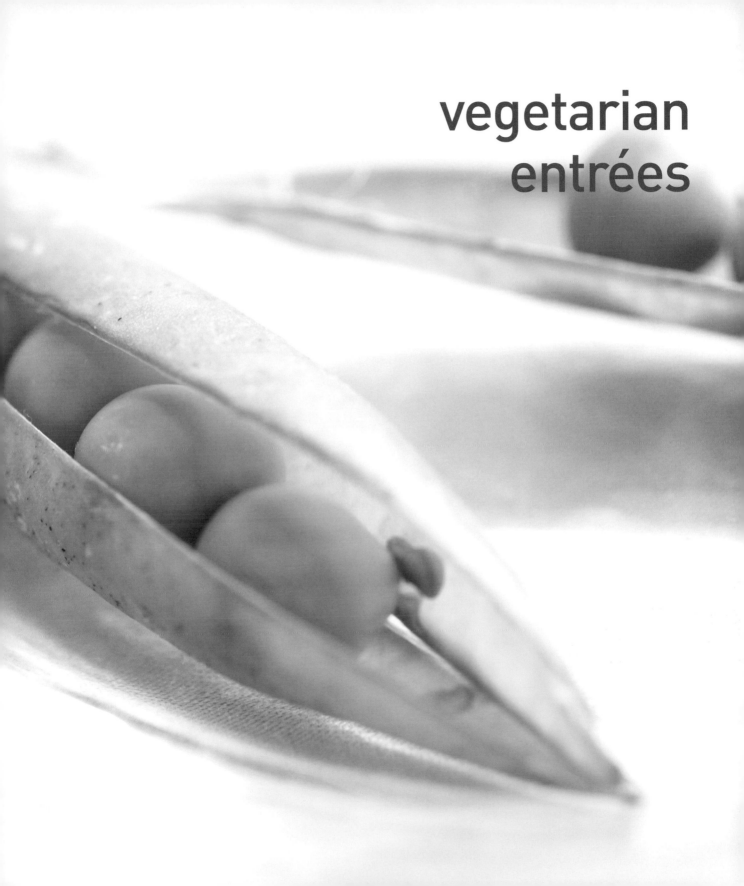

vegetarian entrées

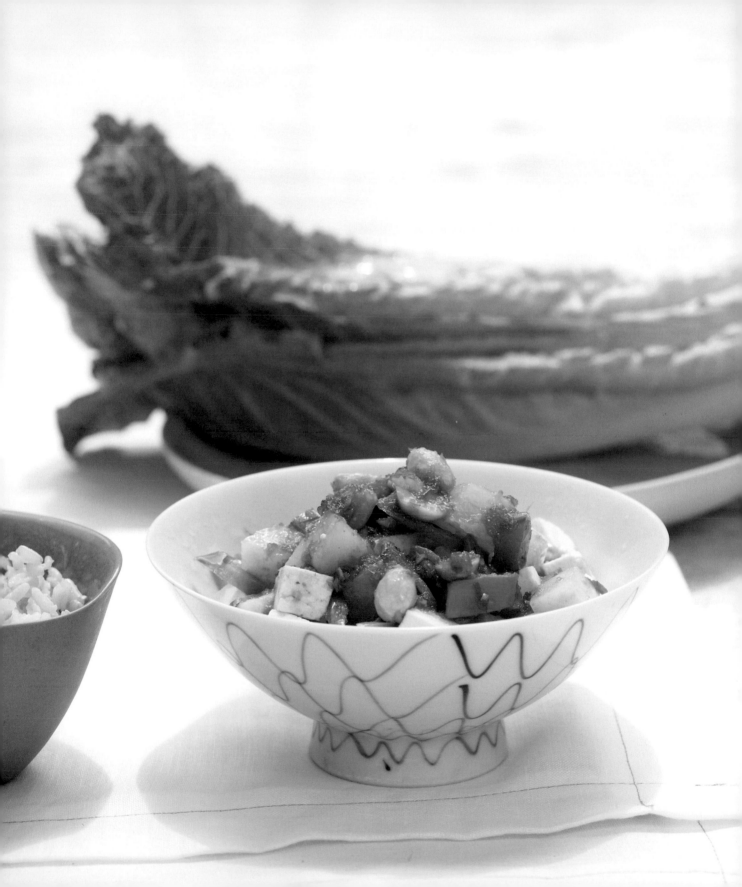

TOFU LETTUCE WRAPS

This recipe also works with chicken. You can precook boneless, skinless chicken breast halves by grilling, poaching, or sautéing them until the internal temperature reaches 165°F. Let the chicken cool, dice, and proceed as for tofu.

MAKES 4 SERVINGS

FOR THE SAUCE

¼ cup low-sodium tamari sauce

1 teaspoon minced garlic

1 tablespoon minced shallots

1 tablespoon firmly packed light brown sugar

1 tablespoon plus 1 teaspoon rice vinegar

¼ cup plus 2 tablespoons water

1 tablespoon plus 1 teaspoon cornstarch

¼ teaspoon crushed red pepper flakes

¾ teaspoon minced fresh ginger

———

½ cup diced carrots

½ cup sugar snap peas, diced

½ cup diced jicama

½ cup diced pineapple

¾ pound extra-firm tofu, diced

¼ cup whole roasted unsalted peanuts

12 romaine leaves

1⅓ cups cooked brown rice

1. Combine the tamari, garlic, shallots, brown sugar, rice vinegar, water cornstarch, red pepper flakes, and ginger in a blender and puree until smooth.

2. Toss together the carrots, snap peas, jicama, and pineapple in a large bowl. Mix in the tofu.

3. Heat a wok or large sauté pan that has been lightly sprayed with canola oil over high heat. Add the tofu mixture and cook for 30 seconds, constantly tossing to cook on all sides. Stir in the sauce and cook for 15 to 20 seconds, or until slightly thickened.

4. On each plate, serve 1 cup tofu mixture garnished with 1 tablespoon peanuts, along with 3 romaine leaves and ⅓ cup brown rice.

n NUTRITION NOTE: *Among its other good qualities, tofu is one of the better sources of magnesium, a mineral lacking in the diets of most adults.*

EACH SERVING CONTAINS

400 calories

51 g carbohydrate

15 g fat

0 mg cholesterol

19 g protein

649 mg sodium

7 g fiber

BUTTERNUT SQUASH TART
WITH ARUGULA SALAD

We serve this as an appetizer in our Superfoods Dinner, pairing it with Salmon with Blueberry Mango Salsa (page 219) as the entrée.

MAKES 16 SERVINGS

FOR THE FLAXSEED CRUST

¼ cup golden flaxseeds

½ cup plus 1 tablespoon unbleached all-purpose flour

⅛ teaspoon sea salt

¼ cup water

1 tablespoon egg whites

———

2½ pounds butternut squash, peeled and cubed

1 medium yellow bell pepper, chopped

1 medium red bell pepper, chopped

1 medium red onion, chopped

¼ cup fresh cilantro, chopped

2 tablespoons Latin Spice Rub (page 187)

3 tablespoons fresh lime juice

8 egg yolks

(continued)

1. Preheat the oven to 350°F.

2. Grind the flaxseeds in a spice grinder or coffee grinder. Combine the flaxseed, flour, and salt in a large bowl. Add the water and stir together until a ball of dough forms.

3. On a lightly floured surface, roll out the dough into a 12-inch circle. Place in a 10-inch tart pan and lightly press into the pan. Brush the dough evenly with the egg whites and bake for 10 minutes. Remove from the oven and set aside. Increase the oven temperature to 400°F.

4. Spread the cubed squash, yellow bell peppers, and red bell peppers evenly on a large baking sheet that has been sprayed with canola oil. Roast for 25 minutes, or until golden brown. Let cool.

5. Combine the roasted squash, bell peppers, onions, cilantro, spice rub, lime juice, and egg yolks in a food processor or blender and process until finely diced and mixed together.

6. Fill the prepared crust with the squash mixture. Bake for 30 to 40 minutes. Let cool slightly. Cut into 16 slices.

7. For the pomegranate dressing, combine the shallots, pomegranate concentrate, and lime juice, and mix well.

8. Serve 1 tart slice with ½ cup arugula topped with 1 tablespoon pomegranate dressing.

FOR THE POMEGRANATE
DRESSING

⅓ cup minced
roasted shallots

¾ cup pomegranate
concentrate

¼ cup plus 2 tablespoons
fresh lime juice

8 cups baby arugula,
washed

n NUTRITION NOTE: *Flaxseed is a rich source of lignans, fiberlike substances that help support beneficial intestinal flora and modulate hormone activity.*

c COOK'S NOTE: *Flaxseed is an excellent source of omega-3 fatty acids; grinding the seeds helps release these compounds. The ground seed has a limited shelf life, so it's best to grind just what you need. Ground flaxseed meal, which can be kept in an airtight opaque container in the refrigerator for up to 30 days, is also available. Whole flaxseed can be kept in the refrigerator in an airtight opaque container for up to 6 months. If the seed or meal develops an off odor, discard it.*

EACH SERVING CONTAINS

135 calories

23 g carbohydrate

4 g fat

87 mg cholesterol

4 g protein

103 mg sodium

4 g fiber

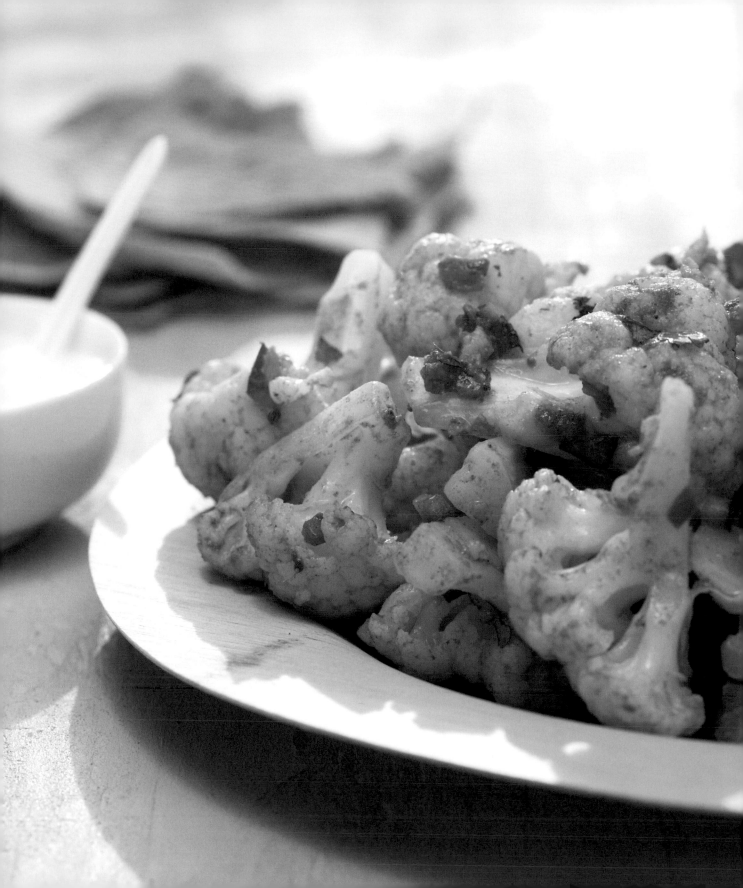

SPICY CURRIED CAULIFLOWER

Traditionally, this would be served with naan bread; we use tortillas instead.

MAKES 4 SERVINGS

2 tablespoons extra virgin olive oil

¼ cup minced fresh ginger

¼ cup diced canned mild green chiles

1 cup diced Roma tomatoes

2 tablespoons plus 1 teaspoon gobi spice mix

4 cups diced cauliflower

½ cup vegetable stock

2 tablespoons chopped fresh cilantro

1½ cups nonfat plain yogurt

¼ teaspoon sea salt

Four 10-inch whole wheat tortillas, warmed

1. Heat the olive oil over medium-high heat in a large saucepan. Sauté the ginger and green chiles for 1 minute. Add the tomatoes and sauté briefly. Add the spice mix and sauté to caramelize the spices.

2. Add the cauliflower and sauté to coat. Add the vegetable stock, cover, and cook for 20 minutes, stirring occasionally, until the cauliflower is soft. Stir in the cilantro.

3. Combine the yogurt and salt in a medium bowl and mix well.

4. Serve 1 cup cauliflower with ⅓ cup yogurt sauce and 1 tortilla.

n NUTRITION NOTE: *Cauliflower is a cruciferous vegetable that is not only high in vitamin C and fiber, but also indoles, a sulfur-containing compound that may protect against breast cancer.*

c COOK'S NOTE: *You'll find gobi spice mix at Middle Eastern markets and online.*

EACH SERVING CONTAINS

330 calories

45 g carbohydrate

12 g fat

2 mg cholesterol

12 g protein

751 mg sodium

7 g fiber

ZUCCHINI FRITTERS
WITH TOMATO FETA RELISH

MAKES 4 SERVINGS

1 tablespoon extra virgin olive oil

2 medium yellow onions, julienned

1 teaspoon minced garlic

1 pound zucchini, julienned

1 large egg

½ cup nonfat milk

½ cup buttermilk

½ cup unbleached all-purpose flour

¾ teaspoon sea salt

½ teaspoon aluminum-free baking powder

2 tablespoons dried parsley flakes

1 tablespoon plus 1 teaspoon dried oregano

⅛ teaspoon freshly ground black pepper

Tomato Feta Relish (page 182)

¼ cup chopped toasted pine nuts

1. Preheat the oven to 350°F. Lightly spray a baking sheet with canola oil spray.

2. Heat the olive oil over medium heat in a large sauté pan. Sauté the onions and garlic until the onions are translucent. Add the zucchini and cook until the zucchini just begins to soften. Remove from the heat and place the mixture in a colander to drain and cool.

3. Using an electric mixer, beat the egg in a large bowl until frothy. Stir in the milk and buttermilk. Add the flour, salt, and baking powder and stir until just mixed. Add the zucchini mixture, parsley, oregano, and pepper and stir until well combined.

4. Heat a large heavy-bottomed sauté pan and lightly spray with canola oil spray. Using a ¼ cup measure, scoop mounds of the zucchini mixture into the pan and flatten with a spatula. Sauté the fritters until golden brown and crispy on each side. Transfer the fritters to a baking sheet and bake for 8 to 10 minutes, or until the fritters are very crispy and there is no moisture in the middle.

5. Top with 2 tablespoons of the tomato feta relish and sprinkle 1 table-spoon chopped pine nuts over the top of each.

EACH SERVING CONTAINS

430 calories

55 g carbohydrate

19 g fat

69 mg cholesterol

15 g protein

782 mg sodium

8 g fiber

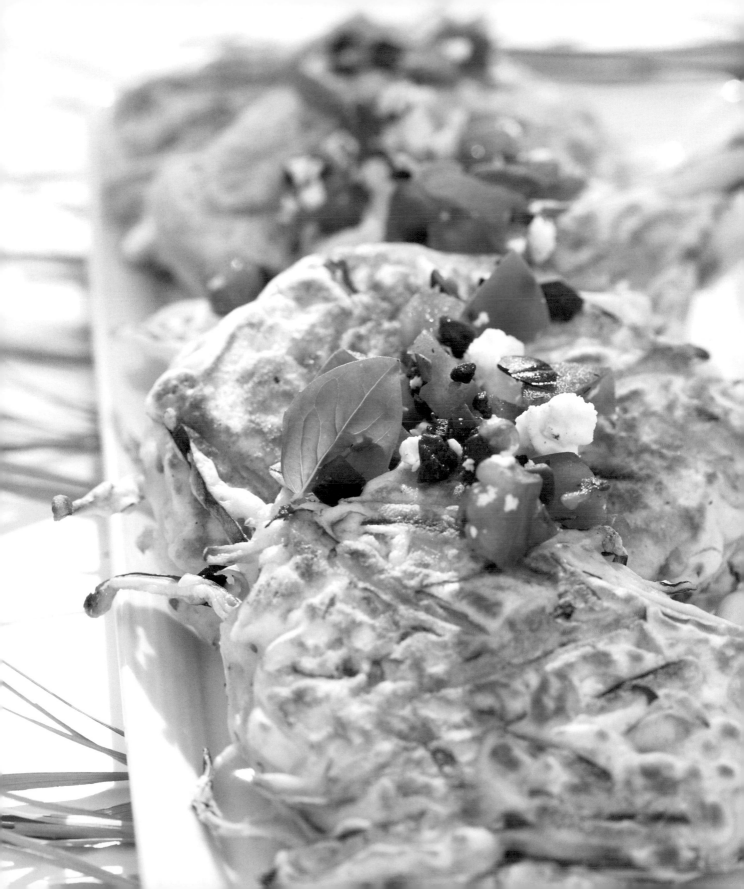

CAULIFLOWER FRITTERS

Look for tapioca starch in health food stores and exceptionally well-stocked supermarkets.

MAKES 4 SERVINGS

1⅓ pounds cauliflower

¾ cup unbleached all-purpose flour

⅓ cup tapioca starch

1 tablespoon plus 1 teaspoon cane sugar

1½ teaspoons minced garlic

¾ teaspoon sea salt

¼ teaspoon freshly ground black pepper

⅓ cup evaporated skim milk

⅓ cup light coconut milk

¼ cup toasted coconut flakes

¼ cup toasted sliced almonds

1. Preheat the oven to 350°F. Lightly spray a baking sheet with canola oil spray.

2. Cut the cauliflower into very small florets and steam for 5 to 8 minutes until soft. Cool.

3. Combine the flour, tapioca starch, cane sugar, garlic, salt, pepper, evaporated skim milk, coconut milk, coconut flakes, and 3 tablespoons of the sliced almonds in a large bowl. Add the cauliflower and toss gently.

4. Heat a large heavy-bottomed sauté pan and lightly spray with canola oil spray. Using a ¼ cup measure, scoop mounds of the cauliflower mixture onto the pan and then flatten with a spatula. Sauté the fritters until golden brown on each side.

5. Transfer the fritters to a baking sheet and bake for 8 to 10 minutes, or until the fritters are very crisp and there is no moisture in the middle.

6. Serve 3 fritters topped with each of the remaining toasted almonds.

EACH SERVING CONTAINS

365 calories

49 g carbohydrate

14 g fat

0 mg cholesterol

12 g protein

433 mg sodium

6 g fiber

CHEESE ENCHILADAS
WITH TOMATILLO SAUCE

Enchiladas are the ubiquitous staff-of-life casserole dish of the Southwest.

MAKES 4 SERVINGS

FOR THE
TOMATILLO SAUCE

1 pound fresh tomatillos, husks and stems removed, washed

¼ jalapeño pepper, minced

½ teaspoon dried oregano

2 tablespoons chopped fresh cilantro

1 tablespoon minced garlic

½ teaspoon sea salt

2 teaspoons fresh lime juice

———————

1¼ cups grated Cheddar

1 cup chopped red onions

8 corn tortillas

2 cups Southwest Green Cabbage Salad (page 102)

1. Preheat the oven to 400°. Lightly spray a baking sheet with canola oil spray.

2. Arrange the tomatillos on the baking sheet and roast for 10 minutes, or until soft and beginning to caramelize.

3. Place the tomatillos, jalapeños, oregano, cilantro, garlic, salt, and lime juice in a food processor and puree until smooth. Set aside. (Wear gloves when handling hot chile peppers, or wash your hands thoroughly before touching your eyes, nose, or mouth.)

4. Increase the oven temperature to broil or preheat the broiler.

5. Combine 1 cup of the Cheddar and the onions i a small bowl.

6. Lay the tortillas on a flat surface. Place ¼ cup cheese mixture onto each tortilla. Roll up burrito style. Place enchiladas in an 8-inch baking pan. (For safety reasons, do not use a glass dish under a broiler.) Pour the tomatillo sauce over the enchilades and top with the remaining ¼ cup Cheddar. Place under the broiler until the cheese is melted.

7. Serve 2 enchiladas with ½ cup cabbage salad.

n NUTRITION NOTE: *The amount of fiber in this delicious enchilada plate is astounding for the calories. It comes mostly from the tomatillos and the cabbage. Both are also high in vitamin C.*

EACH SERVING CONTAINS

325 calories

40 g carbohydrate

14 g fat

34 mg cholesterol

14 g protein

718 mg sodium

8 g fiber

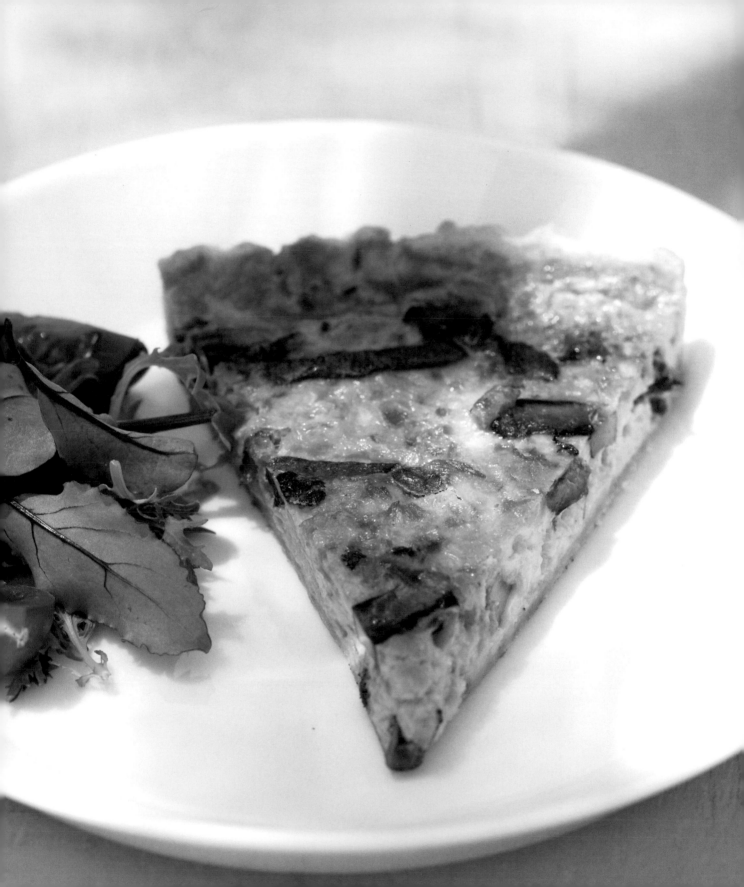

WILD MUSHROOM AND AGED GOUDA TART

This is lovely served with a simple green salad. The aged Gouda is the key here. Look for it at a good cheese shop.

MAKES 8 SERVINGS

FOR THE CRUST

1 cup unbleached all-purpose flour

¼ teaspoon sea salt

4 tablespoons (½ stick) cold unsalted butter

6 tablespoons ice water

¾ cup minced shallots

1 pound thickly sliced mushrooms

4 large eggs

2 large egg whites (about ¼ cup)

¾ cup nonfat milk

½ cup half-and-half

1 cup shredded aged Gouda

½ teaspoon sea salt

¼ teaspoon freshly ground black pepper

⅛ teaspoon ground nutmeg

1 tablespoon unbleached all-purpose flour

1. Preheat the oven to 350°F.

2. Place flour in a medium bowl. Add the salt and mix well. Cut the butter into the flour, using a pastry cutter, until the butter is the size of small peas. Add the water, 1 tablespoon at a time, mixing gently with a fork after each addition. The dough will begin to form a ball when enough water has been added. Gather the dough with dry hands and form it into an even ball. Let rest for 5 minutes.

3. On a lightly floured surface, roll out the dough into a 12-inch circle. Place in a 10-inch tart pan and lightly press into the pan. Bake using pie weights or 1 to 2 cups dried beans in the bottom for 15 minutes.

4. Reduce the oven temperature to 325°F.

5. Lightly spray a large sauté pan with canola oil. Sauté the shallots over medium heat. Add the mushrooms and sauté until cooked through and beginning to dry after giving up their moisture. Allow to cool.

6. Whisk the eggs in a large bowl. Add the egg whites, milk, half-and-half, Gouda, salt, pepper, nutmeg, and flour and mix well. Stir in the mushroom mixture. Pour into the prebaked shell.

7. Bake for 30 minutes, or until the tart has set. Cool slightly, then cut into 8 pieces.

> *n* NUTRITION NOTE: *The generous amount of mushrooms in this savory tart makes it a rich source of the B vitamins niacin and riboflavin.*

EACH SERVING CONTAINS

235 calories

21 g carbohydrate

12 g fat

137 mg cholesterol

13 g protein

397 mg sodium

1 g fiber

THREE-CHEESE-STUFFED PORTOBELLO MUSHROOM

Serve with Chunky Tomato Sauce (page 174) or Fresh Marinara Sauce (page 172) for an even bigger boost of flavor and nutrients.

MAKES 4 SERVINGS

½ cup nonfat ricotta cheese

¼ cup shredded mozzarella

¼ cup freshly grated Parmesan

2 tablespoons fresh chopped basil

1 teaspoon dried oregano

1 tablespoon minced garlic

½ teaspoon sea salt

¼ teaspoon freshly ground black pepper

4 portobello mushroom caps, gills and stems removed

¼ cup panko bread crumbs

2 tablespoons extra virgin olive oil

1. Preheat oven to 400°F. Lightly coat a baking pan with extra virgin olive oil spray.

2. Combine the ricotta, mozzarella, Parmesan, basil, oregano, garlic, salt, and pepper in a medium bowl and mix well.

3. Arrange the portobellos in the baking pan hollow sides up. Place ¼ cup ricotta mixture in each, sprinkle with 1 tablespoon bread crumbs, and drizzle with olive oil.

4. Bake for 5 to 10 minutes, or until the mushrooms are soft and the filling is golden brown.

n NUTRITION NOTE: *With three types of cheese, this dish is a good source of calcium. Ricotta is especially high in this vital mineral.*

EACH SERVING CONTAINS

170 calories

10 g carbohydrate

10 g fat

12 mg cholesterol

11 g protein

422 mg sodium

2 g fiber

MUSHROOM BURGERS

These may seem as if it's a lot of work, but the results are well worth it.

MAKES 4 SERVINGS

2 teaspoons extra virgin olive oil

⅔ cup minced yellow onions

2 tablespoons minced garlic

10 ounces portobello mushrooms, gills and stems removed

⅔ cup chopped oyster mushrooms

⅔ cup chopped shiitake mushrooms, stems removed

¼ teaspoon sea salt

½ teaspoon freshly ground black pepper

2 tablespoons low-sodium tamari sauce

1 tablespoon plus 1 teaspoon Worcestershire sauce

2 teaspoons chili powder

½ cup oat flour

¼ cup roasted, chopped cashews

2 tablespoons brown rice flour

2 teaspoons minced fresh flat-leaf parsley

Four 3-ounce multigrain rolls

4 lettuce leaves

4 slices tomato

4 slices red onion

1. Heat the olive oil over medium heat in a large sauté pan. Sauté the onions and garlic until the onions are translucent.

2. Add all the portobellos, oyster mushrooms, and shiitakes and cook to release their liquids and slightly caramelize them. Add the salt, pepper, tamari, Worcestershire, and chili powder and cook until dry.

3. Remove from the heat and stir in the oat flour, cashews, rice flour, and parsley. Immediately pulse in a food processor, until the mixture comes together.

4. Form the mushroom mixture into 3-ounce patties. Grill the patties on a flat-top grill or in an electric skillet at 350°F until slightly brown on each side.

5. Serve each patty on a roll with lettuce, tomato, and onion.

n NUTRITION NOTE: *Mushrooms, especially the more exotic varieties, have been studied for their beneficial effects on immunity. They are also excellent sources of certain B vitamins.*

c COOK'S NOTE: *Make oat flour by whirling quick or regular oats in a blender until powdered. Look for brown rice flour in natural grocery stores or the specialty sections of most supermarkets.*

EACH SERVING CONTAINS

360 calories

63 g carbohydrate

8 g fat

0 mg cholesterol

13 g protein

587 mg sodium

7 g fiber

SPICY INDIAN GARBANZO BEANS

As in so many classic Indian dishes, a cooling yogurt sauce balances the spicy main event. (Without the yogurt sauce, this is vegan.)

MAKES 5 SERVINGS

2 tablespoons extra virgin olive oil

¼ cup finely minced fresh ginger

½ cup diced red onions

¼ cup diced red bell peppers

4 tablespoons Punjabi spice blend

1 cup diced tomatoes

Two 15-ounce cans garbanzo beans, rinsed and drained

½ cup vegetable stock

½ teaspoon sea salt

1 tablespoon chopped fresh cilantro

1. Heat the olive oil over medium-high heat in a large saucepan. Sauté the ginger, onions, and bell peppers until the onions are translucent. Add the spice mix and sauté to caramelize the spices. Add the tomatoes and sauté briefly.

2. Add the garbanzos and vegetable stock and cook until the liquid is absorbed and the beans are well cooked. Season with the salt and cilantro.

3. Combine the yogurt and salt in a small bowl and mix well.

4. Serve 1 cup garbanzo mixture and ¼ cup yogurt sauce over ⅓ cup brown rice.

n NUTRITION NOTE: *The ginger and turmeric that season most Indian dishes have natural antiinflammatory activity. When eaten regularly, they really do seem to help reduce aches and pains as well as diseases that have an inflammatory component, such as heart disease, insulin resistance, and autoimmune disorders.*

c COOK'S NOTE: *Look for Punjabi spice blend at Middle Eastern markets.*

FOR THE YOGURT SAUCE

1 cup nonfat plain yogurt

¼ teaspoon sea salt

1½ cups cooked brown rice

EACH SERVING CONTAINS

470 calories

77 g carbohydrate

11 g fat

1 mg cholesterol

19 g protein

708 mg sodium

14 g fiber

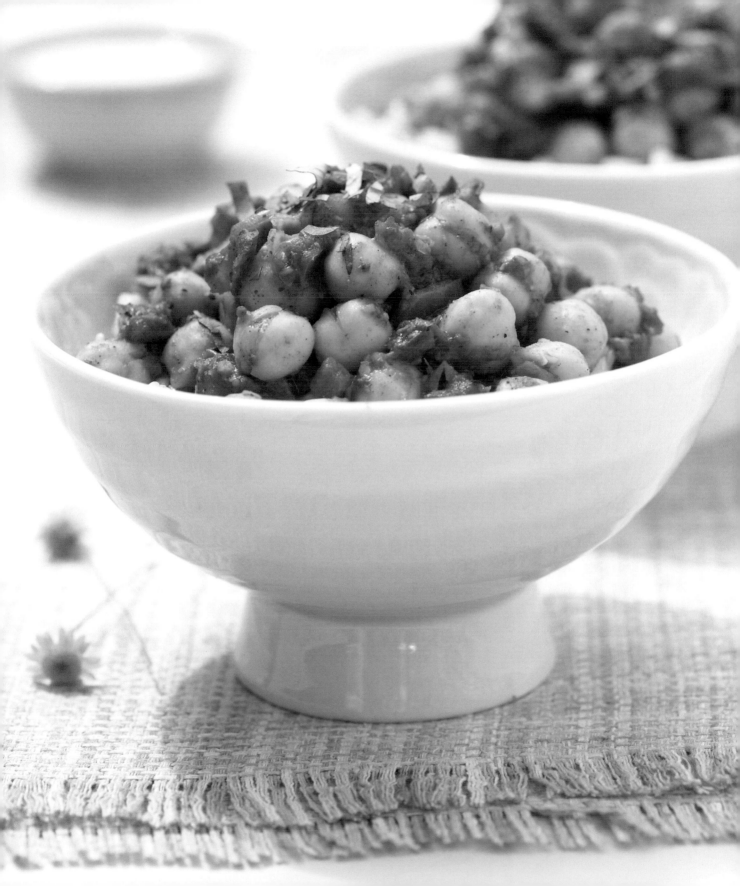

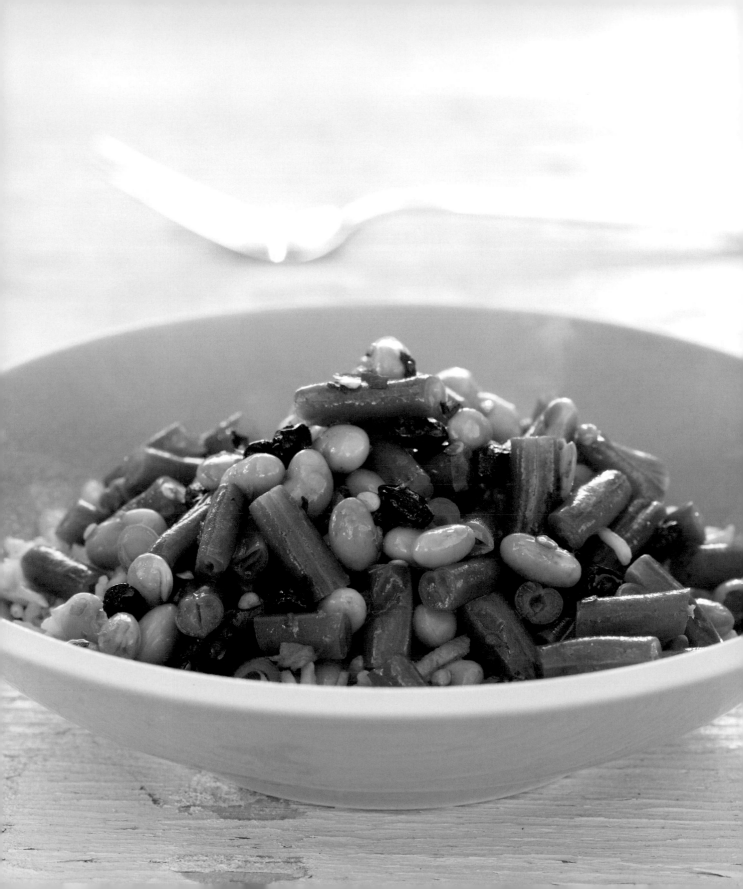

GREEN BEAN AND EDAMAME STIR-FRY

*Fermented black beans are widely available at Asian markets
in the refrigerated section of the store.*

MAKES 4 SERVINGS

1 pound green
beans, trimmed

¼ cup fermented
black beans

½ cup mirin wine

1 tablespoon brown
miso paste

½ cup chopped
scallions, both green
and white parts

1 tablespoon
minced garlic

1 tablespoon minced
fresh ginger

½ teaspoon crushed
red pepper flakes

1 cup thawed shelled
edamame (green
soybeans)

2 teaspoons extra
virgin olive oil

2 cups cooked brown rice

1. Bring 1 gallon water and ½ cup salt to a boil in a large stockpot. Blanch the green beans for 5 to 7 minutes, or until tender but not mushy. Drain and cool.

2. Combine the black beans, wine, miso, scallions, garlic, ginger, and red pepper flakes in a small bowl. Stir until miso dissolves.

3. Cut the green beans into 1-inch pieces. Combine with the edamame in a medium bowl.

4. Add the olive oil, then bean mixture to a cold wok. Turn the heat on high. Stir-fry to heat the green bean mixture, then add the black bean mixture. Cook until the sauce sticks to the beans. Remove from the wok.

5. Evenly divide the beans among four plates and serve with ½ cup brown rice.

n NUTRITION NOTE: *When you combine fresh green beans and edamame, you get a lot of fiber (11 grams!) and, even though this is a vegan meal, a respectable amount of protein.*

EACH SERVING CONTAINS

360 calories

53 g carbohydrate

7 g fat

0 mg cholesterol

16 g protein

716 mg sodium

11 g fiber

RISOTTO CAKES
WITH ROASTED VEGETABLES

Risotto Cakes—crispy on the outside, creamy on the inside—offer a satisfying textural contrast to warm roasted vegetables.

MAKES 4 SERVINGS

1 teaspoon extra virgin olive oil

⅓ cup diced yellow onions

1 teaspoon minced garlic

⅔ cup Arborio rice

½ teaspoon sea salt

1½ cups vegetable stock

1 medium zucchini, cut into ¼-inch strips

1 large portobello mushroom, cut into ¼-inch strips

1 cup peeled and sliced eggplant (¼ inch thick)

½ cup sliced red onions

1 red bell pepper, cut in half

1 teaspoon garlic granules

½ teaspoon dried basil

¼ teaspoon freshly ground black pepper

½ cup shredded mozzarella

1 cup Fresh Marinara Sauce (page 172)

1. Heat the olive oil over medium heat in a large sauté pan. Sauté the onions and garlic until the onions are translucent. Add the rice and sauté for 1 to 2 minutes. Add ¼ teaspoon of the salt and begin adding vegetable stock to the pan ½ cup at a time, stirring constantly until the liquid is absorbed. Continue adding broth ½ cup at a time until all the liquid has been absorbed and the rice is creamy. Allow the risotto to cool for 15 to 20 minutes.

2. Preheat the griddle or electric skillet to 350°F. Lightly spray the griddle with canola oil.

3. For each cake, use ⅓ cup risotto formed into a ball and flattened to ¼ inch thickness. Cook, flipping once, until crisp on each side. Place the cakes on a baking sheet. Set aside.

4. Preheat the oven to 350°.

5. Spread the zucchini, mushrooms, eggplant, onions, and bell peppers evenly on a separate baking sheet. Lightly spray with canola oil.

6. In a small bowl or cup, mix together the garlic granules, basil, the remaining ¼ teaspoon salt and pepper. Dust the vegetables evenly with 1 teaspoon of the garlic seasoning mix.

7. Roast in the oven for 20 minutes, or until slightly browned. Remove the skin from the bell pepper and slice the pepper into strips. Mix with other vegetables.

8. Evenly divide the vegetable mixture over each of the 4 risotto cakes. Top each cake with 2 tablespoons mozzarella. Dust with a pinch of the remaining garlic seasoning mix. Bake for 5 to 10 minutes, or until the cheese melts.

9. Ladle ¼ cup marinara sauce on each plate and top with one risotto cake.

250 calories

43 g carbohydrate

5 g fat

8 mg cholesterol

9 g protein

466 mg sodium

5 g fiber

EACH SERVING CONTAINS

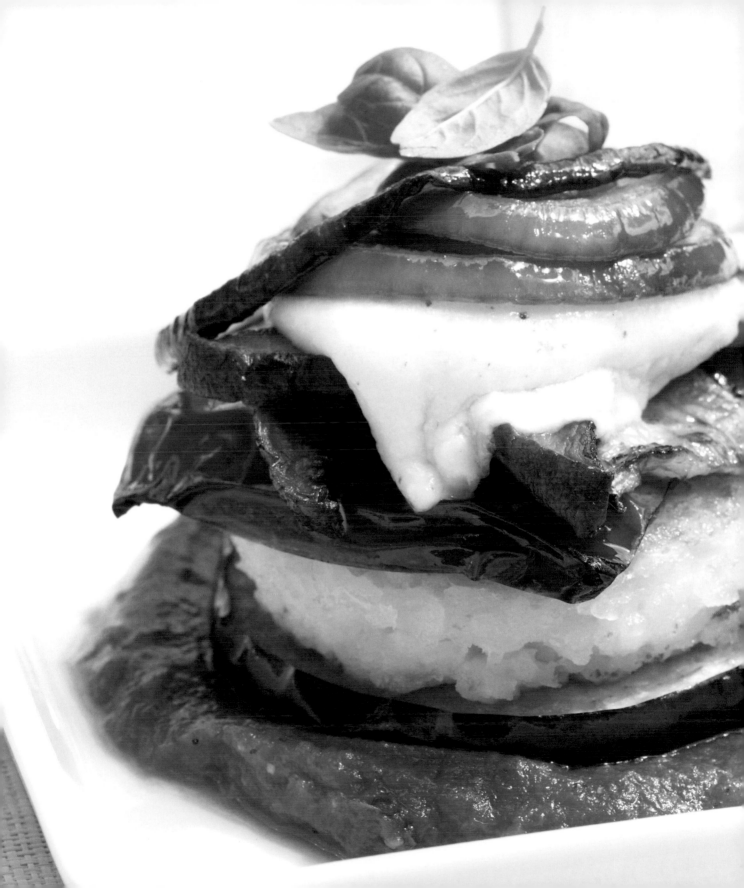

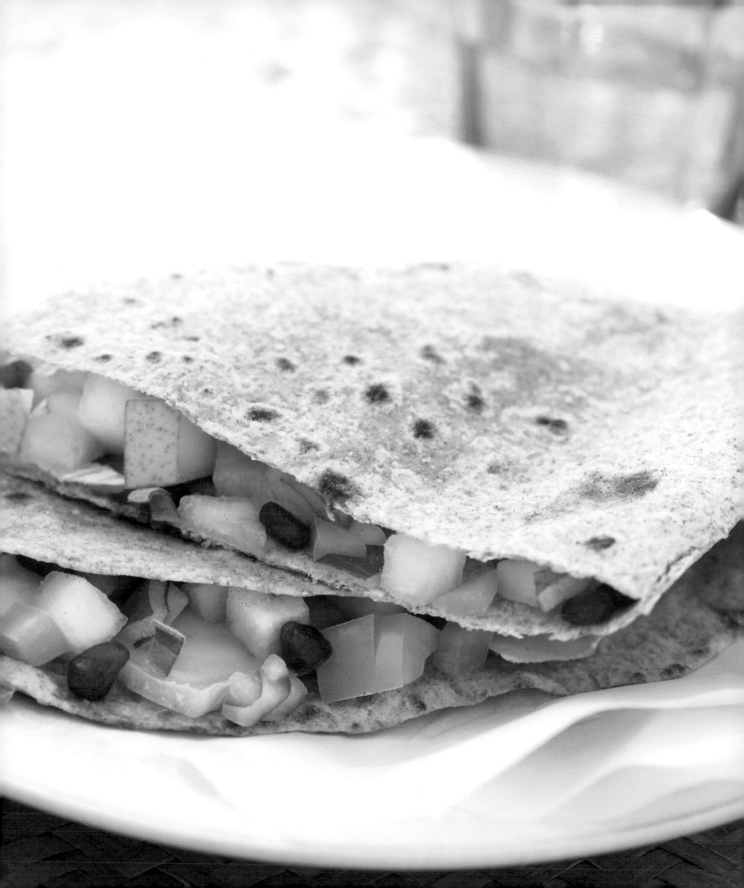

BRIE WITH PEAR
AND POMEGRANATE QUESADILLA

Pomegranate seeds add beautiful color and an antioxidant punch to this elegant variation on a Southwestern staple. Pomegranates—and sometimes just their seeds—are available in the produce sections of some supermarkets.

MAKES 6 SERVINGS

FOR THE PEAR AND
POMEGRANATE SALSA

2 Bartlett pears, cored and minced

¼ cup minced red onions

2 tablespoons minced yellow bell peppers

¼ cup pomegranate seeds

2 tablespoons fresh lemon juice

¼ teaspoon sea salt

1½ teaspoons evaporated cane juice

½ teaspoon dried sage, or 1 teaspoon fresh

6 ounces Brie

Six 10-inch whole wheat tortillas

1. Preheat a heavy-bottomed sauté pan on medium heat.

2. Combine the pears, onions, bell peppers, pomegranate seeds, lemon juice, salt, cane juice, and sage in a small bowl and mix well.

3. Slice the Brie pieces into thin slices.

4. Build the quesadillas one at a time by placing a tortilla in the preheated pan and evenly distributing 1 ounce of cheese and ¼ cup of salsa on half of each tortilla.

5. When the cheese begins to melt, using tongs or a metal spatula, fold the tortilla in half. Remove from the pan when the tortilla is slightly crisp.

n   NUTRITION NOTE: *The fiber in this delightful quesadilla comes primarily from the whole wheat tortillas, but the pear and pomegranate seeds add their share.*

c   COOK'S NOTE: *If you freeze the Brie for 15 to 20 minutes, it is much easier to slice.*

325 calories
—
40 g carbohydrate
—
14 g fat
—
28 mg cholesterol
—
11 g protein
—
476 mg sodium
—
5 g fiber

EACH SERVING CONTAINS

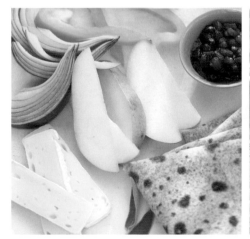
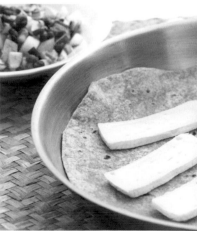

EGGPLANT GYRO

For best flavor, toast the coriander seeds and grind them with a mortar and pestle just before making the yogurt coriander sauce.

MAKES 4 SERVINGS

(continued)

FOR THE GREEK SPICE MIX

½ teaspoon sea salt

1 tablespoon dried oregano

1½ teaspoons garlic granules

1 teaspoon onion powder

1 tablespoon cornstarch

1½ teaspoons freshly ground black pepper

2 tablespoons dried parsley flakes

1½ teaspoons ground cinnamon

½ teaspoon ground nutmeg

1 teaspoon cane sugar

¼ cup unbleached all-purpose flour

2 eggs

1 medium eggplant

1 cup panko bread crumbs

1. Preheat the oven to 375°. Lightly coat a baking sheet with canola oil spray.

2. Combine the Greek spice mix and flour in a small bowl.

3. Beat the eggs in a small bowl.

4. Peel the eggplant and slice into twelve ¼-inch-thick rounds. Dredge the eggplant in the flour mixture, dip in the eggs and dredge in the bread crumbs. Place on the baking sheet. Lightly spray both sides of the coated eggplant with canola oil spray.

5. Bake for 30 minutes until golden, turning once during baking.

6. For the yogurt coriander sauce, combine the coriander, sour cream, yogurt, garlic, cilantro, and salt in a medium bowl.

7. Place 3 slices cooked eggplant in a pita half and top with a quarter each of the diced tomatoes and cucumbers. Serve each gyro with 4 tablespoons yogurt coriander sauce on the side.

¾ teaspoon
coriander seed

½ cup non-fat sour cream

½ cup low-fat plain yogurt

½ teaspoon minced garlic

1 tablespoon chopped
fresh cilantro

½ teaspoon sea salt

———————

2 whole wheat
pitas, cut in half

½ cup diced Roma
tomatoes

½ cup peeled, diced
cucumbers

n NUTRITION NOTE: *Eggplant has a meaty texture and a lot of viscous fiber, the type that lowers both cholesterol and blood sugar.*

EACH SERVING CONTAINS

270 calories

47 g carbohydrate

4 g fat

109 mg cholesterol

13 g protein

626 mg sodium

6 g fiber

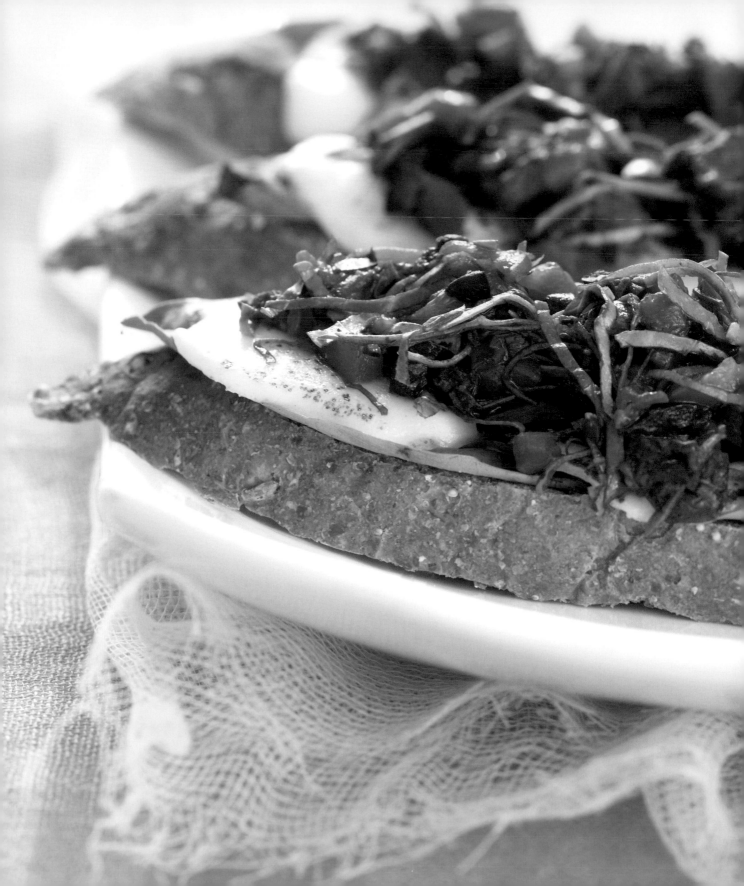

ITALIAN GRILLED CHEESE
WITH ARTICHOKE SALAD

A terrific brunch.

MAKES 4 SERVINGS

FOR THE ROASTED RED
PEPPER RELISH

½ cup minced roasted
red peppers

½ cup chopped
kalamata olives

2 tablespoons
chiffonade of arugula

1 tablespoon red
wine vinegar

¼ teaspoon sea salt

¼ teaspoon freshly
ground black pepper

8 slices whole wheat
baguette (1 to 2
inches thick)

8 fresh basil leaves

½ cup shredded
mozzarella

2 cups Artichoke
Salad (page 144)

1. Combine the red peppers and olives in a small bowl. Fold in the arugula, vinegar, salt, and pepper.

2. Lightly toast bread slices in a toaster oven. Top each slice with 1 basil leaf and 1 tablespoon mozzarella. Place in a toaster oven until the cheese melts.

3. Place 2 baguette slices on each plate and top with 2 tablespoons red pepper relish. Serve each with ½ cup artichoke salad.

n NUTRITION NOTE: *The calories in this entrée are quite low, leaving room for the addition of other menu items such as a bean soup to increase the protein of the meal.*

c COOK'S NOTE: *To increase flavor, brush the bread slices with extra virgin olive oil after toasting. (This will increase the calories and fat.)*

EACH SERVING CONTAINS

210 calories

29 g carbohydrate

7 g fat

4 mg cholesterol

8 g protein

435 mg sodium

4 g fiber

CHAPTER TWELVE | *Hooray for dessert!*

We recommend that our guests enjoy fresh fruit for dessert at least once a day. Sometimes, however, we just want something more, and our chefs have created a wide array of delectable sweet endings using reasonable amounts of wholesome sweeteners. We also limit fats and pay attention to portion sizes. At Canyon Ranch, we enjoy dessert without feeling guilty!

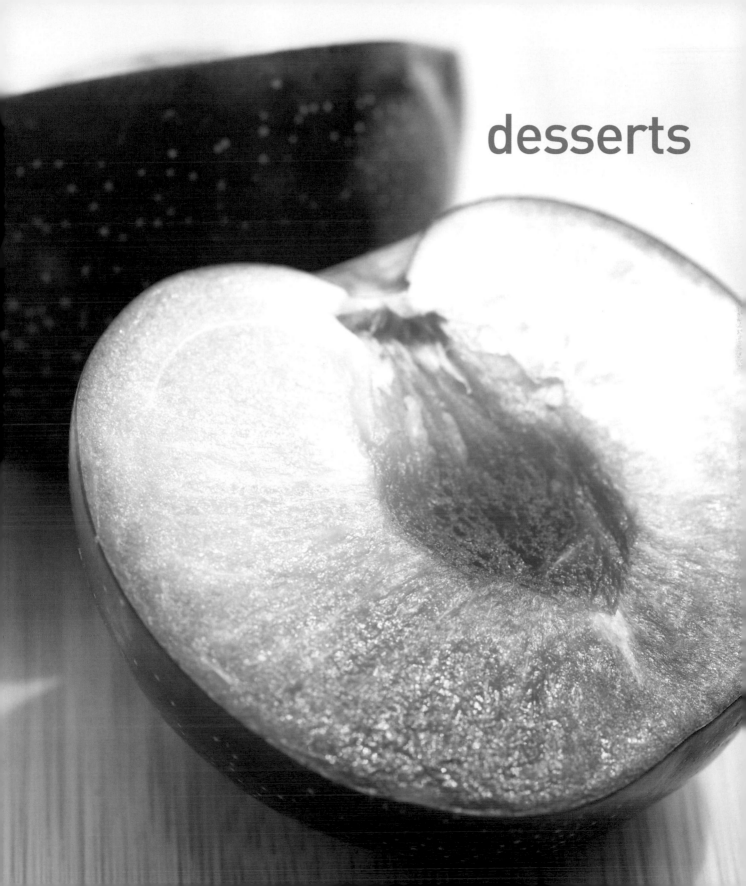

desserts

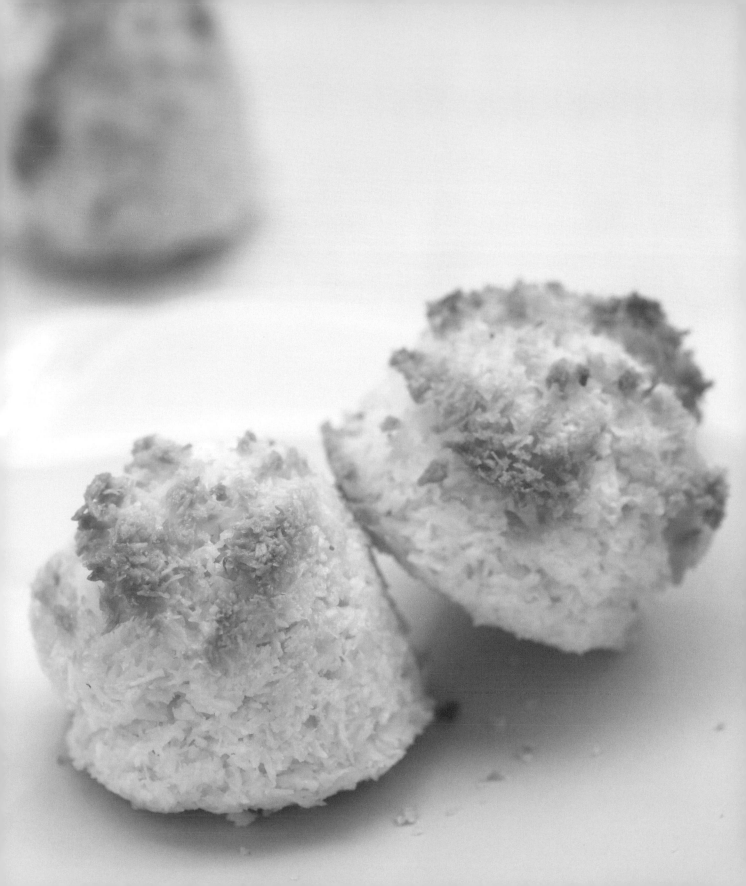

COCONUT MACAROONS

These succulent golden mouthfuls hold together well,
so they're ideal for picnics and potlucks. And they're gluten free!

MAKES 38 MACAROONS

⅓ cup water

1 cup cane sugar

2 tablespoons honey

¼ teaspoon sea salt

¾ teaspoon pure
vanilla extract

1 large egg white

4 cups unsweetened
coconut flakes

1. Preheat the oven to 350°F. Lightly coat a baking sheet with canola oil spray.

2. Combine the water, cane sugar, honey, salt, and vanilla in a small saucepan. Bring to a boil over medium-high heat. Stir for about 30 seconds or until syrup forms. Remove from the heat.

3. Combine the egg white and coconut flakes in a large bowl and mix well. Add the syrup and stir to form a dough. Place 1-tablespoon mounds about 1 inch apart on the baking sheet.

4. Bake for 8 minutes. Rotate the baking pan in the oven and bake for another 4 to 5 minutes, or until light brown and set. Transfer to a cooling rack until completely cooled. Store in a tightly sealed container.

n NUTRITION NOTE: *We are impressed that populations that use unrefined coconut oil as their main cooking fat don't have high rates of heart disease, even though coconut contains saturated fat. We rarely suggest avoiding real food, especially when it tastes as good as coconut.*

EACH SERVING CONTAINS

60 calories

6 g carbohydrate

4 g fat

0 mg cholesterol

1 g protein

21 mg sodium

0 g fiber

ALMOND MACAROONS

For shaped cookies, use a pastry bag with a large tip to make stars, swirls, or whatever shapes strike your fancy.

MAKES 36 COOKIES

2 cups almond paste

1 cup cane sugar

2 large egg whites (about ¼ cup)

1. Preheat the oven to 350°F. Lightly coat a baking sheet with canola oil spray.

2. With an electric mixer on low speed, beat the almond paste with the cane sugar in a large mixer bowl until combined, about 1 minute. Add the egg whites and beat on medium high until the mixture starts to become fluffy. Place heaping tablespoons about 1½ inches apart on the baking sheet.

3. Bake for 8 to 10 minutes, or until the cookies are set and just beginning to turn golden. Transfer to a cooling rack until completely cooled. Store in a tightly sealed container.

n NUTRITION NOTE: *The fat in these little Italian cookies comes totally from the almonds and is largely the healthy monounsaturated type.*

c COOK'S NOTE: *Almond paste is stocked by most supermarkets and specialty food stores. Look for brands without artificial ingredients.*

EACH SERVING CONTAINS

80 calories

12 g carbohydrate

3 g fat

0 mg cholesterol

1 g protein

4 mg sodium

1 g fiber

CHOCOLATE CHIP COOKIES

The legendary Canyon Ranch Chocolate Chip Cookie was created by Chef Scott Uehlein. The dough keeps for several days in the refrigerator if well wrapped, so you can have fresh cookies at a moment's notice. Yum.

MAKES 38 COOKIES

4 tablespoons (½ stick) unsalted butter, cold

⅓ cup low-fat cream cheese, cold

1 cup firmly packed light brown sugar

2 large egg yolks

¾ teaspoon pure vanilla extract

1 cup unbleached all-purpose flour

⅓ cup whole wheat flour

¾ teaspoon baking soda

½ teaspoon sea salt

One (6-ounce) package semisweet chocolate chips

1. Preheat the oven to 350°F. Lightly coat a baking sheet with canola oil spray.

2. With an electric mixer on high speed, cream the butter, cream cheese, and brown sugar. Turn the mixer to low and add the egg yolk and vanilla and mix until combined.

3. Combine the all-purpose flour, whole wheat flour, baking soda, salt, and chocolate chips in a medium bowl. Add to the butter mixture and mix by hand until combined.

4. Drop rounded heaping teaspoonfuls onto the baking sheet about 1½ inches apart.

5. Bake for 7 minutes. Lightly flatten cookies with a finger. Rotate the baking sheet in the oven and bake for 3 minutes more, or until golden. Cool on a baking sheet until the cookies are set. Transfer to a cooling rack until completely cooled. Store in a tightly sealed container.

n NUTRITION NOTE: *Dark semisweet chocolate chips provide more immune-boosting antioxidants than milk chocolate chips.*

EACH SERVING CONTAINS

85 calories

13 g carbohydrate

3 g fat

16 mg cholesterol

1 g protein

58 mg sodium

0 g fiber

OATMEAL COOKIES

Chewy and satisfying. Truly better than the original.

MAKES 38 COOKIES

4 tablespoons (½ stick)
unsalted butter, softened

⅓ cup low-fat
cream cheese

1 cup firmly packed
light brown sugar

1 large egg yolk

¾ teaspoon pure
vanilla extract

¾ cup unbleached
all-purpose flour

1½ cups regular
rolled oats

¾ teaspoon aluminum-
free baking powder

¾ teaspoon ground
cinnamon

½ teaspoon sea salt

½ cup raisins

1. Preheat the oven to 350°F. Lightly coat a baking sheet with canola oil spray.

2. With an electric mixer on high speed, cream the butter, cream cheese, and brown sugar. Turn the mixer to low and add the egg yolk and vanilla and mix until combined.

3. Combine the all-purpose flour, rolled oats, baking powder, cinnamon, salt, and raisins in a medium bowl. Add to the butter mixture and mix by hand until combined.

4. Drop rounded heaping teaspoonfuls onto the baking sheet about 1½ inches apart.

5. Bake for 7 minutes. Lightly flatten the cookies with a finger. Rotate the baking sheet in the oven and bake for 4 minutes more, or until golden. Cool on a baking sheet until the cookies are set. Transfer to a cooling rack until completely cooled. Store in a tightly sealed container.

n   **NUTRITION NOTE:** *The only revision our chefs made to this great oatmeal raisin cookie recipe is the substitution of low-fat cream cheese for some of the butter. Otherwise, they are the real thing, complete with healthy oats and raisins.*

EACH SERVING CONTAINS

75 calories

13 g carbohydrate

2 g fat

15 mg cholesterol

1 g protein

49 mg sodium

1 g fiber

DOUBLE CHOCOLATE BROWNIES

These are lower in fat and higher in fiber than most brownies, but they're still a real chocolate fix.

MAKES 16 SERVINGS

¾ cup semisweet chocolate chips

4 tablespoons (¼ cup) unsalted butter

¼ cup nonfat sour cream

¾ cup firmly packed light brown sugar

1 teaspoon pure vanilla extract

2 large eggs

¼ cup unbleached all-purpose flour

¼ cup whole wheat flour

1 tablespoon unsweetened cocoa powder

¼ teaspoon aluminum-free baking powder

¼ teaspoon sea salt

1.   Preheat the oven to 325°F. Lightly coat an 8-inch square baking pan with canola oil spray.

2.   Melt the chocolate chips, butter, and sour cream in a medium saucepan over low heat. Remove from the heat. Stir in the brown sugar and vanilla. Stir in the eggs one at a time. Stir in the all-purpose flour, whole wheat flour, cocoa, baking powder, and salt and mix well. Pour the batter into the prepared pan.

3.   Bake for 20 to 25 minutes, or until a toothpick inserted into the center comes out clean. Cool completely on a wire rack. Cut into 16 servings. Store in a covered container.

n   NUTRITION NOTE: *The flavonols in chocolate are particularly powerful antioxidants and cell-signaling regulators. One recent study using a cocoa-rich beverage showed beneficial effects on the appearance and feel of skin.*

EACH SERVING CONTAINS

140 calories

17 g carbohydrate

7 g fat

35 mg cholesterol

2 g protein

53 mg sodium

Trace fiber

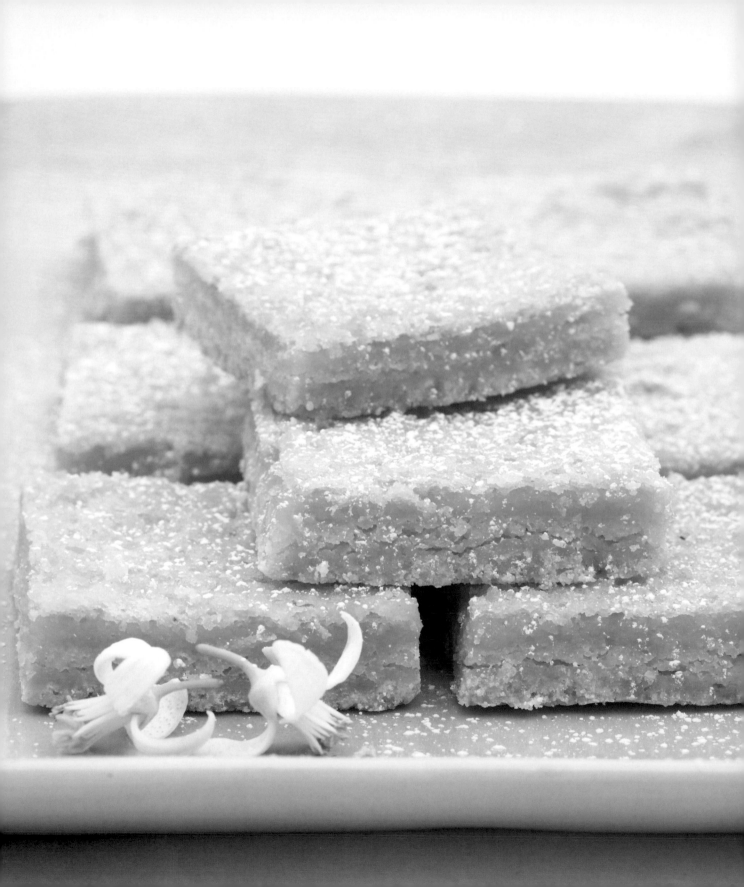

LEMON BARS

These classic bars are elegant and quick and easy to transport right in their baking pan. Lovely with tea.

MAKES 32 SERVINGS

FOR THE CRUST

½ cup plus 3 tablespoons unsalted butter, at room temperature

⅓ cup cane sugar

1 tablespoon minced lemon zest

1⅔ cups unbleached all-purpose flour

———

1½ cups cane sugar

¼ cup unbleached all-purpose flour

½ teaspoon aluminum-free baking powder

5 large eggs

3 tablespoons minced lemon zest

⅔ cup fresh lemon juice (approximately 4 medium lemons)

1½ teaspoons pure vanilla extract

1. Preheat the oven to 350°F.

2. Blend the butter, cane sugar, and lemon peel in a food processor. Gradually add in flour to form soft crumbs.

3. Evenly press the mixture into a 9 x 13-inch baking pan to form a crust. Bake for 15 minutes. Set aside.

4. Stir together the cane sugar, flour, and baking powder in a small bowl.

5. With an electric mixer on high speed, beat the eggs well in a large bowl. Reduce the speed to low. Gradually add the flour mixture.

6. Stir in the lemon zest, lemon juice, and vanilla. Pour the lemon mixture over the baked crust.

7. Bake for 20 minutes, or until the top is golden around the edges. Allow to cool for at least 30 minutes. Cut into 32 squares, about 2 x 1½ inches. Store wrapped in a refrigerator.

n **NUTRITION NOTE:** *We didn't feel the need to make any major modifications to this recipe, but we're careful to cut the bars into fairly small portions. We also recommend using organic citrus when you plan to use the peel.*

EACH SERVING CONTAINS

120 calories

18 g carbohydrate

5 g fat

45 mg cholesterol

2 g protein

24 mg sodium

Trace fiber

ALMOND LEMON TART

Almond and cherry is one of the great flavor combinations.

MAKES 16 SERVINGS

FOR THE CRUST

1 cup unbleached
all-purpose flour

½ teaspoon sea salt

½ teaspoon evaporated
cane juice

2 tablespoons cold
unsalted butter, cubed

2 to 4 tablespoons ice water

———

¾ cup chopped almonds

3 tablespoons almond paste

⅓ cup evaporated cane juice

½ teaspoon fresh lemon juice

2 tablespoons lemon zest,
minced (about 3 lemons)

2 large eggs

⅓ cup buttermilk

½ teaspoon pure
almond extract

½ teaspoon pure lemon extract

FOR THE CHERRY COMPOTE

¾ cup fresh cherries, pitted

3 tablespoons water

1 tablespoon fresh lime juice

2 tablespoons evaporated
cane juice

1 teaspoon cornstarch

1 teaspoon Grand Marnier

1. Preheat the oven to 350°F.

2. Combine the flour, salt, and cane juice in a medium bowl and mix well. Cut the butter into the flour, using a pastry cutter, until the butter is the size of small peas. Add the water, 1 tablespoon at a time, mixing gently with a fork after each addition. The dough will begin to form a ball when enough water has been added. Gather the dough with dry hands and form into a ball. Let rest for 5 minutes.

3. On a lightly floured surface, roll out the dough to form a 12-inch circle. Lightly press into a 10-inch tart pan.

4. Place the almonds, almond paste, and cane juice in a food processor and process until the nuts are finely ground, taking care not to liquefy. Stop the food processor to add the lemon juice, lemon zest, eggs, buttermilk, almond extract, and lemon extract. Process until well blended. Pour the mixture into the prepared tart pan.

5. Bake for 20 to 25 minutes until set. Cool completely on a wire rack.

6. Combine the cherries, water, lime juice, and cane juice in a medium saucepan over medium heat. Bring to a boil. Reduce the heat to medium low and simmer for 15 minutes, stirring occasionally.

7. Combine the cornstarch and Grand Marnier in a small bowl.

8. Stir the cornstarch mixture into the cherries and return to a boil. Cook for 1 minute while stirring. Reduce the heat to low and simmer until thickened, about 4 minutes. Remove from the heat and allow to cool.

9. Cut the tart into 16 pieces. Serve each slice topped with 1 teaspoon cherry compote.

EACH SERVING CONTAINS

135 calories

16 g carbohydrate

6 g fat

32 mg cholesterol

4 g protein

67 mg sodium

1 g fiber

> **NUTRITION NOTE:** *Once again, the trick for healthy desserts is including wholesome ingredients such as fruit and nuts and careful portioning.*

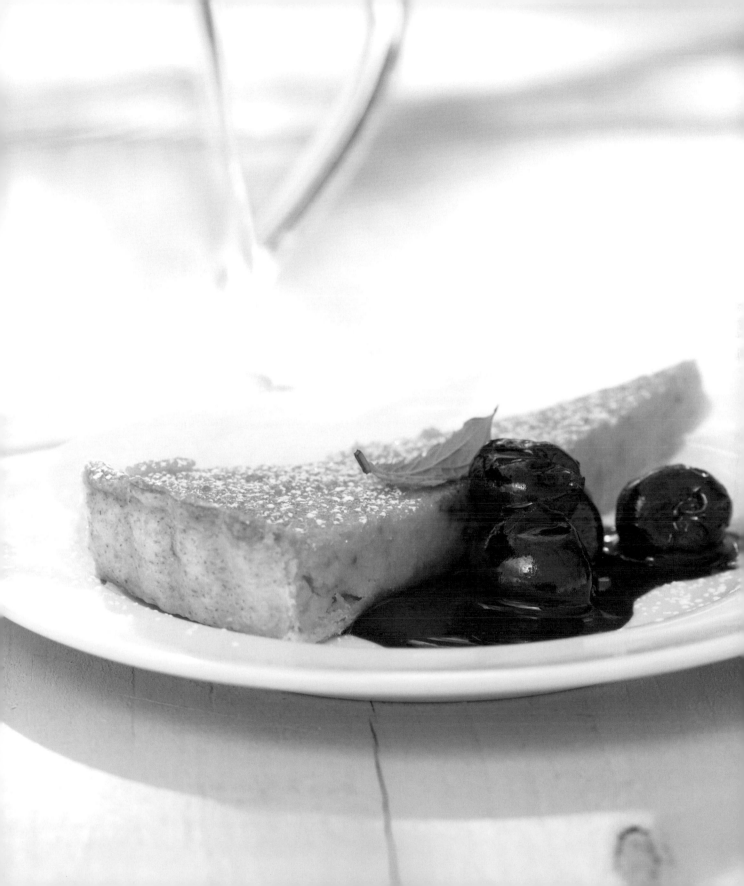

SWEET POTATO TARTLETS
WITH BLUE CORN CRUST

*These delightful little desserts showcase the
goodness of the native foods of the Southwest.*

MAKES 12 SERVINGS

FOR THE BLUE CORN CRUST

**2¼ cups blue corn cereal
flakes (available in natural-
foods supermarkets)**

¼ cup toasted pecans

1 tablespoon cane sugar

**1 tablespoon unsalted
butter, melted**

**1 tablespoon egg white (about
half a large egg white)**

**¾ pound sweet potatoes, peeled
and large diced (about 1 large)**

3 tablespoons unsalted butter

**⅓ cup firmly packed
light brown sugar**

**3 large egg whites
(6 tablespoons)**

¼ teaspoon ground nutmeg

½ teaspoon ground cinnamon

1 teaspoon pure vanilla extract

⅛ teaspoon sea salt

FOR THE SWEETENED
WHIPPED CREAM

¼ cup heavy cream

1 teaspoon cane sugar

½ teaspoon pure vanilla extract

1. Preheat the oven to 350°F. Lightly spray a 12-cup muffin pan with canola oil spray.

2. Grind the corn flakes, pecans, and cane sugar in a food processor. Add the butter and egg whites and mix until well combined. Firmly press 1½ tablespoons corn flake mixture into the bottom of each muffin cup to form a crust.

3. Steam the sweet potatoes in a large covered saucepan for 50 minutes until soft. On medium speed, break up the sweet potatoes into small pieces in the bowl of an electric mixer fitted with a paddle attachment. Add the butter and continue mixing. Add the brown sugar, egg whites, nutmeg, cinnamon, vanilla, and salt and continue mixing until smooth. Place 2 tablespoons sweet potato mixture in each muffin cup.

4. Bake for 20 to 25 minutes, or until set or a toothpick inserted into the center comes out clean. Cool on a wire rack for 20 minutes. Carefully remove the tartlets from the muffin pan by running a knife along the edges of the crusts. Cool completely on the wire rack.

5. Just prior to serving, combine the cream, cane sugar, and vanilla in a small chilled bowl. Whip with a whisk until soft peaks form.

6. Serve each sweet potato tartlet with 2 teaspoons whipped cream.

n   NUTRITION NOTE: *Vegetables for dessert! Get them any way you can.*

EACH SERVING CONTAINS

175 calories

24 g carbohydrate

7 g fat

17 mg cholesterol

2 g protein

75 mg sodium

2 g fiber

KEY LIME PIE

A scrumptious classic that's fantastically easy to make. If you can't find Key limes, you can use standard limes for a slightly different but still lovely result.

MAKES 12 SERVINGS

1 cup crushed
graham crackers

4 large egg yolks

½ cup fresh Key lime juice
(about 10 Key limes)

One 14-ounce
can sweetened
condensed milk

1.   Preheat the oven to 325°F.

2.   Spread the graham cracker crumbs in the bottom of a 9-inch pie pan. Wet with a little water and press the graham crackers firmly into the pie pan to form a crust.

3.   With an electric mixer on high speed, beat the egg yolks and lime juice in a large bowl until lemon yellow in color and doubled in volume. Add the condensed milk and mix on low speed until just well combined. Do not over-mix. Pour the mixture into the prepared crust.

4.   Bake for 15 to 20 minutes, or until a knife inserted into the center comes out clean. Let cool for 30 minutes and refrigerate for 1 hour or until set before serving.

n   NUTRITION NOTE: *A graham cracker crust made without extra sugar and melted butter saves loads of calories.*

EACH SERVING CONTAINS

170 calories

25 g carbohydrate

6 g fat

128 mg cholesterol

5 g protein

89 mg sodium

0 g fiber

NEW ENGLAND APPLE PIE

As good as Mom's, but created by our pastry chef at Canyon Ranch in Lenox, Massachusetts.

MAKES 12 SERVINGS

FOR THE CRUST

2 cups unbleached all-purpose flour

½ teaspoon sea salt

⅓ cup evaporated cane juice

8 tablespoons cold unsalted butter, cubed

12 tablespoons ice water

4 Red Delicious apples, cored, peeled, and thinly sliced

4 Granny Smith apples, cored, peeled, and thinly sliced

½ cup evaporated cane juice

1½ teaspoons ground cinnamon

1 large egg white (about 2 tablespoons), lightly beaten

1. Preheat the oven to 350°F.

2. Place flour in a medium bowl. Add salt and evaporated cane juice and mix well. Cut the butter into the flour, using a pastry cutter, until the butter is the size of small peas. Add the water, 1 tablespoon at a time, mixing gently with a fork after each addition. The dough will begin to form a ball when enough water has been added. Gather the dough with dry hands and form into a ball. Let rest for 5 minutes.

3. Divide the dough in half. On a lightly floured surface, roll out each half into a circle to fit a 10-inch pie pan. Line the pie pan with one circle of dough. Evenly spread the apple slices over the dough.

4. Mix the cane juice and cinnamon in a small bowl or cup. Sprinkle the mixture over the apples.

5. Place the remaining circle of dough over the top of the pie and pinch the edges together. Cut 5 slits in the center of the top crust. Brush the crust with the egg white.

6. Bake for 40 to 50 minutes, or until the crust is golden and the filling is bubbling. Cool for 30 minutes before serving.

n NUTRITION NOTE: *Apples are a leading source of quercetin, a bioflavonoid known to counter inflammation.*

c COOK'S NOTE: *In our kitchens, we use a mandoline to slice apples easily and uniformly.*

EACH SERVING CONTAINS

175 calories

33 g carbohydrate

4 g fat

10 mg cholesterol

2 g protein

46 mg sodium

2 g fiber

SPICE CAKES WITH APPLE COMPOTE

An autumn classic.

MAKES 18 INDIVIDUAL CAKES

1 cup unbleached
all-purpose flour

¾ cup evaporated cane juice

1 tablespoon aluminum-
free baking powder

1 teaspoon ground cinnamon

½ teaspoon baking soda

⅛ teaspoon sea salt

¼ teaspoon ground cloves

2 large eggs

1¾ cups unsweetened
applesauce

¼ cup canola oil

FOR THE APPLE COMPOTE

6 cups peeled, cored,
and chopped Red
Delicious apples (6 to
7 medium apples)

½ teaspoon ground cinnamon

½ cup firmly packed
light brown sugar

FOR THE SWEETENED
WHIPPED CREAM

¾ cup heavy cream

¼ cup confectioners' sugar

1 teaspoon pure
vanilla extract

Fresh mint sprigs

1. Preheat the oven to 350°F. Lightly coat 18 muffin cups with canola oil spray.

2. Sift together the flour, cane juice, baking powder, cinnamon, baking soda, salt, and cloves in a large bowl. Stir in the eggs, applesauce, and canola oil until well combined. Spoon ¼ cup batter into each muffin cup.

3. Bake for 15 to 20 minutes, or until a toothpick inserted in the center comes out clean. Cool for 10 minutes, or until the cake pulls away from the sides of the pan.

4. Combine the apples, cinnamon, and brown sugar in a large saucepan. Cook over medium heat for 5 to 10 minutes, or until soft but not mushy. Set aside.

5. With an electric mixer on high speed, whip the heavy cream, confectioners' sugar, and vanilla in a medium chilled bowl until soft peaks form.

6. Place one cake on each plate, and top with 2 tablespoons apple compote and a heaping teaspoon whipped cream. Garnish with a mint sprig.

n NUTRITION NOTE: *Replacing some of the oil with applesauce cuts calories and results in a wonderfully moist cake. This is an old technique worth keeping.*

EACH SERVING CONTAINS

175 calories

28 g carbohydrate

7 g fat

36 mg cholesterol

2 g protein

144 mg sodium

2 g fiber

WARM CHOCOLATE CAKES
WITH COFFEE CRÈME ANGLAISE

Small, sinfully rich-tasting little cakes topped with a fabulous sauce.

MAKES 8 SERVINGS

2 large eggs, separated

¼ cup evaporated cane juice

½ cup chopped bittersweet chocolate

⅓ cup nonfat plain yogurt

FOR THE COFFEE CRÈME ANGLAISE

1 cup 2% milk

¼ cup evaporated cane juice

½ vanilla bean

¼ cup brewed coffee

3 large egg yolks

1. Lightly coat eight 4-ounce individual aluminum molds or ramekins with canola oil spray and dust with confectioners' sugar.

2. Combine the egg yolks with 1 tablespoon of the evaporated cane juice in a small bowl. Beat with a whisk until very pale and thick.

3. With an electric mixer on high speed, beat the egg whites in a medium bowl until foamy. Add the cane juice, 1 teaspoon at a time, beating on high until stiff peaks form.

4. Melt the chocolate in the top of a double boiler. Remove from the heat and stir in the yogurt. While stirring, add a small amount of the chocolate mixture to the egg yolk mixture to temper the yolks. Add the yolks to the chocolate mixture and mix well. Carefully fold in the egg whites. Spoon ¼ cup into each mold and refrigerate for at least 30 minutes.

5. Combine milk, cane juice, vanilla bean, and coffee in a large saucepan. Bring to a simmer over medium heat, stirring constantly. Immediately remove vanilla bean, cut it open lengthwise with a sharp knife, and scrape the seed paste into the milk mixture. Stir. Discard the bean.

6. Place the egg yolks in a small bowl. While stirring, add about ½ cup of the hot milk mixture to the egg yolks to temper. Add the yolks to simmering milk. Cook for 1 more minute. Remove from the heat and let cool. When the crème anglaise reaches room temperature, cover and refrigerate for at least 1 hour.

7. Preheat the oven to 325°F.

8. Remove the molds from the refrigerator. Bake for 12 to 15 mintes, or until the cakes spring back when lightly touched. Cool for 2 to 3 minutes.

9. Invert the cakes onto eight plates and serve each with 2 tablespoons crème anglaise.

n **NUTRITION NOTE:** *We are so happy to tell you again how healthy chocolate is. Pick a high-quality dark chocolate with a relatively high percentage of cocoa solids.*

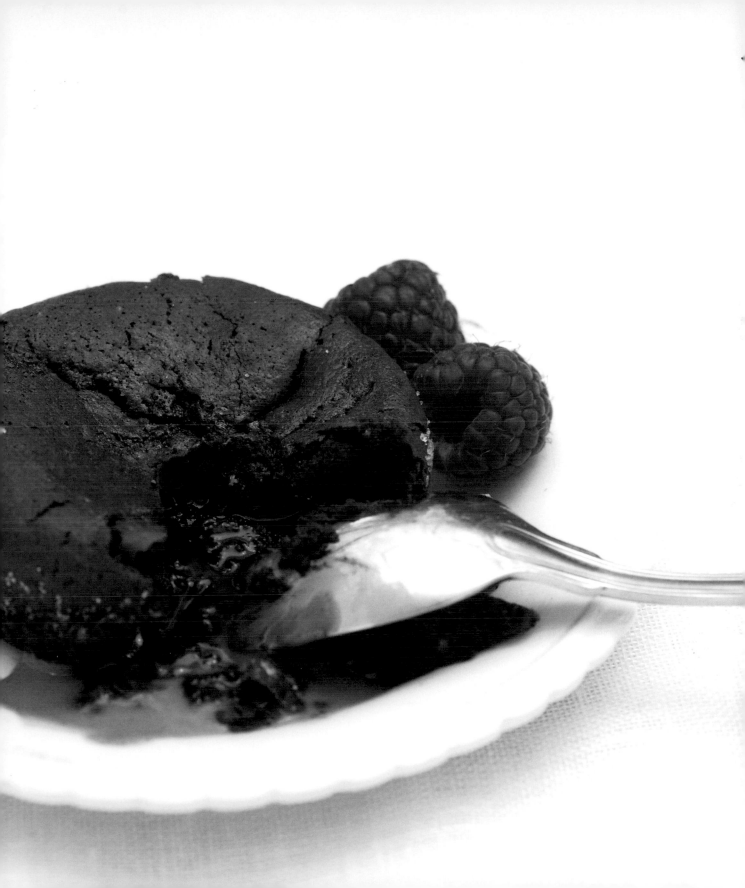

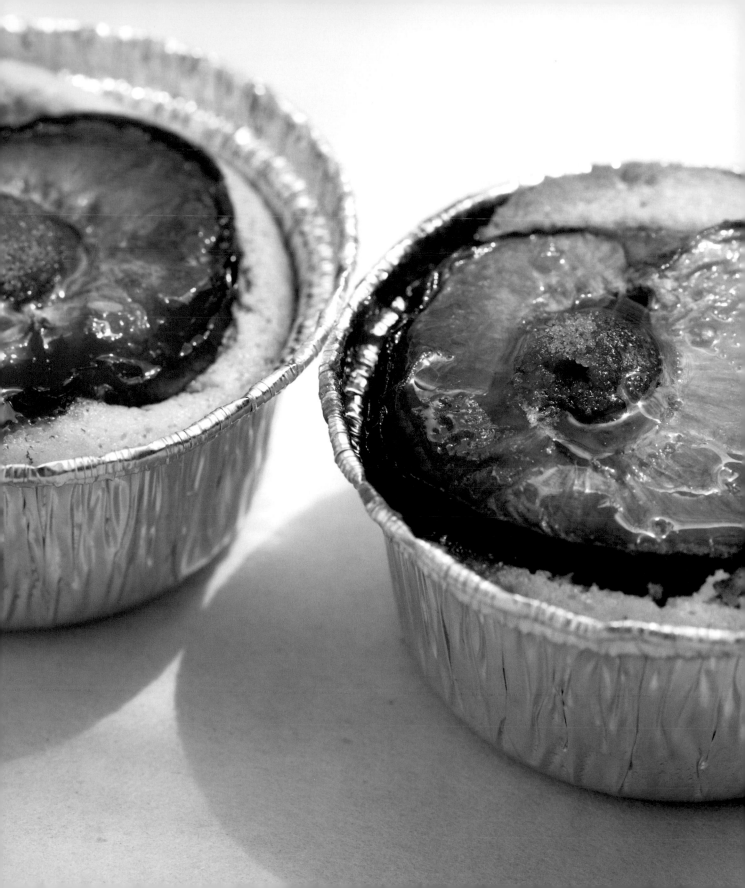

ALSATIAN PLUM CAKES

Dense and lovely marzipan cake cradles warm, juicy fruit in these delightful individual desserts. You can substitute apricots for the plums, if you like.

MAKES 6 SERVINGS

2 tablespoons (⅛ cup) unsalted butter

¼ cup almond paste

2 tablespoons nonfat sour cream

1 large egg

1 teaspoon pure vanilla extract

¼ cup unbleached all-purpose flour

4 tablespoons evaporated cane juice

3 fresh plums

2 tablespoons firmly packed light brown sugar

1. Preheat the oven to 350°F.

2. Melt the butter in a small saucepan over low heat.

3. Cream together the butter, almond paste, and sour cream in a medium bowl. Scrape down the sides of the bowl. Stir in the egg and vanilla. Gradually stir in the flour and cane juice. Set aside.

4. Cut the plums in half and remove the pits.

5. Lightly spray six 4-ounce aluminum cups or ramekins with canola oil. Scoop 3 tablespoons almond paste mixture into each ramekin. Place ½ plum cut side up in the center of the paste, and top each with 1 teaspoon brown sugar.

6. Bake for 30 to 35 minutes, or until the plum is soft and a toothpick inserted in the center of the cake comes out clean. Cool a minimum of 15 mintes and serve.

n NUTRITION NOTE: *Choose a "clean" nonfat sour cream with no thickeners or unnecessary ingredients, organic if possible.*

EACH SERVING CONTAINS

170 calories

24 g carbohydrate

7 g fat

53 mg cholesterol

3 g protein

18 mg sodium

1 g fiber

LINZER CAKE

MAKES 12 SERVINGS

½ cup whole wheat
pastry flour

¼ cup unbleached
all-purpose flour

½ teaspoon aluminum-
free baking powder

½ teaspoon sea salt

½ cup toasted hazelnuts

2 tablespoons 2% milk

2 tablespoons canola oil

1 teaspoon pure
almond extract

4 large eggs

¾ cup evaporated
cane juice

⅓ cup raspberry
preserves

1 tablespoon
confectioners' sugar

Fresh raspberries
(optional)

165 calories
—
23 g carbohydrate
—
7 g fat
—
71 mg cholesterol
—
4 g protein
—
124 mg sodium
—
2 g fiber

EACH SERVING CONTAINS

1. Preheat the oven to 325°F. Lightly coat two 9-inch round cake pans with canola oil spray and dust with all-purpose flour.

2. Whisk together the whole wheat flour, all-purpose flour, baking powder, and salt in a small bowl. Set aside.

3. Grind the hazelnuts in a food processor until finely ground. (Do not overgrind; you don't want nut butter.) Add the milk, canola oil, and almond extract and pulse to combine.

4. Separate the eggs, putting the whites in a medium bowl and the egg yolks in a large bowl.

5. With an electric mixer on high speed, beat the egg whites until soft peaks form. Beat in ¼ cup of the cane juice in a slow, steady stream. Continue beating until stiff peaks form.

6. Clean the beaters, then beat the egg yolks with the remaining ½ cup cane juice until pale yellow in color and doubled in volume.

7. Gently stir the hazelnut mixture into the egg yolk mixture. Slowly add the flour mixture and gently stir until mixed. Fold 1 cup egg whites into the batter until combined. Gently fold the remaining whites into the batter using long strokes until no white streaks remain. Divide the batter between the two prepared cake pans.

8. Bake for 18 to 20 minutes, or until lightly browned and a toothpick inserted in the center comes out clean. Cool on wire racks for 10 to 15 minutes. Remove from the pans and place on wire racks to cool completely.

9. Place one layer top side down on a plate. Spread raspberry preserves evenly over the top. Cover with the second layer top side down. Sift the confectioners' sugar over the top. Decorate with raspberries.

_n_ **NUTRITION NOTE:** _A serving of cake with 2 grams of fiber shouldn't be taken for granted. This recipe gets that from whole wheat pastry flour, nuts, and raspberries._

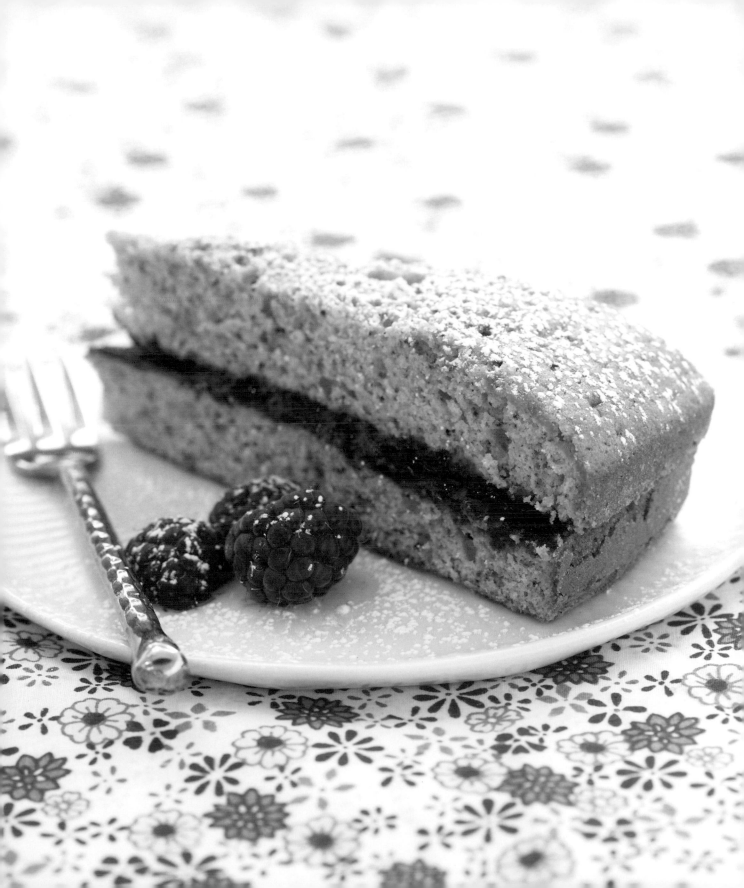

PEAR CURRANT CAKE

Extra virgin olive oil, unsweetened applesauce, and ripe fruit make this cake wonderfully moist—and healthful!

MAKES 16 SERVINGS

¼ cup extra virgin olive oil

¾ cup unsweetened applesauce

4 large eggs

1 tablespoon pure vanilla extract

¾ cup evaporated cane juice

⅓ cup white grape juice

¾ cup unbleached all-purpose flour

¾ cup pastry flour

½ cup whole wheat flour

2 teaspoons aluminum-free baking powder

1 tablespoon ground cinnamon

1 teaspoon ground cardamom

1 pound Bartlett pears, peeled, cored, and thinly sliced

¼ cup dried currants

1. Preheat the oven to 350°F. Lightly coat a 9-inch Bundt pan with canola oil spray and dust with all-purpose flour.

2. Combine the olive oil, applesauce, eggs, vanilla, cane juice, and white grape juice in a large bowl and mix until just combined.

3. Sift together the all-purpose flour, pastry flour, whole wheat flour, baking powder, cinnamon, and cardamon in a medium bowl.

4. Add the flour mixture to the applesauce and mix well. Stir in the pears and currants. Pour the batter into the Bundt pan.

5. Bake for 55 to 60 minutes, or until a knife inserted in the center comes out clean. Cool and cut into 16 slices.

EACH SERVING CONTAINS

170 calories

29 g carbohydrate

5 g fat

53 mg cholesterol

4 g protein

80 mg sodium

2 g fiber

MOCHA POUND CAKE

Coffee and chocolate—and delicious.

MAKES 20 SERVINGS

⅓ cup unsalted butter, softened

¼ cup low-fat cream cheese

¾ cup cane sugar

1 large egg

1¾ cups unbleached all-purpose flour

½ cup unsweetened natural cocoa powder

2 teaspoons aluminum-free baking powder

½ teaspoon baking soda

½ teaspoon sea salt

¾ cup buttermilk

1 teaspoon pure vanilla extract

¼ cup brewed coffee

⅓ cup fruit-juice-sweetened, low-fat chocolate sauce (available in natural-foods supermarkets)

FOR THE GANACHE

⅓ cup nonfat evaporated milk

⅔ cup semisweet chocolate chips

1. Preheat the oven to 325°F. Lightly coat a 9-inch Bundt pan with canola oil spray and dust with flour.

2. With an electric mixer on low speed, cream the butter, cream cheese, and cane sugar in a large mixer bowl until the cane sugar is dissolved. Add the egg and mix until combined.

3. Sift together the flour, cocoa, baking powder, baking soda, and salt in a medium bowl.

4. Combine the buttermilk, vanilla, coffee, and chocolate sauce in another bowl.

5. Add one-half the flour mixture to the butter mixture and mix on low speed for 30 seconds. Add one-half the buttermilk mixture to the butter mixture and mix until just combined. Add the remaining flour mixture and mix for 30 seconds. Add the remaining buttermilk mixture and mix briefly until smooth. Pour the batter into the Bundt pan.

6. Bake for 30 to 35 minutes, or until a toothpick inserted in the center comes out clean. Cool for 15 minutes on a wire rack. Invert the cake onto a large plate, remove the pan, and let cool completely.

7. For the ganache, heat the milk over medium heat in a medium saucepan until almost boiling. Stir in the chocolate chips. Cover, turn off the heat, and let sit for 5 minutes until the chocolate melts, then whip well with a wire whisk.

8. Pour the warm ganache over the top of the cake. Cut into 20 slices.

EACH SERVING CONTAINS

170 calories

26 g carbohydrate

7 g fat

21 mg cholesterol

3 g protein

156 mg sodium

1 g fiber

RASPBERRY CHOCOLATE ANGEL FOOD CAKE

An angel food cake with pizzazz.

MAKES 20 SERVINGS

⅓ cup cocoa powder

¾ cup unbleached all-purpose flour

1⅓ cups cane sugar

¼ teaspoon sea salt

1½ cups egg whites (12 egg whites)

1 teaspoon cream of tartar

½ teaspoon almond extract

½ teaspoon pure vanilla extract

FOR THE RASPBERRIES

4 cups fresh or frozen raspberries, slightly thawed

¼ cup cane sugar

FOR THE SWEETENED WHIPPED CREAM

1½ cups heavy cream

1 tablespoon cane sugar

Seeds scraped from ½ vanilla bean

1. Preheat the oven to 325°F. Lightly coat a 9-inch tube or Bundt pan with canola oil spray.

2. Whisk together the cocoa powder, flour, ⅓ cup of the cane sugar, and salt in a small bowl.

3. With an electric mixer on medium low, beat the egg whites with the cream of tartar in a large bowl until the whites are frothy. Slowly add the remaining 1 cup of the cane sugar, the almond extract, and vanilla. Increase the speed to high and beat until firm peaks form. Stop the mixer and slowly sift the cocoa mixture over the egg whites. Fold together by hand. Pour the batter into the tube pan.

4. Bake for 40 to 50 minutes, or until slightly resistant to the touch or until a toothpick inserted in the center comes out clean. Cool on a wire rack. Use a knife to loosen the sides and bottom of the cake. Cool about 1 hour until the sides of the cake come away from the pan. Cut into 20 slices.

5. Combine the raspberries and cane juice in a medium bowl and set aside for 15 to 20 minutes until juicy and well blended.

6. With a wire whisk, whip together the heavy cream, cane sugar, and scraped vanilla seeds in a chilled bowl.

7. Serve each slice of cake with 1 tablespoon raspberries and 1 tablespoon sweetened whipped cream.

EACH SERVING CONTAINS

145 calories

25 g carbohydrate

4 g fat

12 mg cholesterol

3 g protein

58 mg sodium

3 g fiber

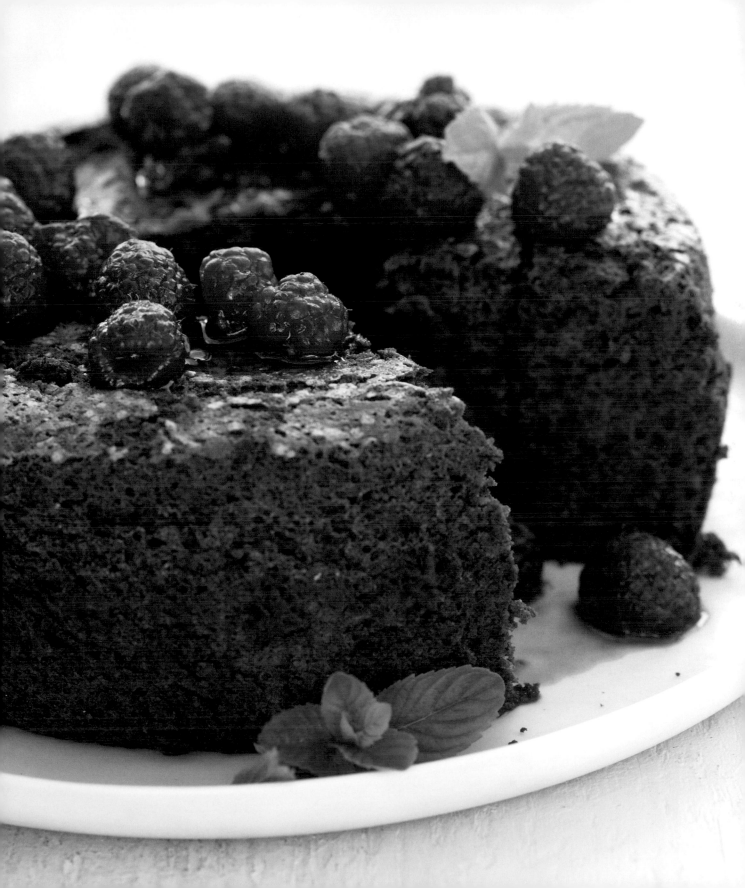

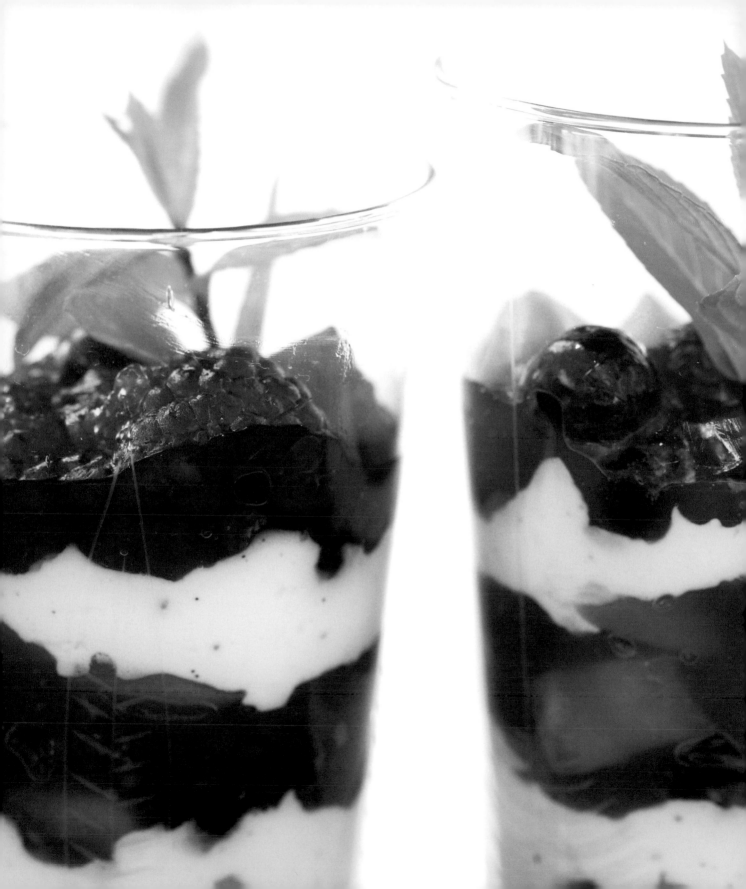

SUMMER FRUIT PARFAIT

All hail midsummer and its bounty of fresh fruit!
Makes a great brunch starter or dessert.

MAKES 8 SERVINGS

3 tablespoons cane sugar

¼ cup cranberry
nectar or juice

1 cup diced peaches

1 cup raspberries

1 cup blueberries

1 cup blackberries

FOR THE CREAMY
VANILLA SAUCE

1 cup plain Greek-
style yogurt

3 tablespoons low-
fat cream cheese

3 tablespoons pure
maple syrup

2 teaspoons cane sugar

½ teaspoon pure
vanilla extract

Seeds scraped from
¼ vanilla bean

1. Combine the cane sugar, cranberry nectar, peaches, raspberries, blue-berries, and blackberries in a large bowl. Lightly crush the fruit while mixing the ingredients together until the cane juice is dissolved.

2. Combine the yogurt, cream cheese, maple syrup, cane sugar, vanilla, and scraped vanilla seeds in a blender and blend until well mixed.

3. Layer ¼ cup fruit with 3 tablespoons vanilla sauce in each of eight small parfait glasses.

EACH SERVING CONTAINS

140 calories

28 g carbohydrate

1 g fat

4 mg cholesterol

4 g protein

125 mg sodium

0 g fiber

COFFEE CRÈME BRÛLÉE

Milk, cream, coffee, vanilla, and egg—nothing could be simpler or tastier.

MAKES 7 SERVINGS

½ cup half-and-half

2½ cups 2% milk

3 tablespoons instant coffee granules

1 vanilla bean, split lengthwise

1 tablespoon pure vanilla extract

6 tablespoons cane sugar

2 large egg yolks

2 large eggs

170 calories

17 g carbohydrate

7 g fat

173 mg cholesterol

7 g protein

65 mg sodium

0 g fiber

EACH SERVING CONTAINS

1. Preheat the oven to 300°F

2. Combine the half-and-half, milk, and coffee granules in a large saucepan over medium heat. Scrape the seeds from the vanilla bean and add to the milk mixture, along with the bean. Add the vanilla extract and stir. Heat the mixture over medium heat to just below a simmer. Add 4 tablespoons of the cane sugar, stir, and heat to a simmer. Remove from the heat. Remove and discard the vanilla bean.

3. Whisk the egg yolks and whole eggs in a medium bowl. While whisking, slowly add half the hot milk mixture to the eggs. Whisk the egg mixture back into the remaining hot milk mixture and return to the heat. Cook, stirring, until thickened. Do not allow to boil. Remove from the heat and let cool, about 10 minutes.

4. Pour approximately ¼ cup custard into each of seven 4-ounce ramekins and arrange in a deep baking pan or casserole dish. Add enough hot water to the baking pan to come up to the level of the custard in the ramekins.

5. Bake for 40 to 45 minutes, or until a knife inserted in the center comes out clean. Cool about 1 hour and refrigerate seven hours.

6. When ready to serve, preheat the broiler.

7. Sprinkle 1 teaspoon evaporated cane juice on top of each ramekin. Place under the broiler for 1 minute (or flame with a torch) until the cane juice is caramelized. Be careful not to burn.

n NUTRITION NOTE: *Most desserts are much higher in carbohydrate than this creamy custard, which has been lightened by incorporating both egg whites and low-fat milk with the traditional higher-fat ingredients.*

BANANA PUDDING
WITH VANILLA WAFERS

Kids' food for grown-ups.

MAKES 8 SERVINGS

FOR THE VANILLA WAFERS

½ cup cane sugar

2 tablespoons cornstarch

2 tablespoons (⅛ cup) very soft unsalted butter

1 large egg

1 tablespoon pure vanilla extract

¾ cup unbleached all-purpose flour

½ teaspoon aluminum-free baking powder

⅛ teaspoon sea salt

FOR THE PUDDING

½ cup cane sugar

3 tablespoons cornstarch

¼ teaspoon sea salt

3 cups 1% milk

2 large egg yolks

1 tablespoon unsalted butter

1½ teaspoons pure vanilla extract

Seeds scraped from 2 vanilla beans

1 teaspoon pure banana extract

2 medium ripe bananas

1. Preheat the oven to 350°F. Lightly spray a baking sheet with canola oil spray.

2. Combine the cane sugar, cornstarch, butter, and egg in a large bowl and beat well with a wire whisk. Add the vanilla, flour, baking powder, and salt and stir until smooth to form a dough.

3. Roll the dough into 14 tablespoon-size balls and place about 1½ inches apart on the baking sheet.

4. Bake for 10 to15 minutes, or until lightly golden. Remove the wafers from the pan and cool on wire racks.

5. Combine the cane sugar, cornstarch, salt, and milk in a large saucepan over medium heat. Heat to just below boiling.

6. Whisk the egg yolks in a small bowl. While whisking, slowly add half the hot milk mixture to the eggs. Whisk the egg mixture back into the remaining hot milk mixture and return to the heat. Cook, stirring, until thickened. Do not allow to boil. Remove from the heat and add the butter, vanilla extract, vanilla seeds, and banana extract. Cool quickly at room temperature by pouring the pudding into a large, shallow pan.

7. Cut the bananas into rounds. Layer ½ cup banana pudding and about ⅛ of the banana slices in each of eight parfait glasses. Top each with half a crumbled vanilla wafer.

EACH SERVING CONTAINS

175 calories

28 g carbohydrate

4 g fat

64 mg cholesterol

4 g protein

109 mg sodium

1 g fiber

BUTTERMILK PANNA COTTA

Panna cotta means "cooked cream." This version reflects an authentically Italian appreciation of lightness and simplicity.

MAKES 4 SERVINGS

FOR THE FRUIT COMPOTE

¾ cup orange segments, peeled and pith removed

½ cup blueberries

1½ tablespoons cane sugar

———————

1 teaspoon unflavored gelatin

2 teaspoons warm water

½ cup buttermilk

2 tablespoons cane sugar

1 large egg white (about 2 tablespoons)

¼ cup heavy cream

1. Combine the oranges, blueberries, and cane sugar in a small bowl and mix well. Set aside.

2. Dissolve the gelatin in the water in a small bowl or cup.

3. Combine the buttermilk and 1 tablespoon of the cane sugar over medium heat in a small saucepan. Warm just until the cane juice dissolves. Add the dissolved gelatin, stir well, and strain the mixture into a small bowl. Place the bowl in a larger bowl or pan filled with ice and let the mixture set up for about 1 hour, or until the consistency of yogurt.

4. Whisk together the egg white and the remaining 1 tablespoon cane sugar until stiff peaks form. Fold into the gelatin mixture.

5. Whip the cream with a whisk in a small chilled bowl until soft peaks form. Fold into the gelatin mixture.

6. Scoop ¼ cup panna cotta into four serving dishes and spoon ¼ cup fruit compote over each.

> **C** **COOK'S NOTE:** *Buttermilk sounds rich, but is actually a low-fat milk. If you don't have any on hand, clabber nonfat milk by adding 2 teaspoons fresh lemon juice to enough nonfat milk to equal ½ cup. Let stand for 5 minutes. Since the egg white never cooks, use a pasteurized egg white in this recipe.*

EACH SERVING CONTAINS

140 calories

20 g carbohydrate

6 g fat

21 mg cholesterol

3 g protein

51 mg sodium

1 g fiber

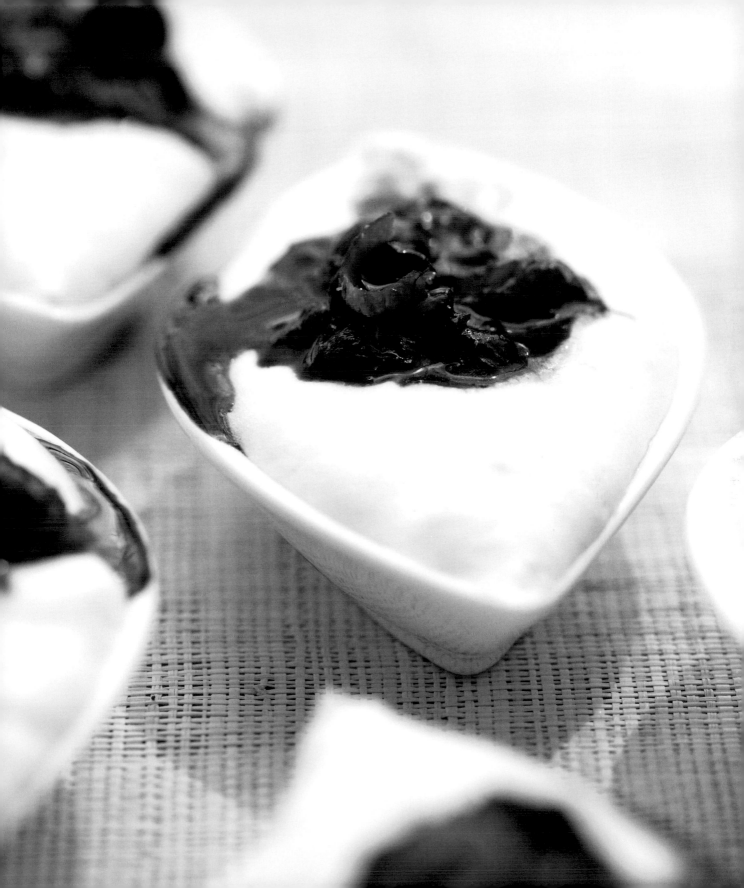

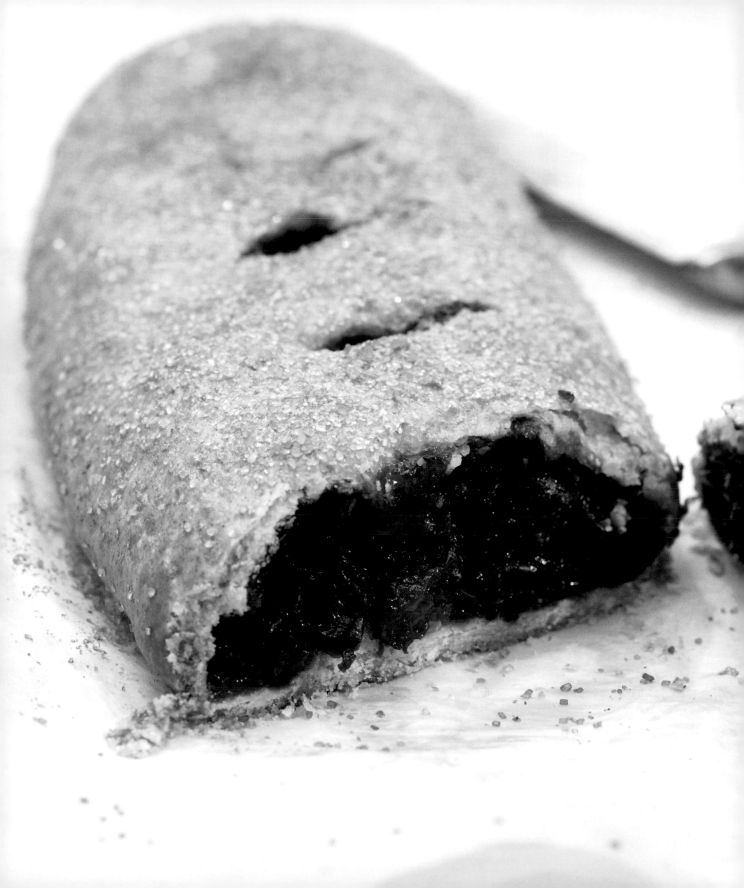

CHERRY STRUDEL

MAKES 10 SERVINGS

3 tablespoons cornstarch

¼ cup water

1½ pounds fresh or frozen pitted cherries, thawed if frozen

3 tablespoons cane sugar

½ cup dried tart cherries

FOR THE CRUST

1 cup unbleached all-purpose flour

¼ teaspoon sea salt

3 tablespoons evaporated cane juice

4 tablespoons (½ stick) cold unsalted butter, diced

4 to 6 tablespoons ice water

1 large egg white (about 2 tablespoons), lightly beaten

1 teaspoon cane sugar

1. Preheat the oven to 375°F. Lightly coat a baking sheet with canola oil spray.

2. Mix the cornstarch and 2 tablespoons of the water in a small bowl or cup to form a slurry. Set aside.

3. Lightly coat a medium sauté pan with canola oil spray. Sauté the fresh or thawed cherries, cane sugar, and the remaining 2 tablespoons water over medium heat. When the cherries are tender, stir in the dried cherries. Stir in the slurry and cook until thickened. Remove from the heat and cool completely until thick.

4. Place the flour in a medium bowl. Add the salt and cane sugar and mix well. Cut the butter into the flour, using a pastry cutter, until the butter is the size of small peas. Add the water, 1 tablespoon at a time, mixing gently with a fork after each addition. The dough will begin to form a ball when enough water has been added. Gather the dough with dry hands and form into a ball. Let rest for 5 minutes.

5. On a lightly floured surface, roll the dough into an 8 x 12-inch rectangle. Spoon the cherries along the long edge of the dough, about 1 inch from the edge. Roll the dough and filling over themselves and seal the ends to form a strudel. Score the top into ten 1-inch slices.

6. Brush the top of the strudel with the egg white and sprinkle with cane sugar. Place on a baking sheet and refrigerate for 5 to 10 minutes.

7. Remove the strudel from the refrigerator. Bake for 35 to 40 minutes, or until lightly browned. Allow to cool for 15 to 20 minutes and trim any extra pastry off the ends. Cut into 10 slices.

n NUTRITION NOTE: *Cherries are similar to raspberries, blueberries, and pomegranates in flavonoid content—the color is the key.*

EACH SERVING CONTAINS

180 calories
—
37 g carbohydrate
—
3 g fat
—
6 mg cholesterol
—
2 g protein
—
30 mg sodium
—
2 g fiber

BAKED VANILLA PEARS IN PASTRY

Make this when you want to show off.

MAKES 8 SERVINGS

1 cup unbleached all-purpose flour

¼ teaspoon sea salt

4½ teaspoons cane sugar

2 tablespoons cold unsalted butter, diced

4 to 6 tablespoons ice water

FOR THE FILLING

¼ cup chopped toasted walnuts

¼ cup dried cranberries

2 teaspoons cane sugar

2 teaspoons firmly packed light brown sugar

¼ teaspoon ground cinnamon

4 medium pears, peeled, cored, and cut in half lengthwise

1 large egg white (about 2 tablespoons), lightly beaten

2 teaspoons ground cinnamon

2 tablespoons cane sugar

½ cup apple cider, warmed

1. Preheat the oven to 375°F.

2. Place the flour, salt, and cane sugar in a medium bowl and mix well. Cut the butter into the flour, using a pastry cutter, until the butter is the size of small peas. Add the water, 1 tablespoon at a time, mixing gently with a fork after each addition. The dough will start to form a ball when enough water has been added. Gather the dough with dry hands and form into a ball. Let rest for 5 minutes.

3. Combine the walnuts, cranberries, cane sugar, brown sugar, and cinnamon in a small bowl and mix together.

4. Fill the cored area of each pear half with 1 tablespoon of walnut filling.

5. Divide the dough into 8 portions and form into balls. On a lightly floured surface, roll out each ball into a circle about ⅛ inch thick and big enough to fully enclose a pear half.

6. Set each filled pear half cut side up in the center of a pastry circle and gather up the edges. Pinch together the edges of the pastry over the center of the fruit. Brush each wrapped pear with the egg white and sprinkle lightly with cinnamon and cane sugar. Place on a baking sheet.

7. Bake for 30 to 35 minutes, or until the fruit is tender (test with a skewer) and the pastry crust is lightly browned.

8. While still warm, place each wrapped pear on a plate and garnish with a tablespoon of warm apple cider.

NUTRITION NOTE: *Serve this beautiful dessert in the autumn or winter, when pears are in season. Note the 3 grams of fiber—a solid benefit of fruit and nuts.*

EACH SERVING CONTAINS

190 calories

30 g carbohydrate

6 g fat

8 mg cholesterol

3 g protein

67 mg sodium

3 g fiber

BANANA BREAD PUDDING

If you like chocolate-dipped bananas, you'll love this.

MAKES 12 SERVINGS

1 cup evaporated skim milk

½ cup half-and-half

½ cup 2% milk

1 large egg

4 large egg yolks

3 tablespoons cane sugar

2 ripe bananas, peeled and chopped into bite-size pieces

Pinch sea salt

6 slices multigrain bread

¼ cup fruit-juice-sweetened, low-fat chocolate sauce (available in natural-foods supermarkets)

1. Preheat the oven to 325°F. Lightly coat an 8-inch square baking pan with canola oil spray.

2. Combine the evaporated milk, half-and-half, 2% milk, egg, egg yolks, cane sugar, bananas, and salt in a large bowl.

3. Break up the slices of bread into small pieces and spread out on the bottom of the baking pan. Pour the banana mixture over the bread and let soak for 15 minutes only.

4. Bake for 45 minutes, or until a knife inserted into the center comes out clean. Remove from oven and cool slightly on a wire rack.

5. Cut the bread pudding into twelve 2 x 2½-inch pieces and serve each one topped with 1 teaspoon chocolate sauce.

EACH SERVING CONTAINS

150 calories

24 g carbohydrate

4 g fat

88 mg cholesterol

6 g protein

120 mg sodium

1 g fiber

CRANBERRY PEAR CRISP

*A wonderful fall dish. Make extra and enjoy warm or cold,
topped with a big dollop of yogurt, as a quick breakfast.*

MAKES 6 SERVINGS

3 cups peeled, cored, and diced pears

½ cup dried cranberries

2 tablespoons cane sugar

¼ teaspoon ground nutmeg

¼ teaspoon ground cinnamon

FOR THE TOPPING

1 tablespoon unsalted butter, softened

¼ cup whole wheat flour

1 tablespoon firmly packed light brown sugar

1 tablespoon canola oil

½ teaspoon ground nutmeg

½ teaspoon ground cinnamon

1½ teaspoons honey

½ cup steel-cut oats

1. Preheat the oven to 400°F. Lightly coat six 4-ounce ceramic ramekins with canola oil spray.

2. Mix together the pears, cranberries, cane sugar, nutmeg, and cinnamon in a large bowl until well combined.

3. Mix together the butter, flour, brown sugar, canola oil, nutmeg, cinnamon, honey and oats in a small bowl.

4. Fill each ramekin with ½ cup pear mixture, then sprinkle with 2 tablespoons topping.

5. Bake for 8 to 10 minutes, or until light golden brown. Serve warm.

n NUTRITION NOTE: *This streusel topping is really healthy because of the steel-cut oats, canola oil, and whole wheat flour. Use it on any type of fruit.*

EACH SERVING CONTAINS

175 calories

33 g carbohydrates

3 g fat

5 mg cholesterol

3 g protein

2 mg sodium

5 g fiber

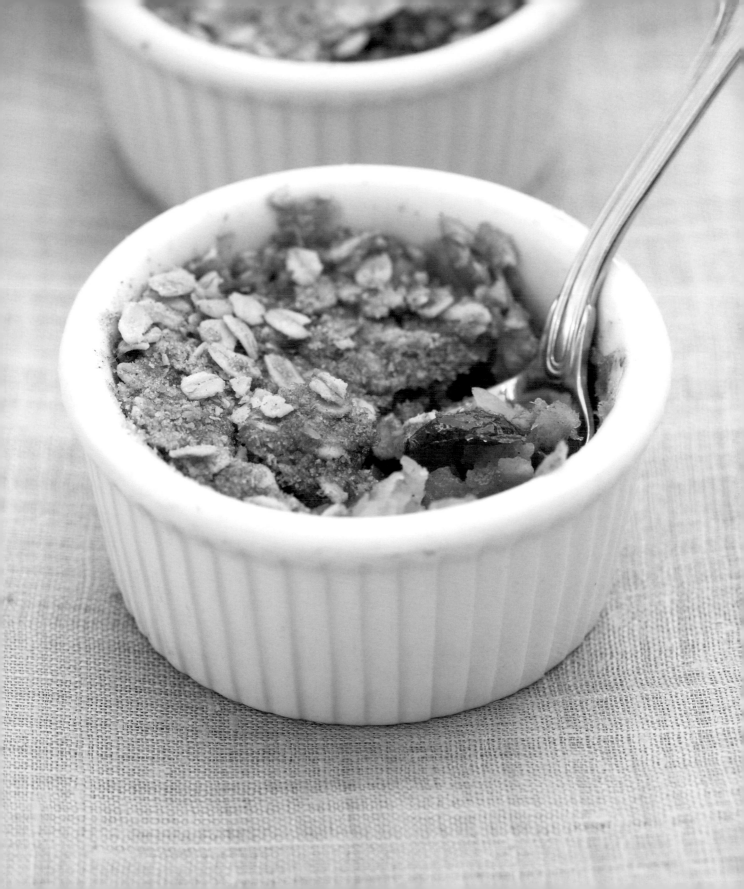

STRAWBERRY SHORTCAKE

MAKES 12 SERVINGS

FOR THE SHORTCAKE
BISCUITS:

1¼ cups unbleached
all-purpose flour

¾ cup whole wheat flour

1¼ teaspoons sea salt

1 tablespoon plus 1
teaspoon aluminum-
free baking powder

3 tablespoons cold
unsalted butter, cubed

⅓ cup low-fat cream cheese

¾ cup buttermilk

———————

3 cups strawbwerries,
hulled and sliced

3 tablespoons cane sugar

1½ teaspoons orange
zest, minced

2 teaspoons fresh
orange juice

6 tablespoons heavy cream

1. Preheat the oven to 400°F. Lightly coat a baking sheet with canola oil spray.

2. Sift together the all-purpose flour, whole wheat flour, salt, and baking powder in a large bowl.

3. Cut the butter and cream cheese into the flour mixture, using a pastry cutter, until the butter is the size of small peas. Add the buttermilk and mix with a fork until just combined.

4. On a lightly floured surface, knead the dough gently just until a dough forms. Roll it out to ¾ inch thick. Using a 2½-inch round cutter, form 12 biscuits and place about 1 inch apart on the baking sheet. Lightly spray the tops of the biscuits with canola oil.

5. Bake for 10 minutes, or until golden in color and cooked through. Cool slightly.

6. Combine the strawberries, cane sugar, orange zest, and orange juice in a medium bowl. Cover and refrigerate until ready to use.

7. Pour the cream into a small chilled bowl and whip with a wire whisk until soft peaks form. Chill.

8. Cut the biscuits crosswise in half and place ¼ cup strawberry mixture on each bottom half. Cover with the top halves and garnish each shortcake with 1 heaping teaspoon whipped cream.

n **NUTRITION NOTE:** *We suggest organic strawberries (that's all we'll serve at Canyon Ranch). We also suggest you keep this classic dessert as a springtime exclusive when strawberries are in season.*

EACH SERVING CONTAINS

165 calories

23 g carbohydrate

7 g fat

21 mg cholesterol

4 g protein

412 mg sodium

2 g fiber

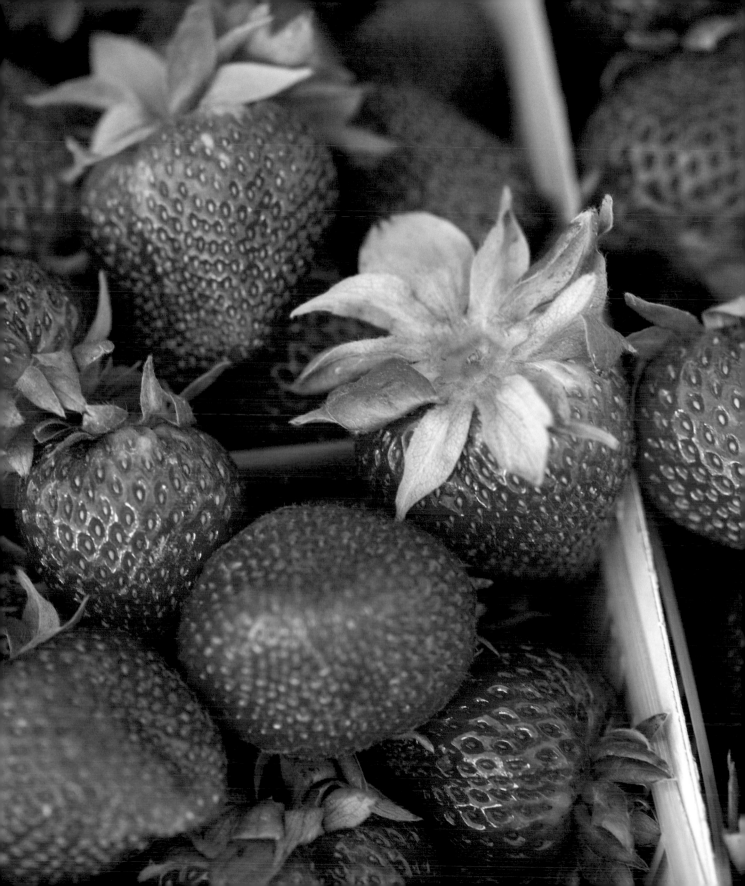

INGREDIENT CONVERSIONS

FOOD	AMOUNT	EQUIVALENT
Almonds	1 pound, shelled	4 cups
Apples, fresh	1 pound, 3 medium	2½ cups, chopped; 3 cups, sliced
Apples, dried	1 pound	4 cups
Apricots, fresh	1 pound, 12 medium	2 cups, sliced
Apricots, dried	1 pound	2½ cups
Asparagus, fresh	1 pound, 16 medium spears	3½ cups, chopped
Avocado	8 ounces, 1 large	1¼ cups, chopped; peeled and pitted, 1 cup, pureed
Bananas	4 ounces, 1 medium	¾ cup, sliced; ½ cup, pureed
Barley	1 cup, dry	3¾ cups, cooked
Beans		
adzuki	1 pound, dried	2½ cups, dried
	1 cup, dried	2½ cups, cooked
anasazi	1 pound, dried	2 cups, dried
	1 cup, dried	2 cups, cooked
black	1 pound, dried	2¼ cups, dried
	1 cup, dried	2½ cups, cooked
fava	1 pound, dried	2 cups, dried
	1 cup, dried	2 cups, cooked
garbanzo	1 pound, dried	2 cups, dried
	1 cup, dried	2½ cups, cooked
kidney	1 pound, dried	2 cups, dried
	1 cup, dried	2½ cups, cooked
lima	1 pound, dried	2 cups, dried
	1 cup, dried	2½ cups, cooked
navy	1 pound, dried	2¼ cups, dried
	1 cup, dried	2½ cups, cooked
pinto	1 pound, dried	2 cups, dried
	1 cup, dried	2½ cups, cooked
Beets	1 pound, fresh	2 cups, chopped or sliced

FOOD	AMOUNT	EQUIVALENT
Blackberries	1 pint, fresh 10-ounce bag, frozen	2 cups, fresh 2 cups, frozen
Blueberries	1 pint, fresh 10-ounce bag, frozen	2 cups, fresh 1½ cups, frozen
Bread	1-pound loaf 1 slice	About sixteen ½-inch slices; 7 cups fresh crumbs ½ cup fresh crumbs
Broccoli	1 pound, fresh, 10-ounce bag, frozen	2 cups, chopped 1½ cups, chopped
Brussels sprouts	1 pound fresh, about 20 sprouts 10-ounce bag, frozen	3 cups, fresh 2½ cups, frozen
Bulgur wheat	1 cup dry	3¾ cups, cooked
Butter	1 pound	2 cups, 4 sticks
Cabbage	1 pound, fresh	4 cups, shredded
Cantaloupe	1 medium, 2 pounds	3 cups, diced
Carrots	1 pound, trimmed, 4 medium 10-ounce bag, frozen	3 cups, chopped; 2 cups, grated 2 cups, frozen, sliced
Cashews	1 pound, shelled	3½ cups
Cauliflower	1 pound, fresh 10-ounce bag, frozen	3 cups florets; 2 cups, chopped 1½ cups, chopped
Celery	1 pound 2 medium ribs	3 cups, chopped ½ cup chopped

Cheese
  blue, feta, goat
  cheddar, Jack, mozzarella
  Parmesan
  Romano
	
	4 ounces
	1 pound
	1 pound
	¼ ounce
		
		1 cup crumbled
		4 cups shredded
		4 cups grated
		1 tablespoon

Cherries	1 pound, fresh 10-ounce bag, frozen	3 cups pitted 1 cup, frozen
Chestnuts	1 pound, shelled	2½ cups

FOOD	AMOUNT	EQUIVALENT
Chicken	½ breast, 4 ounces	¾ cup, cooked, diced
Chocolate, all types	8 ounces chips 1 ounce, melted, or 1 square	1 cup 2 tablespoons
Clams, canned	1 pound, drained	2 cups
Clams, fresh	3 dozen, in shell	4 cups, shucked
Cocoa powder	8 ounces	2¾ cups
Coconut	8 ounces, shredded	3½ cups
Corn	2 medium ears, fresh 10-ounce bag, frozen	1 cup kernels 1¾ cups, frozen
Cornmeal	1 pound, dry	3 cups, dry
Cornstarch	1 pound	3 cups
Corn syrup, light or dark	16 fluid ounces	2 cups
Cottage cheese	8 ounces	1 cup
Couscous	1 cup, dry	2½ cups, cooked
Crab	1 pound cooked meat	3 cups, cooked
Crackers, Graham	15 squares	1 cup crumbs
Cranberries	12 ounces, fresh	3 cups, fresh

Cream
  half-and-half
  heavy, whipping
  sour
	
	1 pint
	1 pint
	1 pint
		
		2 cups
		2 cups; 4 cups, whipped
		2 cups

Cream cheese	8 ounces	1 cup
Cucumber	1 medium	1½ cups, chopped
Currants	1 pound, dried	3¼ cups, dried
Dates	1 pound, pitted	2½ cups, pitted
Eggplant, fresh	1 pound, fresh	3½ cups, diced; 2 cups, cooked, diced
Egg roll wrappers	1 pound	14 wrappers

FOOD	AMOUNT	EQUIVALENT
Eggs, whole, large	1 dozen 5 eggs 1 egg	2⅓ cups 1 cup 3 tablespoons
Eggs, whites, large	1 dozen 8 whites 2 whites	1½ cups 1 cup 2½ cups, stiffly beaten
Eggs, yolks, large	1 dozen yolks 1 yolk	1 cup 1½ tablespoons
Eggs, hard-cooked	1 whole egg	⅓ cup, chopped
Figs	1 pound, fresh	12 medium 3 cups, chopped

Flour
    all-purpose, bread, hi-gluten
    pastry, cake
    potato
    rice
    rye
    tapioca
    whole wheat
	
	1 pound
	1 pound
	1 pound
	1 pound
	1 pound
	1 pound
	1 pound
		
		3 cups, sifted
		4½ cups, sifted
		3 cups, sifted
		3½ cups, sifted
		3½ cups, sifted
		3½ cups, sifted
		3½ cups, unsifted

Garlic	1 large head 1 large clove	12 cloves; 4 tablespoons, minced 1 teaspoon, minced
Gelatin, unflavored	¼-ounce packet	1 tablespoon
Ginger, fresh	2-inch piece	2 tablespoons, minced; 1 tablespoon juice
Grapefruit	1 pound fresh	1 medium; 1½ cups segments; ¾ cup juice
Grapes	1 pound	3 cups
Green beans (haricots verts)	1 pound, fresh	3½ cups, whole, trimmed
Greens kale, chard, mustard	 1 pound fresh	 1½ cups, cooked
Hazelnuts	1 pound, shelled	1½ cups

FOOD	AMOUNT	EQUIVALENT
Herbs	1 tablespoon, fresh	1 teaspoon, dried, chopped, crumbled
Honey	16 ounces	2 cups
Horseradish	1 pound, fresh	3 cups, grated
Ketchup	16-ounce bottle	2 cups
Kiwi	1 pound, 6 medium	2¼ cups, chopped
Leeks	1 pound	2½ cups, chopped 1 cup, cooked
Lemons	1 pound, 6 medium 1 medium	1 cup juice 3 tablespoons juice; 1 tablespoon grated peel
Lentils	1 pound, dried 1 cup, dried	2¼ cups, dried 2 cups, cooked
Lettuce, all types	1 pound	6 cups, chopped or torn; 4 cups, shredded
Limes	1 pound, 8 medium 1 medium	¾ cup juice 1½ tablespoons juice; 1½ teaspoons grated peel
Lobster	1 pound	2½ cups meat
Mango, fresh	12 ounces, 1 medium	1 cup, chopped
Maple syrup	16 fluid ounces	2 cups
Meat, ground	1 pound	2 cups

Milk
    evaporated skim
    sweetened condensed, skim
	1 quart
	12-ounce can
	14-ounce can
		4 cups
		1½ cups
		1¾ cups

Millet	1 cup	3½ cups, cooked
Molasses	16 fluid ounces	2 cups
Mushrooms, all types	1 pound fresh	6 cups, chopped; 5½ cups, sliced
Mussels, fresh	1 pound, medium	1 cup meat 12 mussels

FOOD	AMOUNT	EQUIVALENT
Mustard, all types	16 ounces 1 tablespoon, prepared	2 cups, prepared 1 teaspoon, dried
Nectarines	1 pound, 3 to 4 medium	2 cups, chopped 2½ cups, sliced
Oats, rolled	1 pound, dry 1 cup, dry	5 cups, dry 1¾ cups, cooked
Oil, all types	8 ounces	1 cup
Okra	1 pound, fresh 10-ounce bag, frozen	2¼ cups, chopped, cooked 1¼ cups, chopped
Onions green, scallions white, yellow, or red	1 medium, bulb and top 1 pound, fresh, 4 medium	⅓ cup, chopped 4 cups, chopped
Oranges	1 pound, 3 medium 1 medium	1¼ cups juice ¾ cup segments, sliced; 1½ tablespoons grated orange peel
Oranges, mandarin	11-ounce can	1¼ cups segments, drained
Oysters	8 ounces, 16 oysters	1 cup, shucked
Papaya	12 ounces, 1 medium	1½ cups, chopped; 2 cups, sliced
Parsnips	1 pound, fresh, 4 medium	2 cups, chopped; 2½ cups, sliced
Pasta macaroni noodles, 1-inch pieces spaghetti	2 ounces, dry 1 cup, dry 2 ounces, dry 1 cup, dry 2 ounces, dry	1 cup, cooked 1¾ cups, cooked 1 cup, cooked 1¾ cups, cooked 1 cup, cooked
Peaches	1 pound, fresh, 4 medium 10-ounce bag, frozen 1 pound, dried	2½ cups, chopped; 2¾ cups, sliced 1½ cups, sliced 2¾ cups, dried
Peanut butter	16-ounce jar	1½ cups
Peanuts	1 pound, shelled	3½ cups

FOOD	AMOUNT	EQUIVALENT
Pears	1 pound, fresh, 3 medium 1 pound, canned, drained 1 pound, dried	2 cups, sliced 2 cups, sliced 2¾ cups, dried
Peas, black-eyed	1 pound, dried 1 cup, dried 10-ounce bag, frozen	2 cups, dried 2 cups, cooked 1½ cups
Peas, green	1 pound, fresh, in pod 10-ounce bag, frozen	1 cup, shelled 2 cups
Peas, split	1 pound, dried 1 cup, dried	2¼ cups, dried 2 cups, cooked
Pecans	1 pound, shelled	4 cups halves; 3½ cups, chopped
Peppers, bell	1 pound, 2 large 1 medium	2½ cups, chopped; 3 cups, sliced 1 cup, chopped
Phyllo	1-pound package	24 sheets
Pineapple	1 medium, fresh 15-ounce can	5 cups, cubed 1½ cups, drained pineapple and juice
Pine nuts	1 pound, shelled	3 cups
Pistachios	1 pound, shelled	3½ cups
Plums	1 pound, fresh	2 cups, chopped; 2½ cups, sliced

Potatoes
  red bliss
  russet
  sweet
  Yukon gold
	
	1 pound, 4 medium
	1 pound, 2 large
	1 pound, fresh, 3 medium
	1 pound, 4 medium
		
		3½ cups, chopped; 4 cups, sliced
		3½ cups, chopped; 4 cups, sliced
		3½ cups, chopped; 4 cups, sliced
		3½ cups, chopped; 4 cups, sliced

Prunes	1 pound, dried	2½ cups, dried; 4 cups, cooked
Pumpkin	1 pound, fresh 15-ounce can	1 cup, cooked, mashed 1¾ cups, mashed
Quinoa	1 pound, dried 1 cup, dried	2½ cups, dried 3 cups, cooked
Radishes	1 pound, fresh, 24 radishes	1½ cups, sliced

FOOD	AMOUNT	EQUIVALENT
Raisins	1 pound, dried	2½ cups, dried
Raspberries	1 pint, fresh 10-ounce bag, frozen	2 cups, fresh 1¾ cups, frozen
Rhubarb	1 pound, fresh 10-ounce bag, frozen	2 cups, chopped, cooked 1¼ cups, chopped, frozen
Rice	1 cup, white basmati 1 cup, brown 1 cup, wild	3 cups, cooked 3 cups, cooked 3 cups, cooked
Ricotta cheese	7½ ounces	1 cup
Rutabaga, fresh	1 pound, fresh	2½ cups, cubed
Sauerkraut	1 pound	2 cups
Scallops	1 pound, medium	2 cups
Shallots	1 pound	2½ cups, chopped
Shrimp	1 pound, shelled 1 pound, unshelled	2 cups, cooked 12 jumbo 16 large 30 medium 36 small
Soybeans, fresh (edamame)	1 pound, shelled	2 cups, shelled
Spinach	1 pound, fresh 10-ounce bag, frozen	10 cups, fresh; 2 cups, cooked 1½ cups, frozen

Squash
  acorn, yellow, zucchini
  butternut
	
	1 pound, 3 medium
	1 pound, fresh
		
		3 cups, chopped; 3½ cups, sliced
		1 cup, cooked, mashed

Strawberries	1 pint, fresh 10-ounce bag, frozen	2 cups, sliced 1½ cups

Sugar
  brown
  granulated
  powdered
	
	1 pound
	1 pound
	1 pound
		
		2¼ cups, packed
		2 cups
		4 cups

Tangerines	1 pound, 4 medium	2 cups, segments

FOOD	AMOUNT	EQUIVALENT

Tofu
  firm
  silken
	
	1 pound
	1 pound
		
		2¾ cups, cubed
		2½ cups, cubed

Tomatoes	1 pound, 3 medium 15-ounce can	1½ cups, chopped; 2 cups, sliced 1¾ cups, whole or diced with juice; 2 cups, pureed
Tomato paste	6-ounce can	¾ cup
Tuna	6-ounce can	¾ cup
Turkey	12 pounds, raw	16 cups cooked meat
Turnips	1 pound, 3 medium	2½ cups, cooked, chopped
Walnuts	1 pound, shelled	3¾ cups, halved; 3½ cups, chopped
Watermelon	10 pounds	20 cups, cubed
Wheat germ	16 ounces	4 cups
Wine	750 ml bottle	3¼ cups
Wonton skins (wrappers)	1 pound	60 wrappers
Yeast	¼-ounce package	1 tablespoon
Yogurt	8 ounces	1 cup

GLUTEN-FREE RECIPES

Gluten-free recipes contain no wheat, barley, rye, or spelt. We include recipes with oats because current research indicates the oats are gluten free.

Beverages and Snacks

Almosjito

Canyon Ranch Granola

Chocolate Espresso Soda

Crispy Roasted Garbonzo Beans

Dirty Apple Chini

H_2-Tini

Limeade

Pomatini

Pumpkin Crunch

Roasted Edamame

Sparkling Fruit Soda

Trail Mix with Almonds and Chocolate Chips

Breakfast

Breakfast Rellenos

Eggs Zydeco

Frittata with Bell Peppers and Onion

Homemade Fruit Preserves

Southwest Scrambled Eggs

Starters and Sides

Braised Red Cabbage

Broccolini with Garlic and Olive Oil

Parsnip Carrot Puree

Chilled Green Bean Salad

Coconut Black Rice

Curried Mussels

Grits Cake

Mashed Butternut Squash with Maple Syrup

Mashed Lima Beans

Mashed Potatoes

Mashed Sesame Soybeans

Oat Cakes

Potato Medley

Rainbow Vegetable Salad

Roasted Acorn Squash

Roasted Fennel

Roasted Tomatoes with Radicchio

Sautéed Kale

Sautéed Spinach and Garlic

Soft Corn Polenta

Southwest Green Cabbage Salad

Vegetable Nori Rolls

Soups

Ajiaco Soup

Chilled Cucumber Soup with Arugula

Chipotle Black Bean Soup

Cream of Mushroom Soup

Cream of Parsnip Soup

Cream of Tomato Tarragon Soup

Italian Vegetable Soup with Cannellini Beans

Puree of White Bean and Celery Root Soup

Spelt Berry Gazpacho with Cilantro Lime Shrimp

Sweet 100 Tomato Soup

Yellow Gazpacho

Yellow Split Pea and Potato Soup

Salads

Apple-Cranberry Salmon Salad

Artichoke Salad

Arugula Pear Salad

Frisée Salad with Sherry Shallot Vinaigrette

Grilled Caesar Salad

Hearts of Palm Salad

Mixed Greens with Pineapple Vinaigrette

Napoleon of Heirloom Tomatoes and Mozzarella

Paprika-Lemon Chicken Salad

Quinoa Walnut Salad

Salmon Citrus Salad

Smoked Salmon, Spinach, and Mushroom Salad

Spinach and Candied Pecan Salad

Turkey Pineapple Salad

Salsas and Sauces

BBQ Sauce

Béchamel Sauce

Bolognese Sauce

Chunky Tomato Sauce

Creamy Parmesan Sauce

Creamy Pesto Sauce

Cucumber, Dill, and Goat Cheese Relish

Fennel and Garlic Salsa

Fresh Marinara Sauce

Ginger Peach Hot Sauce

Green Curry Paste

Guacamole

Latin Spice Rub

Mongolian BBQ Sauce

Olive Salsa

Pico de Gallo

Ponzu Sauce

Roasted Red Pepper Relish

Thai Peanut Sauce

Tomato and Feta Relish

Beef and Lamb

Asian Braised Flank Steak with Bok Choy and Brown Rice

Beef Short Ribs

Beef Tenderloins with Bourbon Cherries

Grilled Beef Tenderloins with Tomato-Blue Cheese Salsa

London Broil

Pot Roast

Za'atar-Crusted Lamb Chops with Pomegranate Molasses

Fish and Shellfish

Ahi Tuna with Shrimp Jicama Salsa

Broiled Salmon with Cucumber Lemongrass Salsa

Chili-Rubbed Tequila Shrimp

Grilled Marinated Trout

Grouper with Tomatillo Salsa

Orange-Glazed Salmon with Screamin' Ginger
Salsa

Red Curry-Crusted Grouper with Rainbow
Vegetable Salad

Salmon with Blueberry Mango Salsa

Scallops with Mashed Artichokes and Tomato
Confit

Seared Scallops with Cranberry Ginger
Vinaigrette

Snapper with Kumquat Vinaigrette

Wasabi-Crusted Mahi-Mahi with Ponzu Sauce

Poultry

Cashew Chicken Stir-fry

Chicken Medallions with Mushroom Tarragon
Sauce

Chicken with Artichoke-Sun-Dried Tomato Pesto

Chicken with Black Bean-Chipotle Sauce

Peppered Chicken Medallions with Mushrooms

Spinach-Stuffed Chicken with Artichoke Caper
Sauce

Turkey Medallions with Honey Chipotle Sauce

Vegetarian

Green Bean and Edamame Stir-fry

Risotto Cakes with Roasted Vegetables

Spicy Indian Garbanzo Beans

Tofu Lettuce Wraps

Desserts

Almond Macaroons

Buttermilk Panna Cotta

Coconut Macaroons

Coffee Crème Brûlée

Summer Fruit Parfait

Sweet Potato Tartlets with Blue Corn Crust

Warm Chocolate Cakes with Coffee Crème
Anglaise

DAIRY-FREE RECIPES

Dairy free means no milk or milk products, including butter.

Beverages and Snacks

Almosjito

Canyon Ranch Granola

Chocolate Espresso Soda

Crispy Roasted Garbonzo Beans

Dirty Apple Chini

H_2-Tini

Limeade

Pomatini

Pumpkin Crunch

Roasted Edamame

Sparkling Fruit Soda

Trail Mix with Almonds and Chocolate Chips

Breakfast

Apple Cinnamon-Crusted Oatmeal

Eggs Zydeco

Homemade Fruit Preserves

Starters and Sides

Braised Red Cabbage

Broccolini with Garlic and Olive Oil

Chicken Pot Stickers

Chilled Green Bean Salad

Cold Noodle Salad

Curried Mussels

Mashed Sesame Soybeans

Pomegranate Couscous

Potato Medley

Rainbow Vegetable Salad

Roasted Acorn Squash

Roasted Fennel

Sautéed Kale

Sautéed Spinach and Garlic

Southwest Green Cabbage Salad

Vegetable Nori Rolls

Whole Wheat Croutons

Soups

Ajiaco Soup

Potato Vegetable Bisque

Puree of White Bean and Celery Root Soup

Spelt Berry Gazpacho with Cilantro Lime Shrimp

Sweet 100 Tomato Soup

Yellow Gazpacho

Yellow Split Pea and Potato Soup

Salads

Apple-Cranberry Salmon Salad

Chicken Panzanella

Chopped Salad with Lox

Fatoosh Salad

Hearts of Palm Salad

Paprika-Lemon Chicken Salad

Quinoa Walnut Salad

Salmon Citrus Salad

Shrimp Salad with Mango Vinaigrette

Smoked Salmon, Spinach, and Mushroom Salad

Spinach and Candied Pecan Salad

Strawberry, Chicken, and Arugula Salad

Turkey Pineapple Salad

Salsas and Sauces

BBQ Sauce

Bolognese Sauce

Chunky Tomato Sauce

Fennel and Garlic Salsa

Fresh Marinara Sauce

Ginger Peach Hot Sauce

Green Curry Paste

Guacamole

Latin Spice Rub

Mongolian BBQ Sauce

Olive Salsa

Pico de Gallo

Ponzu Sauce

Roasted Red Pepper Relish

Thai Peanut Sauce

Beef and Lamb

Asian Braised Flank Steak with Bok Choy and
Brown Rice

Beef Short Ribs

Beef Tenderloins with Bourbon Cherries

London Broil

Pot Roast

Spicy Thai Beef Wrap

Steak Pizzaiola

Za'atar-Crusted Lamb Chops with Pomegranate
Molasses

Fish and Shellfish

Ahi Tuna with Shrimp Jicama Salsa

Broiled Salmon with Cucumber Lemongrass
Salsa

Chili-Rubbed Tequila Shrimp

Coconut-Crusted Mahi-Mahi with Horseradish
Orange Marmalade

Cod with Cauliflower Tomato Broth

Crab Soufflés with Caramelized Carrot Sauce

Grilled Marinated Trout

Grouper with Tomatillo Salsa

Orange-Glazed Salmon with Screamin' Ginger
Salsa

Red Curry-Crusted Grouper with Rainbow
Vegetable Salad

Salmon with Blueberry Mango Salsa

Seared Scallops with Cranberry Ginger
Vinaigrette

Shrimp Cocktail Wrap

Shrimp Fritters with Cucumber Pineapple Salad

Shrimp Salad Sandwich

Snapper with Kumquat Vinaigrette

Wasabi-Crusted Mahi-Mahi with Ponzu Sauce

Poultry

Vegetarian

Desserts

INDEX

peanut butter and banana
    sandwich, grilled, 64
peanut sauce, Thai, 183
pear(s):
    arugula salad, 146
    baked vanilla, in pastry, 342
    and blue cheese flatbreads, 80
    cranberry crisp, 344
    currant cake, 330
    and pomegranate quesadilla,
        Brie with, 303
pecan:
    candied, and spinach salad,
        153
    waffles, 61
peppers:
    bell, for steak pizzaiola, 199
    bell, frittata with onions and, 58
    chipotle-black bean sauce,
        chicken with, 266
    chipotle black bean soup, 138
    chipotle honey sauce, turkey
        medallions with, 278
    poblano, for breakfast rellenos,
        53
    poblano, and crab quesadilla,
        246
    roasted red, relish, 181
pesto:
    artichoke-sun-dried tomato,
        chicken with, 264
    sauce, creamy, 177
pico de gallo, 189
pie:
    Key lime, 321
    New England apple, 322
pineapple:
    cucumber salad, shrimp fritters
        with, 251
    turkey salad, 163
    vinaigrette, mixed greens with,
        151
pita chips, for fatoosh salad,
    156
pizzaiola, steak, 199

plum cakes, Alsatian, 327
polenta, soft corn, 115
pomatini, 37
pomegranate:
    couscous, 112
    molasses, za'atar-crusted lamb
        chops with, 214
    and pear quesadilla, Brie with,
        303
ponzu sauce, 185
potato(es):
    mashed, 105
    medley, 113
    vegetable bisque, 141
    and yellow split pea soup, 136
pot pies, chicken, 270–71
pot roast, 203
pot stickers, chicken, 85
preserves, homemade fruit, 71
pumpkin crunch, 49

Q

quesadillas:
    Brie with pear and
        pomegranate, 303
    crab and poblano, 246
quinoa walnut salad, 152

R

radicchio, roasted tomatoes with,
    88
raspberry chocolate angel food
    cake, 332
red curry-crusted grouper with
    rainbow vegetable salad,
    230
reducing, 24
relishes:
    cucumber, dill, and goat
        cheese, 191
    olive spread, for turkey
        muffaletta, 276
    roasted red pepper, 181
    tomato feta, 182
rice, see grains

risotto cakes with roasted
    vegetables, 300
roasting, 17–18
rustic chicken, 269

S

salads, 142–69
    apple-cranberry salmon, 161
    artichoke, 144
    arugula, butternut squash tart
        with, 284–85
    arugula pear, 146
    chicken, sandwiches, 274
    chicken panzanella, 158
    chilled green bean, 93
    chopped, with lox, 159
    classic egg, sandwich, 169
    cold noodle, 108
    cucumber pineapple, shrimp
        fritters with, 251
    fatoosh, 156
    frisée, with sherry shallot
        vinaigrette, 147
    grilled Caesar, 150
    hearts of palm, 149
    mixed greens with pineapple
        vinaigrette, 151
    napoleon of heirloom tomatoes
        and mozzarella, 155
    paprika-lemon chicken, 162
    quinoa walnut, 152
    rainbow vegetable, 98
    salmon citrus, 167
    shrimp, with mango vinaigrette,
        164
    shrimp, sandwich, 252
    smoked salmon, spinach and
        mushroom, 166
    Southwest green cabbage, 102
    spinach and candied pecan, 153
    strawberry, chicken, and
        arugula, 168
    turkey pineapple, 163
    zucchini tomato, baked haddock
        with, 225

tomato(es) *(cont.)*
    confit, scallops with mashed
        artichokes and, 242
    feta relish, 182
    for fresh marinara sauce, 172
    heirloom, and mozzarella,
        napoleon of, 155
    roasted, with radicchio, 88
    sauce, chunky, 174
    soup, sweet 100, 132
    sun-dried, and artichoke pesto,
        chicken with, 264
    tarragon soup, cream of, 126
    in yellow gazpacho, 121
    zucchini salad, baked haddock
        with, 225
tortilla soup, 134
trail mix with almonds and
    chocolate chips, 44
trout, grilled marinated, 241
tuna melt with mustard sauce,
    253
turkey, 254
    apple wrap, 275
    and asparagus sandwich,
        warm, 277
    medallions with honey-chipotle
        sauce, 278
    muffaletta, 276
    pineapple salad, 163

V

vanilla:
    pears in pastry, baked, 342
    wafers, banana pudding with,
        337
vanilla beans, scraping of, 25
vegetable nori rolls, 86
vegetable potato bisque, 141
vegetables, 6–8, 10, 17–18, 142

roasted, risotto cakes with, 300
    see also side dishes; *specific
        vegetables*
vegetable salad, rainbow, 98, 230
vegetable soup with cannellini
    beans, Italian, 129
vegetarian entrées, 283–307
    Brie with pear and
        pomegranate quesadilla,
        303
    butternut squash tart with
        arugula salad, 284–85
    cauliflower fritters, 290
    cheese enchiladas with
        tomatillo sauce, 291
    eggplant gyro, 304–5
    green bean and edamame
        stir-fry, 299
    Italian grilled cheese with
        artichoke salad, 307
    mushroom burgers, 295
    risotto cakes with roasted
        vegetables, 300
    spicy curried cauliflower, 287
    spicy Indian garbanzo beans,
        296
    three-cheese-stuffed portobello
        mushroom, 294
    tofu lettuce wraps, 283
    wild mushroom and aged
        Gouda tart, 293
    zucchini fritters with tomato
        feta relish, 288
vinaigrettes:
    cranberry ginger, seared
        scallops with, 243
    kumquat, snapper with, 233
    mango, shrimp salad with, 164
    pineapple, mixed greens with,
        151

rosemary, for arugula pear
    salad, 146
sherry shallot, frisée salad with,
    147

W

waffles, pecan, 61
walnut quinoa salad, 152
wasabi-crusted mahi-mahi with
    ponzu sauce, 236
Worcestershire sauce, 31
wraps:
    green curry shrimp, 248
    Mediterranean chicken, 273
    poached salmon, with yogurt
        dill sauce, 224
    shrimp cocktail, 249
    spicy Thai beef, 213
    tofu lettuce, 283
    turkey apple, 275

Y

yellow split pea and potato soup, 136
yogurt:
    coriander sauce, for eggplant
        gyro, 5
    dill sauce, poached salmon
        wrap with, 224

Z

za'atar-crusted lamb chops with
    pomegranate molasses, 214
zesting, 25
ziti, baked, 204
zucchini:
    fritters with tomato feta relish,
        288
    tomato salad, baked haddock
        with, 225
zydeco, eggs, 57